New Technologies
in
REPRODUCTIVE MEDICINE,
NEONATOLOGY
and GYNECOLOGY

New Technologies
in
REPRODUCTIVE MEDICINE,
NEONATOLOGY
and GYNECOLOGY

The Proceedings of the
1st International Symposium, March 1998
Folgaria, Italy

Edited by
Ermelando V. Cosmi
University 'La Sapienza', Rome, Italy

Associate editors
E. Marinoni and R. Di Iorio

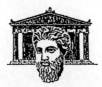

The Parthenon Publishing Group
International Publishers in Medicine, Science & Technology

NEW YORK   LONDON

Published in the USA by
The Parthenon Publishing Group Inc.
One Blue Hill Plaza
PO Box 1564, Pearl River,
New York 10965, USA

Published in the UK and Europe by
The Parthenon Publishing Group Limited
Casterton Hall, Carnforth,
Lancs LA6 2LA, UK

ISBN 1-85070-065-6

Printed and bound by Antony Rowe Ltd., Chippenham, Wiltshire, UK

Contents

3-D imaging

Computerized CTG

Infections

Labor and delivery

Neonatology

Diagnosis, prevention and treatment of IRDS

Oncology

Diagnostic and operative hysteroscopy and laparascopy

Menopause and osteoporosis

Breast

Section 2   Free Communications and Posters 295

Preface

In light of the technological revolution that was moving ahead quickly at the World Conference on Primary Health Care in Alma Alta, 1978, a working understanding of the term 'technology' was formulated. This stands on a base of scientific veracity and must include the interchange and interaction of interrelated relevant methodology among those responsible for its development and those who apply it in the diagnosis and management of health problems. The inevitable natural interdependence of the disciplines of reproductive medicine, neonatology and gynecology has profited enormously by this approach in the service of patient and science alike. A number of interim Conferences, the last in Rome in 1995, have attested to this success.

The present International Symposium on New Technologies in Reproductive Medicine, Neonatology and Gynecology marks another step forward. The exchange among clinical and basic scientists, as recorded in this book, reveals continued accomplishment in the revolution to elevate the health care of women, children and fetuses to a state of art and science that succeeds *pari passu* with the integration of advanced technologies.

The present Symposium was convened in Folgaria, Trento, Italy from March 1 to March 8. It was supported by the Alps-Adria Society of countries of central Europe, including Northern Italy, Germany, Croatia, Slovenia, Austria and Hungary. The co-sponsorship of C.N.R. of Italy and of the International Society for New Technology in Gynecology, Reproduction and Neonatology is also acknowledged. For their invaluable efforts in developing the present Symposium, I am also grateful to Mother and Child International (IAMANEH); the International Association for the Study of Lung Surfactant System; the World and European Associations of Perinatal Medicine; the Italian Societies of Perinatal Medicine, Neonatology, Gynecology and Obstetrics, Elderly Women, and Menopause; the Croatian Society for Ultrasound in Medicine; the Slovenian Association of Obstetrics and Gynecology; and the European Commission on Biomedical Research Programmes (BIOMED 2, Research Project on EURAIL, Europe Against Immature Lung).

I am confident that this book will serve as a prolog to what will be achieved in the 21st century. We are looking forward to continuing along this line also by promoting new meetings; the International Congress on New Technologies in Reproductive Medicine, Neonatology and Gynecology will take place on Sardinia Island, one of the most beautiful places of the world, on September 18–23, 1999.

Ermelando V. Cosmi, M.D., Ph.D.
Director of the 2nd Institute of Obstetrics and
Gynecology
University 'La Sapienza', Rome, Italy

Section 1

Plenary Papers

Prostasome-sperm fusion: possible involvement in fertility

G. Arienti*, E.V. Cosmi** and C.A. Palmerini***

*Istituto di Biochimica e Chimica Medica, Via del Giochetto,Perugia, Italy, ** II Istituto di Ostetricia e Ginecologia, Universita la Sapienza, Roma, Italy and *** Dipartimento di Biologia Cellulare e Molecolare, Via del Giochetto, 06100 Perugia, Italy*

Prostasome are vesicles secreted by the prostate gland and present in the human semen[1]. They can easily be isolated from this material by differential centrifugation and possess a number of catalytically active proteins and a peculiar lipid composition. In addition, they can fuse to sperm in suitable conditions[2].

We expect that after fusion with prostasomes the properties of sperm may be functionally altered.

PROSTASOME FUNCTIONS

Prostasomes are formed by a membrane surrounding a non-organized core and have been claimed to take a part in semen liquefaction[3], in sperm motility and viability[4,5] and in the regulation of the immune response[6,7]. Although the reported possible roles of prostasomes are of primary interest for the reproductive ability of sperm, their mechanisms of action are practically unknown.

PROSTASOME TO SPERM FUSION

Prostasomes may interact with sperm in several ways. Among these, we consider the possibility that prostasome fuse to sperm membrane, so releasing the lipid and protein contents of its membrane and possibly also its content[2]. The lipid composition of prostasomes is quite peculiar because they are very rich in cholesterol and sphingomyelin and comparatively poor in phosphatidylcholine. In addition we found in prostasomes several enzymes (such as some proteases) that are not present in sperm[8,9]. Obviously the transfer of material form prostasome to sperm or vice-versa is bound to deeply affect the spermatozoon. Yet, it is difficult to foresee the nature and/or the extents of the variations of sperm function for two main reasons: several components are expected to be simultaneously transferred and the lipid plasma membrane of the spermatozoon is organized in hardly movable patches.

Table 1 Properties of the sperm to prostasome fusion

Property	Comments
It depends on pH	fusion is absent at pH 8, and increases upon pH lowering. It can be detected at pH 7.5, but it is higher at lower pH. Usually, we worked at pH 5
It is rapid	few minutes (2–3 min) of contact were enough to elicit most of the possible fusion. Usually prostasomes and sperm were kept in contact for 15 min to have the maximal fusion
It does not depend on Ca2+ concentration	
It depends on protein	to inactivate fusion completely, it is necessary to destroy with a protease the protein of both sperm and prostasome membranes. However, if sperm were intact, boiled prostasomes and liposomes prepared with prostasomal lipid could also fuse.
It depends on the relative amounts of prostasomes and sperm	fusion was well evident with a sperm to prostasome protein ratio of about 0.5 (physiological value)

HOW MEMBRANE FUSION CAN BE STUDIED

Several methods have been claimed to indicate the fusion between membranes. The fact that sperm are whole cells and not vesicles as are liposomes, limits the possibility of using a number of techniques. We found the method using octadecylrhodamine was suitable for our purpose[10]. The lipophylic probe shows a fluorescence self-quenching that decreases upon dilution, as may happen when a labelled membrane fuses to an unlabelled membrane. We observed prostasome to sperm fusion in certain conditions (Table 1). It is possible that prostasomes exert at least some of their biological function through the fusion mechanism. The pH values are extremely important in this connection. Indeed, although the vaginal milieu is acidic, we expect that the high buffering capacity of seminal fluid may intervene to limit the decrease of pH. It has been reported[11] that the average pH of human seminal fluid is 7.6, and, therefore, just at the upper limit for fusion to occur. A slight decrease of pH may trigger fusion. In addition, since the fusion, as detected by us, is rapid, even a short exposure of sperm to a slightly acidic milieu in the vagina may allow fusion to occur under physiological conditions.

CONSEQUENCES OF LIPID TRANSFER

The transfer of lipid-form prostasome to sperm has important consequences on the sperm membranes. The fluidity of prostasomes is very low, when compared to other membranes, because of their high cholesterol content. Upon fusion with prostasomes in physiological ratios, the viscosity of sperm increases dramatically[12]. As yet, it is impossible to say how the sperm function may be affected by this phenomenon, but it is reasonable to suppose that a variation of membrane fluidity must have consequences on membrane functions. The lipid composition of membrane is believed to affect membrane-bound enzymes and receptors.

CONSEQUENCES OF POROTEIN TRANSFER

Prostasomes contain a number of enzymatic activities that can be transferred to sperm upon fusion, so modifying the catalytic properties of sperm membranes. Among these are some proteases connected to the CD class of antigens (CD 13 and CD 26)[8,9]. It may be interesting to observe that these peptidases are absent in sperm before fusion. Apart from this consideration, the transfer of aminopeptidases that are integral proteins to the prostasomal membrane, is a further proof of the exchange of material between prostasome and sperm through the pH-stimulated fusion. The data obtained by measuring protein transfer strictly paralleled those obtained by the relief of fluorescence self-quenching of octadecylrhodamine.

CONCLUSIONS

From the above reported data we may propose that at least some of the physiological actions of prostasomes are due to the fusion of these vesicles to sperm.

REFERENCES

1. Ronquist G, Frithz GG. Prostasomes in human semen contain ADP and GDP. *Acta Eur.Fertil.* 1986;17(4):273-6.
2. Arienti G, Carlini E, Palmerini CA. Fusion of human sperm to prostasomes at acidic pH. *J.Membr.Biol.* 1997;155(1):89-94.
3. Lilja H, Laurel CB. Liquefaction of coagulated human semen. *Scand.J.Clin.Lab.Invest.* 1984;44:447-52.
4. Fabiani R, Johansson L, Lundkvist O, Ronquist G. Enhanced recruitment of motile spermatozoa by prostasome inclusion in swim-up medium. *Hum.Reprod.* 1994;9(8): 1485-9.
5. Fabiani R, Johansson L, Lundkvist O, Ulmsten U, Ronquist G. Promotive effect by prostasomes on normal human spermatozoa exhibiting no forward motility due to buffer washings. *European Journal of Obstetrics Gynecology and Reproductive Biology* 1994;57(3):181-8.
6. Kelly RW. Immunosuppressive mechanisms in semen: implications for contraception. *Hum.Reprod.* 1995;10(7):1686-93.
7. Skibinski G, Kelly RW, Harkiss D, James K. Immunosuppression by human seminal plasma–extracellular organelles (prostasomes) modulate activity of phagocytic cells. *Am.J.Reprod.Immunol.* 1992;28(2):97-103.
8. Arienti G, Carlini E, Verdacchi R, Cosmi EV, Palmerini CA. Prostasome to sperm transfer of CD13/aminopeptidase N (E.C. 3.4.11.2). *Biochim.Biophys.Acta* 1997;1336:533-8.
9. Arienti G, Polci A, Carlini E, Palmerini CA. Transfer of CD26/dipeptidyl peptidase IV (EC 3.5.4.4.) from prostasomes to sperm. *FEBS Lett.* 1997;410(23):343-6.

10. Hoekstra D, de Boer T, Klappe K, Wilschut J. Fluorescent method for measuring the kinetic of fusion between biological membranes. *Biochemistry* 1984;23 :5675-81 .
11. Raboch J, Skakova J. The pH of human ejaculates. *Fertil.Steril.* 1965;16:252-6.
12. Carlini E, Palmerini CA, Cosmi EV, Arienti G. Fusion of sperm with prostasomes: effects on membrane fluidity. *Arch.Biochem.Biophys.* 1997;343(1):6-12.

UTERINE PERFUSION IN FERTILE AND INFERTILE PATIENTS

Sanja Kupesic and Asim Kurjak

Department of Obstetrics and Gynecology, Medical School University of Zagreb,

Sveti Duh Hospital, Zagreb, Croatia

ANGIOGENESIS OF THE UTERUS

The majority of the blood supply to the uterus is from the uterine arteries, with only slight additional contributions from the ovarian arteries. The uterine arteries give rise to the arcuate arteries, which are oriented circumferentially in the outer third of the myometrium. These vessels give rise to the radial arteries, which, after crossing the myometrium-endometrium border, further branch and give rise to the basal arteries and the spiral arteries. The basal arteries, which are relatively short, terminate in a capillary bed that serves the stratum basalis of the endometrium. The spiral arteries, on the other hand, project further into the endometrium and terminate in a vast capillary network that serves the stratum functionalis of the endometrium.

Interestingly, only the spiral arteries undergo substantial anatomical changes during the menstrual cycle[1]. At the time of menstruation, probably as a result of decreasing estrogen and progesterone levels, the spiral arteries constrict, producing local hypoxia, ischemia, and eventually cell death within the stratum functionalis. The distal portion of the arteriolar system, as well as the capillary and venous beds, are then shed with the functionalis. The basal arteries, which are insensitive to decreasing estrogen and progesterone titers[2], are relatively unaffected and serve to maintain the integrity of the stratum basalis throughout the menstrual cycle. As the endometrium thickens three to five-fold during the next menstrual cycle, the remnants of the spiral arteries in the basalis must undergo substantial growth and give rise to a completely new capillary bed in order to maintain the integrity of the rapidly growing stroma. This process in initiated by the growth of new capillaries from the existing vasculature in the basalis[2]. These capillaries eventually differentiate into arteries and arterioles as the elastic and vascular smooth muscle components develop around the new capillaries[3]. Uterine angiogenesis during the proliferative and secretory phases provides an existing vascular supply for the trophoblast to invade if fertilization of the ovum occurs[4].

Following fertilization, the first stage of implantation is the adhesion of the blastocyst to the endometrial epithelium. This is followed by the penetration of the trophoblast through the epithelial lining. With further invasion of the trophoblast, maternal capillaries are encountered, surrounded, and induced to undergo profound physiological and architectural changes[5]. One of the first changes is an increase in vascular permeability at the site of implantation[6]. This is followed by metabolic activation of the endothelium in preparation for angiogenesis, and then vascular remodeling[6]. The subsequent remodelling of the maternal vasculature facilitates placentation. More about these events an interested reader can find in chapter on Doppler assessment of early placentation and embryonic circulation.

UTERINE PERFUSION CHANGES DURING THE MENSTRUAL CYCLE

More than any other available technique, transvaginal color Doppler affords detailed delineation of the uterus, its myometrium, endometrium and vessels[7-10].

It is well known that uterine perfusion is largely dependent on the patient's age, phase of the menstrual cycle, and other specific conditions (e.g. pregnancy, tumor)[11]. In this chapter we analyze them in detail.

There are complex relationships between the concentration of the ovarian hormones in peripheral venous plasma and uterine artery blood flow parameters[12-15]. In most women, there is a small amount of end-diastolic flow in the uterine arteries in the proliferative phase. The resistance index (RI) hovers around 0.88±0.04 until day 13 of the 28-day menstrual cycle. Steer and co-workers[14] reported that diastolic flow in the uterine arteries disappeared during the day of ovulation. Goswamy and Steptoe[12] found increasing resistance index and systolic/diastolic ratio during the postovulatory drop in the serum estradiol concentration. Increased uterine artery impedance was reported 3 days after the peak in luteinizing hormone (LH), and Scholtes and colleagues[16] recorded the highest value for the pulsatility index (PI) in the uterine arteries on cycle day 16.

These findings may be explained by increased uterine contractility[17] and compression of the vessels traversing the uterine wall, which decrease their diameter and consequently cause higher resistance to flow. During the normal menstrual cycle, there is a sharp increase in end-diastolic velocities between the proliferative and secretory phases[8]. It is particularly interesting that the lowest blood flow impedance occurs during the time of peak luteal function (resistance index (RI)=0.84±0.04), during which implantation is most likely to occur. It is logical that blood supply to the uterus should be high in the late luteal phase, as has been reported by Kurjak and associates[8], Goswamy and associates[12,13], Steer and associates[14], and Battaglia and associates[18]. The persistently lower RI in the luteal phase suggests that the relaxation effects on the uterine arteries persist until the onset of menstruation. Zaidi et al[19] obtained that there is circadian rhythm in uterine artery blood flow during the periovulatory period which appears to be independent from hormonal changes.

Similar circulatory changes to those observed in the main uterine arteries have been seen in the minute arteries (radial and spiral) with the introduction of transvaginal color and pulsed Doppler[20]. Our results show an increase of the RI in the myometrial vessels after ovulation, during the postovulatory drop in the serum estradiol concentration. Increased uterine contractility has been shown to coincide with decreased endometrial blood flow[17]. It is well known that the endometrium has an exceptional capacity to undergo changes in structure and function during the menstrual cycle. The histological changes include striking development of the blood vessels. The spiral arteries become more developed during the menstrual cycle. The increased endometrial vascularity is highly dependent upon the uterine, arcuate and radial artery blood flow. Blood flow velocity waveform changes in the spiral arteries during normal ovulatory cycles are characterized by lower velocity ($p<0.05$) and lower impedance to blood flow ($p<0.05$) than are those observed in the uterine arteries, with larger diameter[21]. It seems that features of endometrial blood flow may be used to predict the implantation success rate and to reveal unexplained infertility problems more precisely than evaluation of the main uterine artery alone.

UTERINE PERFUSION IN INFERTILE PATIENTS

The expanding experience with transvaginal color and pulsed Doppler sonography has established this technique as an additional tool in the management of infertile patients. In anovulatory cycles, a continuous increase of the uterine artery RI has been detected[8] Moreover, in some infertile patients, and end-diastolic flow is absent[13]. There are not enough data to speculate whether absent diastolic flow is associated with infertility and poor reproductive performance.

The uterine artery blood flow could be used to predict a hostile uterine environment prior to embryo transfer. Steer et al[14] calculated the probability of pregnancy by using PI values obtained from the uterine artery on the day of embryo transfer. With the use of these measurements, the highest probability of becoming pregnant was obtained in those patients with medium values of uterine artery PI. A mean PI of more than 3.0 before the transfer can predict up to 35% of failures to become pregnant. Tsai et al[22] evaluated the prognostic value of uterine perfusion on the day of human chorionic gonadotropin (hCG) administration in patients who were undergoing intrauterine insemination. They calculated pulsatility index of the ascending branch of the uterine arteries on the day of administration of hCG, and compared the uterine artery vascular resistance to the outcome of intrauterine insemination. No pregnancy occurred when the pulsatility index of the ascending branch of the uterine arteries was more than 3. The fecundity rate was 18% when the pulsatility was less than 2, and was 19.8% when the pulsatility index was between 2 and 3. Their data suggest that the measurement of uterine perfusion on the day of hCG administration may have predictive value regarding fecundity in patients undergoing intrauterine insemination. Zaidi et al[23] tried to asses whether measurement of the uterine artery blood flow impedance on the day of hCG administration can predict pregnancy and implantation rates in patients undergoing IVF procedure. They investigated 135 patients undergoing 139 IVF cycles. Their study suggest that the measurement of the uterine artery pulsatility index (PI) can predict subsequent implantation rate, since the highest pregnancy rates (34,7%) were when the uterine artery PI was between 2 and 3. Furthermore, the administration of hCG should be deferred until uterine artery PI falls to <3, which may result in improved implantation rates. However, more studies are necessary to establish the precise relationship between uterine artery perfusion and the probability of pregnancy. Those women with poor uterine perfusion could be advised to have their embryos cryopreserved for transfer at a later date.

An improvement of the uterine blood flow may be achieved by administration of estradiol[24] and perhaps even progesterone[25]. One of the major problems associated with current practice in *in vitro* fertilization is the necessity to use multiple embryo transfer to increase the pregnancy rate. This leads to an increased incidence of multiple pregnancy. This may contribute to increased obstetric risk and poorer perinatal outcome, when compared to singleton pregnancies. It is well known that the probability of pregnancy is strongly related to embryo quality and uterine receptivity. Instead of doing endometrial biopsy, which may cause trauma and bleeding at the implantation site, uterine receptivity should be assessed by color Doppler ultrasound[26]. Zaidi et al[27] evaluated 96 women undergoing in vitro fertilization treatment on the day of hCG administration by transvaginal color Doppler. They assessed endometrial thickness, endometrial morphology, presence or absence of subendometrial or intraendometrial color flow, and intraendometrial vascular penetration on the day of hCG administration and related the results to pregnancy rates. The overall pregnancy rate was 32.3% and there was no significant difference between the pregnant and non-pregnant groups with regard to endometrial thickness, subendometrial peak systolic blood flow velocity and subendometrial index. However, the absence of subendometrial blood flow was always related with failure of implantation. Transvaginal color and pulsed Doppler examination is easily repeatable, rapid, simple to perform and may predict the likelihood of implantation, minimizing the risk of multiple pregnancy. Studies of uterine blood flow might become a non-invasive assay of uterine receptivity, giving us more information on the pathophysiology of infertility, especially in the group of patients with unexplained causes.

UTERINE PERFUSION IN SPONTANEOUS AND INDUCED OVARIAN CYCLES WITH CONFIRMED OVULATION

Kupesic and Kurjak[19] measured the flow velocity of the uterine, radial and spiral arteries during the periovulatory period in spontaneous and induced ovarian cycles with confirmed ovulation. They studied daily measurements of 78 patients attending an infertility clinic, because of the male factor in infertility.

In spontaneous cycles, the uterine flow velocity had a PI of 3.16, 2 days before ovulation, and started to decrease the day before ovulation (PI=2.22). In stimulated cycles, these changes did not occur, and the mean PI of 3.06 remained at that level during the periovulatory period. Clear flow velocity waveforms were obtained from the endometrium and myometrium at around the time of ovulation. The pulsatility indices of radial and spiral arteries showed significantly higher values in stimulated than in spontaneous cycles.

Clomiphene citrate is known to deplete estrogen receptors in estrogen-sensitive tissues, influencing endometrial growth and pattern[28]. There was a strong correlation between endometrial thickness and flow velocities. However, this did not apply to the group of patients stimulated with clomiphene citrate/hMG and normal endometrial growth, where the authors demonstrated the absence of diastolic flow in spiral arteries in 55.6% of patients. However, no difference in endometrial thickness and perfusion was observed between hMG-stimulated patients and those in spontaneous cycles. Indeed, spiral artery blood flow changes may be used as an accurate predictor of implantation success rate in treatment with IVF/embryo transfer. Those women with poor uterine perfusion in their current treatment cycles could be advised to have their embryos cryopreserved and transferred either in a spontaneous cycle or after correction of the endometrial perfusion by and appropriate treatment.

More about improvements of the uterine blood flow in infertile patients is discussed elsewhere in this book.

REFERENCES:

1. Torry, R. J. and Rongish, B. J. (1992). Angiogenesis in the uterus: potential regulation and relation to tumor angiogenesis. Am. J. Reprod. Immunol., 27, 171-9

2. Kaiserman-Abramof, I. R. and Padykula, H. A. (1989). Angiogenesis in the postovulatory primate endometrium: The coiled arteriolar system. Anat. Rec., 224, 479-89

3. Ramsey, E. M. and Donner, M. E. (1980). Placental Vasculature and Circulation, pp. 1-52. (Philadelphia, PA: Sounders)

4. Khong, T. Y., De Wolf, F., Robertson, W. B. and Brosens, I. (1986). Inadequate maternal vascular response to placentation in pregnancies complicated by pre-

eclampsia and by small-for-gestational age infants. Br. J. Obstet. Gynaecol., 93, 1049-59

5. Ramsey, E. M. and Donner, M. V. (1988). Placental vasculature and circulation in primates. In Kaufmann, P., Miller, R. K. (eds.) Trophoblast Research, Vol. 3: Placental Vascularization and Blood flow, pp. 217-33 (New York, NY: Plenum Press)

6. Christofferson, R. and Nilsson, B. O. (1988). Morphology of the endometrial microvasculature during early placentation in the rat. Cell Tissue Res., 253, 209-20

7. Kurjak, A. and Kupesic-Urek, S. (1992). Normal and abnormal uterine perfusion. In Jaffe, R. and Warsof, L. S. (eds.). Color Doppler Imaging in Obstetrics and Gynecology, pp. 255-63. (New York: McGraw Hill)

8. Kurjak, A., Kupesic-Urek, S., Schulman, H. and Zalud, I. (1991). Transvaginal color flow Doppler in the assessment of ovarian and uterine blood flow in infertile women. Fertil. Steril., 56, 870-3

9. Du Bose, T. J., Hill, L. W. and Henningan, J. W. Jr. (1985). Sonography of arcuate uterine blood vessels. J. Ultrasound Med., 4, 229-33

10. Jurkovic, D., Jauniaux, E., Kurjak, A. and Cambell, S. (1991). Transvaginal color Doppler assessment of the uteroplacental circulation in early pregnancy. Obstet. Gynecol., 77, 365-9

11. Long, M. G., Boultbee, J. E., Hanson, M. E. and Begent, J. H. R. (1989). Doppler time velocity waveform studies of the uterine artery and uterus. Br. J. Obstet. Gynaecol., 96, 588-93

12. Goswamy, R. K. and Steptoe, P. C. (1988). Doppler ultrasound studies of the uterine artery in spontaneous ovarian cycles. Hum. Reprod., 3, 721-3

13. Goswamy, R. K., Williams, G. and Steptoe, P. C. (1988). Decreased uterine perfusion a cause of infertility. Hum. Reprod., 3, 955-8

14. Steer, C. V., Mills, C. V. and Campbell, S. (1991). Vaginal color Doppler assessment on the day of embryo transfer (ET) accurately predicts patients in an *in*

vitro fertilization programme with suboptimal uterine perfusion who fail to become pregnant. Ultrasound Obstet. Gynecol., 1, 79-82

15. Bourne, T. H., Jurkovic, D., Waterstone, J., Campbell, S. and Collins, W. P. (1991). Intrafollicular blood flow during human ovulation. Ultrasound Obstet. Gynecol., 1, 53-7

16. Scholtes, M. C. W., Wladimiroff, J. W., van Rijen, H. J. M. and Hop, W. C. J. (1989). Uterine and ovarian flow velocity waveforms in the normal menstrual cycle: a transvaginal study. Fertil. Steril., 52, 981-5

17. Haukson, A., Akerlund, M. and Melin, P. (1988). Uterine blood flow and myometrial activity at menstruation, and the action of vasoprossin and a synthetic antagonist. Br. J. Obstet. Gynaecol., 95, 898-904

18. Battaglia, C., Larocca, E., Lanzani, A., Valentini, M. and Genanzzani, A. R. (1990). Doppler ultrasound studies of the uterine arteries in spontaneous and IVF cycles. Gynecol. Endocrinol., 4, 245-50

19. Zaidi, J., Jurkovic, D., Campbell, S., Pitroff, R., McGregor, A. and Tan, S. L. (1995). Description of carcadian rhythm in uterine artery blood flow during the peri-ovulatory period. Hum. Reprod., 10(7), 1642-6

20. Kupesic, S. and Kurjak, A. (1993). Uterine and ovarian perfusion during the periovulatory period assessed by transvaginal color Doppler. Fertil. Steril., 60, 439-43

21. Kupesic, S., Kurjak, A. and Stilinovic, K. (1994). The assessment of female infertility. In Kurjak, A. (ed.) An Atlas of Transvaginal Color Doppler, pp. 171-99. (Carnforth, UK: Parthenon Publishing)

22. Tsai, Y. C., Chang, J. C., Tai, M. J., Kung, F. T., Yang, L. C. and Chang, S. Y. (1996). Relationship of uterine perfusion to outcome of intrauterine insemination. J. Ultrasound Med., 15, 633-6

23. Zaidi, J., Pitroff, R., Shaker, A., Kyei-Mensah, A., Campbell, S. and Tan, S. L. (1996). Assessment of uterine artery blood flow on the day of human chorionic

gonadotropin administration by transvaginal color Doppler ultrasound in an in vitro fertilization program. Fertil. Steril., 5(2), 377-81

24. Ford, S. P., Reynolds, R. P. and Farley, D. B. (1984). Interaction of ovarian steroids and periarterial alpha-1-adrenergic receptors in altering uterine blood flow during the estrous cycle of gilts. Am. J. Obstet. Gynecol., 150, 480-4

25. de Ziegler, D., Bessis, R. and Frydman, R. (1991). Vascular resistance of uterine arteries: physiological effects of estradiol and progesterone. Fertil. Steril., 55, 775-8

26. Kupesic, S., Kurjak, A., Vujisic, S. and Petrovic, Z. (1997). Luteal phase defect: comparison between Doppler velocimetry, histological and hormonal markers. Ultrasound Obstet. Gynecol., 9, 105-112

27. Zaidi, J., Campbell, S., Pitroff, R. and Tan, S. L. (1995). Endometrial thickness, morphology, vascular penetration and velocimetry in predicting implantation in an in vitro fertilization program. Ultrasound Obstet. Gynecol., 6(3), 191-8

28. Glissant, A., de Mouzon, J. and Frydman, R. (1985). Ultrasound study of the endometrium during in vitro fertilization cycles. Fertil. Steril., 44, 786-90

ASSISTED PROCREATION IN PRIVATE PRACTICE

Funduk-Kurjak B, Mihaljević D

Modern Medical Centre, Zagreb, Croatia

ABSTRACT

Procedure parameters were studied in 812 couples treated for infertility in Modern Medical Centre from January 1995 till December 1997. Four hundred thirty five couples were included in the procedure of insemination, and 377 couples in IVF/ICSI /ET procedure. The age of female patients ranged from 24 to 46 years, while 60% were above 35. Combined male and female factor was the indications for the IVF procedure in more than 50%.The indications for insemination were quality of sperm and anovulatory cycles. Induction of ovulation in the patients for insemination was performed with Clomid+hCG, Clomid+HMG+hCG, or HMG+hCG. Stimulation of ovulation with HMG/FSH, GnRH/ HMG or GnRH/FSH was protocol for IVF patients. Four hundred thirty five couples were included in the procedure of insemination with 460 stimulated cycles. It resulted with 87 pregnancies (18,9%), 11 spontaneous abortions (2,3%), and 2 ectopic pregnancies (0,4%). There were 74 (16,1%) term deliveries, 68 (91,8%) singleton pregnancies, 5 (6,7%) twins and 1 (1,35%) multiple pregnancy. Three hundred seventy seven couples were included in the procedure of IVF with 404 stimulated cycles. The number of punctions was 392 and the number of the cycles with ET 389 (96,35%). Pregnancy rate was 20,6%, spontaneous abortions 7 (1,75%), ectopic pregnancies 2 (0,5%), term deliveries 71 (18,4%), singleton pregnancies 66 (92,95%),twins 5 (7,1%). Endometrial thickness varied from 9 to 14 mm while

RI in spiral arteries was 0,42-0,54 in 80% of the patients. In about 20% patients were with poor endometrial receptivity. The therapy with Gn RH analogues (Decapeptyl 0,1 through 21 days) was helpful in patients with lower endometrial receptivity and resulted with appropriate endometrial secretory transformation.

INTRODUCTION

Methods of assisted reproduction (AIH, IVF, ICSI,) are commonly used in treatment of human infertility, and significantly improve the quality of life by offering a couple a chance to conceive. Indications for assisted human reproduction are: tubal and male factor of infertility, endometriosis, immunological factors and other factors of unknown etiology.

AIH is a procedure which performs isolation of sperm and injection of so treated sperm in female reproductive system.

IVF treatment does include isolation of oocytes and progressive motile sperm, cultivation and fertilization in laboratory conditions. In vitro fertilization (IVF) is used in treatment of human infertility which is caused by tubal factor infertility, endometriosis and milder forms of male infertility (1).

The ICSI technique uses the mechanical insertion of a single sperm into the oocyte cytoplasm. By introducing ICSI technique a significant improvement in assisted human reproduction has been achieved (2). Intracytoplasmic sperm injection (ICSI) method is preferred in severe cases of male infertility.

In this study we wanted to present our experiences in field human assisted reproduction in private practice in Croatia.

MATERIALS AND METHODS

Procedure parameters were studied in 812 couples treated for infertility in Modern Medical Centre from January 1995 till December 1997.

Four hundred thirty five couples were included in the procedure of insemination, three hundred seventy seven couples in IVF/ICSI/ET procedure. The age of female patients ranged from 24 to 46 years, while 60% were above 35.

The indications for insemination were quality of semen and anovulatory cycles, while combined male and female factor was the indications for the IVF procedure in more than 50%. Induction of ovulation in the patients for insemination was performed following three different protocols:

(1) Clomid /hCG; (2) Clomid/ HMG/ hCG ; (3) HMG / hCG

Induction of ovulation in the patients for IVF/ICSI was performed following protocols for IVF/ICSI procedures: (1) HMG /FSH /hCG;

(2) Gn RH /HMG /hCG; (3) Gn RH /FSH /hCG, (4) contraceptives/ Buserelin / HMG /hCG

The induction of ovulation for insemination procedures (AIH) was performed with clomiphene tablets (100mg) once a day from the thirth till the fifth day of menstrual cycle. The next three days the patient was given two ampoules of Pergonal parenterally. The first ultrasound was performed on the seventh day of the menstrual cycle, and the following administration of further therapy depended on the ultrasound finding.

Ovarian stimulation protocols involved hypophysis desensibilization with a short-acting gonadotropin releasing hormone (GnRH) analogue (Decapeptyl - Ferring, Kiel, Deutschland) from 21th day of the previous cycle. Stimulation was achieved by administering 225 IU human menopausal gonadotropines – HMG (Pergonal, Serono, Aubonne, Switzerland) or FSH (Metrodyn, Serono,

Aubonne, Switzerland) per day from day 2 to 4 and 150 IU HMG or FSH Metrodyn, Serono, Aubonne, Switzerland) per day from day 5 to 6 day. Ultrasound monitoring and adjustment of HMG levels began on day 7. Ovulation was triggered by the administration of 10000 of human chorionic gonadotropin – hCG (Primogonyl, Schering AG, Berlin, Deutschland) when the largest follicle was over 16 mm and with a mean estradiol (E2) level of 300 pg/ml per large follicle. Oocytes were retrieved 36 hours after hCG injection by vaginally using ultrasound guidance aspiration follicles. After recovery, oocytes were washed free of follicular fluid and preincubated 3 hr in Quinn's HTF Medium with EDTA and glutamine (Advanced Reproductive Technologies, USA) with 5% Human serum albumin (Advanced Reproductive Technologies, USA) at 37°C in 5% CO_2 in humidified air . Within 2 h oocytes were inseminated with $40x10^3$ to $80x10^3$ motile sperm. Fertilization was checked at about 20 hours after insemination. If oocytes did not contain pronuclea we rechecked fertilization once more after another 24 hours. Embryo transfer was performed 48 -72 after punction and aspiration follicles. Intracytoplasmic sperm injection was performed 4 hours after oocyte recovery, by using hyaluronidase and PVP. The procedure was performed with micropipetes (Humagen Fertility Diagnostics Inc, Charlotottesville, Virginia USA) in drop of HTF buffered by HEPES .(Advanced Reproductive Technologies, USA).

.

RESULTS

Four hundred thirty five couples were included in the procedure of insemination with 460 stimulated cycles. Eighty seven pregnancies were obtained (18,9% of number of total stimulated cycles) after procedure of insemination. Eleven out of 87 pregnancies resulted spontaneous abortions (2,3%), while 2 were ectopic pregnancies (0,4%) (table 1).

TABLE 1: Results of insemination procedure

	N°	%
total couples	435	
total stimulated cycles	460	100,0
total pregnancies	87	18,9
spontaneous abortions	11	2,3
ectopic pregnancies	2	0,4

Eighty seven pregnancies were resulted by 74 term deliveries (16,1% of number of total stimulated cycles). Sixty eight of them (91,8% of number of term deliveries) were singleton pregnancies, five (6,7%) were twins and one (1,3%) was a multiple pregnancy (table 2).

TABLE 2: Outcome of pregnancies after insemination

	N°	%
term deliveries	74	100,0
singleton pregnancies	68	91,8
twins pregnancies	5	6,7
multiple pregnancies	1	1,3

Three hundred seventy seven couples were included in the IVF procedure with 404 stimulated cycles. The results of 392 retrieval cycles were 80 pregnancies (19,8% of number of stimulated cycles). Seven out of 80 pregnancies resulted in spontaneous abortions (1,7%), while two were ectopic pregnancies (0,5%) (table 3).

TABLE 3: Results of IVF procedure

	N°	%
total couples	377	
total stimulated cycles	404	100,0
retrieval cycles	392	
transfer cycles	389	96.3
total pregnancies	80	19.8
spontaneus abortions	7	1,7
ectopic pregnancies	2	0,5

The results of 80 pregnancies were 71 live birth (18,4%of number of all stimulated cycles in IVF procedure), 66 (92,9% of number of live birth) were singleton pregnancies, and 5 (7,1%) were twins.

TABLE 4: Outcome of pregnancies after IVF procedure

	N°	%
live birth	71	100,0
singleton pregnancies	66	92.9
twins pregnancies	5	7.1

In this study we had 8 preterm deliveries (11,3% of number of live birth) after IVF procedures, low birth weight in 9 cases (12,7%) and cesarean section was performed in 15 cases (21,1%).

DISCUSSION

The most of the authors in their studies showed that the complication rate of pregnancies from IVF/ET cycles was higher than that found in spontaneous pregnancies. Srisombut et al (3) analysed difference between outcome of pregnancies achieved by IVF/ET and spontaneous pregnancies. They included 80 pregnancies obtained after IVF/ET procedures and authors described high rate of abortion (30%), multiple pregnancy (20%), ectopic pregnancy (6,25%), heterotopic pregnancy (1,25%), preterm delivery (11,8%), low birth weight in 35,8% cases and caesarean section in 62,7% cases after IVF/ET. Olivennes et al (4) in their study compared the perinatal outcome of 72 IVF/ET twin pregnancies with 164 spontaneous twin pregnancies and with 82 twin pregnancies following spontaneous conception after ovarian stimulation. Authors did not find significant difference in the data analysed, with the exception of the rate of emergency caesarean sections. In the IVF/ET group the prematurity rate (38,9%), small-for gestation-age (18%), and perinatal mortality (3,47%) were not statistically different with the spontaneous group (39,8%, 22,7% and 4,27%) or to the stimulation group (45,1%, 23,2% and 3,05%).

Authors concluded that perinatal outcome of IVF/ET twin pregnancies does not seem to be increased when compared with spontaneous pregnancies or to pregnancies obtained after ovarian stimulation but without IVF/ET. In our study we also analysed outcome of pregnancies conceived by IVF/ICSI or AIH. We concluded that the use of methods of assisted human reproduction does not significantly increase the risk of complications in pregnancy.

Bernasko et al (5) compared outcome of 105 twin pregnancies conceived by IVF or GIFT and 279 twin pregnancies conceived spontaneously. Authors showed that elective cesarean delivery was more frequent in twin pregnancies conceived by IVF or GIFT. There were no statistically significant differences in the frequency of antepartum or intrapartum complications, preterm delivery or mean gestation age at delivery.

Agustsson et al (6) compared difference between obstetric outcome of 453 natural and 69 assisted conception twin pregnancies. Mean gestational age in both groups was 36 weeks. Authors showed that the birthweight, gestational age and perinatal mortality rates by conventional and extended classification were not different. Cesarean section was used more often in the assisted conception group. Final results did not confirm any major difference in obstetric outcome between twins conceived by natural or assisted route.

Causio et al (7) analysed outcome of 48 multiple pregnancies: 36 twin, 8 triplets, 2 quadruplets and 2 quintuplets conceived by IVF. The mean maternal age was 29,72 years, and the mean gestation age was 36,83 weeks. Of the 36 patients with two babies 20 (55,60%) had cesarean section, whereas 12 were delivered vaginally, All the triplets, quadruplets and quintuples were delivered abdominally.

Devroey et al (8) conducted a study in 1993/94 on 69 couples suffering from azoospermia where testicular sperm extraction and intracytoplasmic sperm injection were performed. In 50 couples with obstructive azoospermia a total of 631 oocytes were injected after TESA yielding a 2-PN fertilisation rate of 57%. So far, eight healthy babies have been born, including two singletons and three twin gestation. In 19 couples with non obstructive azoospermia a total of 264 oocytes were injected after TESA, yielding a 2-PN fertilisation rate of 58%. So far, six healthy babies have been born including one singleton, one twin and one triplet gestation.

The similar studies were performed by Kahrahan et al (9) whose included 32 couples with obstructive and non - obstructive azoospermia. Testicular sperm extraction was performed in 16 obstructive azoospermic cases and 16 non-obstructive azoospermia cases with severe spermatogenetic defect where the testicles were the only source of sperm cells. A total of 288 oocytes was obtained from 32 females and 84% were injected. A total of 15 pregnancies was achieved, nine from the obstructive and six from the non-obstructive group. Four pregnancies resulted in clinical abortion (26,6%). Authors described a high implantation rate (26,6% in non-obstructive and 30% in obstructive azoospermia group).

Obruca et al (10) included in their study 16 couples with ductal obstruction. Testis tissue was obtained by excisional biopsies and ICSI was performed. One healthy boy and two girls (twin pregnancy) were born.

The results of our study clearly show that the use of methods of assisted human reproduction does not significantly increase the risk of complications in pregnancy. Medical assisted procreation success rate in other world centers that is given by percentage of pregnancies on number of transfer cycle and goes from 15% to 25%. Our rate is 20,6% which correlates with data in literature.

REFERENCES:

1 Edwards RG, Brody SA. Principles and Practice of Assisted Human Reproduction. London: W. B. Saunders Company, 1995.

2 Palermo G, Joris H, Devroy P, Van Sterteghem AC. Pregnancies after intracytoplasmic injection of single spermatozoon into an ocyte. Lancet 1992; 340: 17-8.

3 Srisombut C, Rojanasakul A, Choktanasiri W, Weerakiet S, Chinsomboon S. Outcome of pregnancy in IVF/ET cycle at Ramathibodi Hospital. J Med Associate of Thailand 1995; 78(12):657-61.

4 Olivennes F, Kadhel P, Rufal P,Fanchini R,Fernandez H, Frydman R. Perinatal outcome of twin pregnancies obtained after in vitro fertilization: comparison with twin pregnancies obtained spontaneously or after ovarian stimulation. Fertil & Steril 1996; 66(1):105-9.

5 Bernasko J, Lynch L, Lapinski R,Berkowitz RL. Twin pregnancies conceived by assisted reproductive techniques: maternal and neonatal outcomes. Obstet $ Gynecol 1997;89(3):368-72.

6 Agustsson T, Geirsson RT, Mires G. Obstetric natural and assisted conception twin pregnancies is similar. Acta Obstet Scand 1997;76(1):45-9.

7 Causio F,Leoneffi T, Falagario M. Incidence and outcome of multiple pregnancy after in vitro fertilization. Acta Europ Fertil 1995; 26(1): 41-4.

8 Devroey P, Nagy P, Tournaye H, Liu J, Silber S, Van Steitteghe A.Outcome of spermatozoa in obstructive and non-obstructive azoospermia. Hum Reprod 1996;11(5):1015-8 .

9 Kahraman S, Ozgur S,Alatas C, Aksoy S, Balaban B, Evrenkaya T, Nuhoglu A, Tasdemir M, Schoysman R, Vanderzwalmen P, Nijs M. High implantation and pregnancy rates with testicular sperm extraction and intracytoplasmic sperm injection in obstructive and non-obstructive azoospermia. Hum Reprod 1996;11(3):673-6.

10 Obruca A, Mock K, Feichtinger W, Lunglmayr G. Fertilization and pregnancies following intracytoplasmic injection of testicular spermatozoa. J of Assist Reprod &Genet 1995;12(9):627-31.

Computer-aided prognosis of birth after successful treatment of infertility

M. Klimek, M. Bałajewicz, A. Frączek and J. Janeczko

OB./GYN Chairs, Jagiellonian University, Cracow, Poland

Pregnancies after successful treatment of infertility are characterised by cesarean section (1,2). This is result of insufficiency of two basic neuroendocrinological systems: oxytocin-oxitocinase and corticotrophin releasing hormone (CRH) – CRH-binding protein, which is typical in those cases, but rarely diagnosed by obstetricians, who also predicte only statistical time of birth (instead of individual one) with resulting iatrogenic consequences.

Introduction of computer-aided birth-date prediction is based on assessment of the degree and rate of individual foetus maturation on the basis of two ultrasonographic scans of the foetuses performed in advanced pregnancy (3,4,5). It allows to eliminate foetal mortality due to hypothalamic insufficiency syndromes in pregnant women, as well as reducing the infant morbidity after high-risk prehnancies.

The study shows the results of observation of 300 pregnancies and deliveries after treatment of infertility (I group). 203 patients with normal course of pregnancy were enrolled in simultaneous observations as a control group without previous fertility therapy (II group).

MATERIAL AND RESULTS

Characteristics of pregnancy outcomes are summarized in Table 1. Both patient groups had statistically different mean values of mather's age, parity and gestational age as well as distribution of birth weeks, but not significantly different gravity. Nevertheless their actual and computer-aided predicted birth terms were not statistically different in the pretreated women (I group: 268.8±11.6 days after last menstrual period versus 269.2±17.0 predicted days without taken into account LMP, t=1.07, NS) as well as in control ones (II group: 278.9±13.4 days vs 276.7±19.1 days, t=1.65, NS).

Table I. Characteristics (mean±SD, t, p) of pregnancy outcomes with (group I) and without (group II) fertility therapy

Group	I	II	t, p
Number	300	203	
Mother			
age (years)	29.9±4.9	25.9±5.1	8.84
	18-48	19-43	<0.001
gravity	2.3±1.4	2.2±1.5	0.76
	1-8	1-8	NS
parity	1.5±1.0	2.2±1.5	6.03
	1-5	1-8	<0.001
Gestation age			
actual (days)	268.8±11.6	278.9±13.4	8.99
	235-316	215-302	<0.001
predicted (days)	269.2±17.0	276.7±19.1	4.61
	227-303	226-327	<0.001
Birth week	N (%)	N (%)	
<37	49 (16.2)	27 (13.3)	
37	66 (22.0)	24 (11.8)	
38	85 (28.1)	27 (13.3)	χ^2=62.77
			<0.001
39-40	73 (24.3)	70 (34.5)	
41	20 (6.7)	15 (7.4)	
42	6 (2.0)	18 (8.9)	
>42	2 (0.7)	22 (10.8)	

Table II. Characteristics (mean±SD, t, p) of newborns

Group	I	II	t, p
Newborn	300	203	
actual weight (g)	3235±445	3326±485	2.17
	1620-4500	1600-4600	0.05
predicted weight	3377±254	3272±306	4.18
	2414-3900	2048-3814	<0.001
Apgar score	9.7±0.7	9.6±0.9	1.44
	4-10	5-10	NS
actual B-K	37.9±2.8	39.0±1.6	5.06
	26-45	23-48	<0.001
predicted B-K	39.3±1.1	39.0±1.7	2.40
	26-45	32-46	0.01

Also predictions of newborns weight (Table 2) were hrighly correct in both groups (I group: 3235±445g vs 3377±254g, t=2.09, NS; II group: 3326±485g vs 3272±306g, t=1.95, NS), but only in pretreated women the predicted mean of maturity in Ballard-Klimek scale was higher than real one (39.3±1.1 points vs 37.9±2.8 pts, t=2.47). It is worth noting, however, that newborns characteristics were different with exception of theirs Apgar scores.

CONCLUSIONS
Computer-aided prognosis of birth term and newborn state enables correct evaluation of pregnancies at risk, including outcomes of pregnancies after successful treatment of intertility.

REFERENCES
1. Klimek R.: Monitoring of Pregnancy and Prediction of Birth-date. Parthenon Publishing Group, London, Casterton, New York, 1994.
2. Klimek R., Fedor-Freybergh P., Janus L., Walas-Skolicka E.: A Time to Be Born, DREAM Publish. Comp.,Cracow, 1996.
3. Klimek M.: Computer-aided imaging in advanced pregnancy. W: Popkin D. R. and Peddle L.J. (eds) Women's Health Today., 245-250. Parthenon, New York-London, 1994.
4. Klimek M. - Medical prognosis versus statistical prediction of birth in Klimek R., Fedor-Freybergh P., Janus L., Walas-Skolicka E.: A Time to Be Born, DREAM Publishing, Cracow, 1996; 9-33.
5. Cosmi E.V., Klimek R., Di Renzo G.C., Kulakov V., Kurjak A., Maeda K., Mandruzzato G.P., Van Geijn H.P., Wladimiroff J.: Prognosis of birth term: recommendations on current practice and overview of new developments. Archives of Perinatal Medicine, 1997, vol 3(2), 31-50.

TECHNIQUES FOR EARLY DIAGNOSIS OF THE ABNORMAL FETUS

ARIS J. ANTSAKLIS

1st Department in Obstetrics and Gynecology, Division of Fetal Maternal Medicine, University of Athens, «Alexandra» Maternity Hospital, Athens - Greece

At the end of the twenty century a large number of approaches promise to increase the likelihood of a successful pregnancy outcome. In the past decade few areas of medicine have evolved as rapidly as that of prenatal diagnosis.

The objectives of prenatal diagnosis are:

1. To provide the couples with the accurate information about the risks of having children with an abnormality and the possibilities of avoiding it.

2. To provide the couples with the adequate technology at disposal in order to obtain the best possible diagnosis.

3. To provide the parents with objective information about the characteristics and prognosis of the diagnosed defect, in order to enable them to choose the possible alternatives (selective abortion, intrauterine treatment, continuation of the pregnancy).

4. To reduce the level of anxiety associated with reproduction, especially in high risk cases for congenital malformations.

It is widely accepted that at least 3% of all new-borns will present with a significant birth defect or genetic disorder and many more individuals will be found to have some congenital or genetic defect during childhood and early adult years.

Accurate fetal diagnosis become possible by the invasive techniques of amniocentesis, fetal blood sampling, chorion villus sampling (CVS) and embryoscopy while improved image resolution also permits ultrasonographic guidance for all the invasive diagnostic procedures mentioned above.

During the last ten years, biochemical and biophysical screening methods inexpensive and easy to use, have been developed for primary first and second trimester screening, to select those women who independently of their personal characteristics, are more susceptible of carrying a fetus with a chromosomal anomaly.

It has been suggested that using specific 2nd trimester sonographic criteria (nuchal thickening, short femur lenght) within an at risk population; 68% of trisomy 21 fetuses can be diagnosed by offering amniocentesis to 5% of pregnant women. (2)

Invasive procedures were primarily limited to the second and third trimester of pregnancy.

The movement of prenatal diagnosis into the first trimester has been rapidly accepted for several reasons. A first trimester procedure provides earlier reassurance and allows easier and more private, pregnancy termination when necessary.

ULTRASONOGRAPHY

The last five years the role of ultrasonography in the detection of many fetal anomalies is well established, remarkably accurate and continues to evolve rapidly through higher resolution units and the development of transvaginal probes.

It is obvious that present possibilities of prenatal diagnosis using ultrasonography depend on the quality of equipment used but especially on the opetators experience.

Transcervical sonography, with a 12,5MHZ catheter based miniature transducer offers the potential for improving basic knowledge about in vivo human development. (3)

By traditional 2-D ultrasonography many fetal structural malformations can be diagnosed. For complex malformations, a high degree of expertise in training is needed to translate 2-D images into the interpretation of a 3-D structure. 3-D ultrasound technology resolves some of these problems and its application in Obstetrics and Gynecology is growing as technology improves and clinical experience accumulates.

In the first trimester for accumulation of fluid behind the fetal neck the term nuchal translucency (NT) is used, because this is the ultrasonographic feature that is observed. During the second trimester NT usually resolves and in a few cases it evolves into either nuchal oedema or cystic hygromas with or without generalised hydrops. It has been suggested that the fetal NT thickness increased with crown rump length. Therefore in determining whether a given NT is increased it is essential to take gestation age into account. (4)

Measurements of fetal nuchal translucency (NT) at 10-14 weeks of gestation is now to be the most effective method of screening for chromosomal defects. The sensitivity of screening by the combination of maternal age and fetal NT is more than 80% for a false positive rate of 5%. This compares favourably with screening by maternal age alone (30%) or by maternal age and second trimester maternal serum markers (60%).

It has been suggested that between 10-14 weeks the larger the NT measurements the higher the risk for trisomies, the higher the maternal serum hCG the higher is the risk for trisomy 21, and the higher the fetal heart rate the higher the risk for trisomies.

When fetal heart rate and maternal serum free-β hCG are also taken into account the detection rate of chromosomal defects is about 90%.

In conclusion, the combination of maternal age and fetal nuchal translucency thicknes at 10-14 weeks is now proven to be the most effective method of screening for chromosomal abnormalities with a sensitivity for trisomy 21 of more than 80%. If the NT at 10-14 weeks is > 3,5mm and fetal karyotype is normal, a very detailed scan should be carried out at 20 weeks and special attention should be given to the examination of the heart and great arteries and to the detection of major defects and small dysmorphic features.

MAGNETIC RESONANCE IMAGING

Studies in early 80's have tried to determine the value of MRI for the study of fetal anatomy and most of them concluded that ultrasound remained the primary method for fetal screening and diagnosis.

Recently it has been suggested that fetal paralysis is not required for satisfactory imaging, and this simplified considerably the use of MRI in clinical obstetrics. At present MRI has been reserved for second and third trimester prenatal diagnosis. More recent studies have focused on the appearance of early embryonic anatomy through MRI which hold great promise for the non invasive detailed visualisation of the developing fetus. (5)

MATERNAL SERUM SCREENING

Recently there has been increased emphasis on the use of maternal serum alpha - fetoprotein (MS AFP) and other maternal serum metabolites as markers for pregnancies at risk for aneuploidy. Using a combination of maternal serum markers AFP, hCG, UE3, maternal age, 55-60% of fetal Down syndrome can be detected. Future strategies for Down's syndrome screening during the second trimester of pregnancy may include the use of new markers such as dimeric inhibin-A and a urinary b-core fragement of hCG. At a 5% false positive rate, the use of serum AFP, HCG, uE3 and inhibin - A, gave a 70% detection rate for Down's syndrome. Given a 5% false positive rate, the calculated detection rate for fetal Down's syndrome was 79,6% using β-core hCG, and 82,3% using b-core hCG and total estrogen.

Advancing biochemical screening into the first trimester would be highly desirable because patients determined to be at increased risk could be offered either CVS or early amniocentesis, thus avoiding second trimester termination when fetal abnormalities are detected. Early evidence appears that screening in the first trimester, will also allow detection of fetal Down's syndrome with an increased accuracy.

Associations exist between Down's syndrome and low MS AFP, low pregnancy associated placental protein A (PAPP A) and elevated free β-hCG (FβhCG). (6)

In 1996 Wald reported a multicenter study using two markers, PAPPA and Fβ hCG, for first trimester Down's syndrome screening and gave a 62% detection rate with a 5% false positive rate. Studies examining the relationship between maternal PAPP-A or free β-hCG concentrations and fetal NT thickness have demonstrated significant association between biochemistry and ultrasound findings in either the chromosomally normal or the trisomy 21 pregnancies. Therefore, maternal serum PAPP-A and free β-hCG and fetal nuchal translucency can be combined in calculating risks for fetal trisomies and can improve the sensitivity of screening for trisomy 21 by about 5%. (7)

EARLY AMNIOCENTESIS

Early amniocentesis was developed as an extension of midtrimester amniocentesis with suggestions that it had a similar level of safety. The technique is similar to traditional amniocentesis except that less amniotic fluid is removed, usually one ml for each completed week of gestation. (8)

However before the 10th week, less than 5 ml could be, obtained on average. The main limited factor of early amniocentesis is the embryonic membranes which may stop the flow and usually allow no further aspiration. (9)

The high cytogenetic failure rate is a difficulty and despite a high clone count, the culture time is prolonged.

Pseudo mosaicism appears to occur more frequently in early than in late amniocentesis but most probably will be lower than that in CVS.

The safety of early amniocentesis is less well established.

It has been suggested that the procedure may have slight higher rate of loss than midtrimester amniocentesis but they still deem it to be a safe and viable diagnostic option. (10)

Overall the safety profile of early amniocentesis, seems at least comparable with this of CVS.

The risk of limb reduction defects also must be considered and assessed. Other techniques that hold promise for first trimester prenatal diagnosis include coelocentesis and lavage/cytobrush collection of trophoblast. (11)

CHORIONIC VILLUS SAMPLING (CVS)

Chorionic villus sampling (CVS) has been used as a successful and safe first trimester prenatal diagnosis technique for over 12 years and became a primary tool for the fetal cytogenetic molecular and biochemical disorders. CVS is best performed between 70 and 90 days after menstrual period by either the transcervical or the transabdominal approach under ultrasound guidance. Both techniques are equally safe and efficacious in most centers, once equivalent expertise is gained with either approach. (12)

It has been estimated that the procedure related loss rate with CVS range from 1% for less experienced to a level approaching midtrimester amniocentesis for those with greater experience. The learning curve appears to be slower than that for amniocentesis. It appears that the learning curve for both trancervical and tranabdominal CVS may exceed 400 of more cases. Operators having performed fewer than 100 cases may have two to three times the post procedure loss rate of operators who have performed more than 1000 procedures. (13)

Recently randomised trials have suggested that when centers become equivalently experienced, amniocentesis and CVS may have the same risk of pregnancy loss. (14)

CVS has led to an improved understanding of several biological processes including confined placental mosaicism which can occur in up to 3% of CVS samples.

The usual approach to the patients with confined placental mosaicism is to offer a second trimester genetic amniocentesis and serial ultrasonographic examination to assess fetal growth. (15)

The development of CVS has opened up an active debate on the potential of early prenatal diagnostic procedures to cause congenital abnormalities. It has been suggested that CVS may be associated with the occurrence of specific fetal malformations.

There have been additional reports of transverse limp defects following very early CVS by several other groups. They suggested that early gestational sampling and excessive placental trauma, maybe etiologic in the reported clusters of post CVS limp reduction defects.

A review of 140.000 CVS procedures was reported to the WHO registry and demonstrated, no increase in the overall incidence of limp reduction defects following CVS nor in any specific type or pattern of defects.

The mechanisms by which CVS could potentially lead to fetal malformations continue to be disputed.

At the present time the possible association of fetal limb ambormalities and CVS appears to have sufficient credibility that patients should be informed of the controversy prior to having the procedure performed.

Sampling prior to 10 weeks gestation should be limited to exceptional centers. CVS beyond 10 weeks, in experienced hands, continues to have a low (if any) risk of fetal abnormalities and should continue to be routinely offered. (16)

FETOSCOPY EMBRYOSCOPY

Fetoscopy has been available since the late 1960's and used for fetal blood, skin or hepatic tissue sampling for the diagnosis of specific disorders such as dermatoses, hepatic dysfunction or hemoglobinopathies or as a diagnostic tool for fetal visualisation during the second trimester of pregnancy.

Briefly embryoscopy is a technique that a high resolution fiberoptic endoscope can be introduced into the amniotic cavity, either transcervical or tranabdominal through 22 gauge needle. A complete examination of the embryo includes visualisation of the head, face dorsal and ventral walls, limbs, umbilical cord and yolk sac. (17)

Embryoscopy can be performed as early as 3 conceptional weeks gestation. The embryonic period extends from the third through the eighth week following conception. During this period all major external and internal structures develop and during this period between 4 and 8 weeks the embryo is most vulnerable to the effects of teratogens.

Transabdominal thin gauge embryofetoscopy offers a technique that can be carefully identified additional anomalies not recognised by ultrasound, confirming others already detected sonographically and investigating the anatomic and physiologic features of the embryo and fetus in utero during the first trimester of pregnancy.

Another application of embryoscopy, is embryonic blood by cordocentesis and tissue sampling during the first trimester of pregnancy. (18) This application serves as a basis for further studies into the diagnosis and treatment of congenital diseases in early pregnancy. If the concept of human gene and cell therapy becomes a reality, embryoscopy will permit accessibility to the human embryo at a time when embryos are immunologically «naive» and may therefore be receptive to these grafts.

Quinter and co-workers (1995) reported a case of percutaneus fetal cystoscopy and endoscopic fulguration of posterior urethal valves, using a thin embryoscope in male fetus with ultrasonographic evidence of lower urinary tract obstruction at 19 weeks of gestation. (19)

De Lia and co-workers (1995) suggested that fetoscopic laser occlusion of chorioangiopagous vessels is technically feasible and improves the course and outcome of severe twin-twin transfusion syndrome in previabe fetuses. (20)

The possibility of fetal therapy raises complex ethical questions about risks and benefits as well as the rights of the mother and fetus as patients.

In conclusion embryoscopy is expected to have a major impact on fetal medicine in the years to come, and prenatal diagnosis and therapy options will continue to expand with increasing emphasis on first trimester intervention.

The new diagnostic techniques and screening approaches for early diagnosis of genetic disorders are exiting and extremely promising but it becomes critical to assess fully the benefits on new technologies before they are applied widely.

REFERENCES

1. Plouffe L and Donahue J: Techniques for early diagnosis of the abnormal fetus. Clinics in Perinatology 1994, 21:723-741.

2. Benacerraf BR: The use of sonography for the antenatal detection of aneuploidy. In : diagnosis and therapy of fetal anomalies. Ed by JC Hobbins and BR Benacerraf, Chutchill Livingstone 1989, pp 21-54.

3. Regavendra N, Beall MH, McMahon JT et al: Transcervical sonography: An investigation technique for visualisation of the embryo. Obstet Gynecol 1993, 8:155.

4. Pandya PP, Snijders RJM, Johnson SJ, Brizot M, Nicolaides KH: Screening for fetal trisomies by maternal age and fetal nuchal translucency thickness at 10 to 14 weeks of gestation. Br J Obstet Gynecol 1995, 102:957-962.

5. Revel MP, Pons JC, Lelaidier C, Fournet P, Vial M, Musset D, Labrune M, Frydsman R: Magnetic resonance imaging of the fetus. A study of 20 cases performed without curarization. Prenat Diagn 1993, 13:775.

6. Berry E, Aitkin DA, Crossley JA: Analysis of maternal serum alpha-fetoprotein and free beta human chorionic gonadotrophin in the first trimester implications for Down's syndrome screening. Prenat Diagn 1995, 15:555.

7. Noble PL, Abraha HD, Snijders RJM, Sherwood R, Nicolaides KH: Screening for fetal trisomy 21 in the first trimester of pregnancy maternal serum free β-hCG and fetal nuchal translucency thickness. Ultrasound Obstet Gynecol 1996, 6:390-395.

8. Kennerknect I, Baur-Aubels S, Grab D et al: First trimester amniocentesis between the seventh and 13 weeks. Evaluation of the earliest possible genetic diagnosis. Prenat Diagn 1992, 12:, 595.

9. Elejalde BR, Elejalde MM, Acuna JM, Thelen D, Trujillo C, Karrmann M: Prospective study of amniocentesis performed between weeks 9 and 16 of gestation: its feasibility, risks, complications, and use in early genetic prenatal diagnosis. Am J Med Genet 1990, 36:188-196.

10. Hanson FW, Tennant F, Hune S et al: Early amniocentesis. Outcome, risks and technical problems at ≤ 12,8 weeks. AM J Obstet Gynecol 1992, 166:1707.

11. Sunberg K, Bang J, Brocks V et al: Early sonographically guided amniocentesis with filtration technique: follow up on 249 procedures. J Ultrasound Med 1995, 14(8):585-590.

12.Jackson LG, Zachary JM, Fowler SE et al: Randomised comparison of trancervical and abdominal chorionic villus sampling. N Enlg J Med 1992, 327:594-598.

13.Saura R, Gauthier B, Taine L et al: Operator experience and fetal loss rate in transabdominal CVS. Prenat Diagn 1994, 14(1):70.

14.Smidt-Jensen S, Permin M, Philip J et al: Randomized comparison of amniocentesis and trancabdominal and transcervical chorionic villus sampling. Lancet 1992, 340:1237.

15.Wapner RJ, Simson JL, Golbus MJ et al: Chorionic mosaicism: Association with fetal loss but not adverse perinatal outcome. Prenat Diagn 1992, 12:347.

16.Wapner R: Chorionic villus sampling. Obstet Gynecol Cinic North. Am 1997, 24:83.

17.Quintero RA, Abuhanad A, Hobbins JE et al: Transabdominal thin gange embryofetoscopy: A technique for early prenatal diagnosis and its use in the diagnosis of a case of Meckel-Cruber syndrome. Am J Obstet Gynecol 1993, 168:1552.

18.Reece EA, Whetham J., Rotmensch S: Gaining access to the embryonic-fetal circulation in first trimester endoscopy. A step into the future. Obstet Gynecol 1993, 82:876.

19.Quintero R, Hume R, Smith C, Johnson M, Cotton D, Romero R, Evans M: Percutaneous fetal cystoscopy and endoscopic fulguration of posterior urethral valves. Am J Obstet Gynecol 1995, 172:206-209.

20.De Lia J, Kuhlmann R, Harstad T, Gruikshank D: Fetoscopic laser ablation of placental vessels in severe prevable twin-twin transfusion syndrome. Am J Obstet Gynecol 1995, 172:1202-1211.

FETAL CELLS DETECTION IN MATERNAL CIRCULATION

G.Ferranti, F. Mezzanotte, E.V. Cosmi.

2ⁿᵈ. Dept. of Obst. and Gyn., Policlinico Umberto I, "La Sapienza Univerity" Rome-Italy

ABSTRACT
Different types of fetal nucleated cells can be found in maternal blood, providing the possibility for non-invasive prenatal diagnosis of genetic abnormalities. For this purpose we have studied nucleated red blood cells (NRBCs). It was believed that these cells were the best candidates for many reasons: they are not normally present in adult circulation, they are the major component of fetal blood and they epress the transferrin receptor antigen (CD71). We investigate the use of Magnetic Activated Cell Sorter after triple density gradient as tool to enrich NRBCs from peripheral blood of 20 pregnant women carrying male fetuses. The origin of NRBCs was determined by FISH using Y specific probes. NRBCs were foun in 18 of the 20 pregnant women at a range of 1 to 200 per 20 ml of venous blood. Only in one case the signal was detected on 5 of 200 examined. Our finding suggest that NRBCs in maternal circulation are predominantly maternal in origin, additional markers are needed better to identify NRBC of fetal origin.

INTRODUCTION
Nucleated cells of fetal origin have been reported to be present in maternal blood in the majority of pregnancies. Fetal cells in maternal blood offer an alternative source of specimens to those obtained by invasive techniques such as amniocentesis, chorionic villus sampling and percutaneous umbilical blood sampling (1).
The non-invasive recovery of fetal cells from maternal blood has great potential to revolutionize fetal medicine. It has been estimated that up to 80 per cent of Down syndrome infants are conceived by women under 35 years of age. These women are generally not considered candidates for fetal diagnosis, because of the risks of invasive diagnostic procedures. The ability to retrieve fetal DNA information from maternal blood would enable all women to undergo fetal DNA analysis. It is already clear that fetal cells can be isolated from maternal blood by flow sorting or magnetic sorting and can be analyzed by Polymerase Chain Reaction (PCR) or fluorescent in situ hybridization (FISH). Various fetal cell types as nucleated red blood cells (NRBCs), trophoblasts and leucocytes can be isolated from maternal circulation (2-4). Isolation

39

of fetal cells from maternal blood has been particularly challenging because of their rarity in maternal blood. Estimates of the frequency of fetal cells in maternal blood vary, ranging from 1 in 10^5 to 1 in 10^9. We have studied NRBCs for many reasons: they are not normally present in adult circulation, they are the major component of fetal blood and they express the transferrin receptor antigen (CD71). The enrichment techniques we investigated is based on a triple density gradient followed by magnetic activated cell sorting. We analyzed totally 20 peripheral venous blood obtained from 20 pregnant women carrying male fetuses. The origin of fetal NBRCs was determined by FISH using Y specific choromosome probe.

MATERIALS AND METHODS

Samples: 20 ml of heparinized venous blood from 20 male pregnant wemen between 16th and 19th weeks of gestation.

Triple density gradient: specimens were diluted 1:3 with Phosphate Buffered Saline. The diluted blood was divided into 6 ml aliquots and each sample was layered on a gradient containing 2 ml of Ficoll-Isopaque 1077, 1110 and 1119. After centrifugation for 30 minutes at 550 g, four distinct bands containing cells were visible, the second band from the top bearing predominantly NRBCs together with neutrophilic granulocytes. The band containing NRBCs was removed for subsequent antibody labeling.

Antibody labeling and MACS: the cells of the second band from pregnant woman blood were incubated with anti-CD45 and then with goat anti-mouse IgG magnetic microbeads and on a mini magnetic activated cell sorting (MACS) column to deplete the sample of most of maternal leucocytes. The negative fraction was then incubated with anti-CD71 magnetic microbeads as above.

FISH: the positive fraction after magnetic cell separation was hybridized with Y-chromosome specific DNA specific probe (DYZ1, Oncor) Hybridization was performed according to the manufacturer' instruction. The slides were observed under a Leica TCS 40 confocal lase scanning microscope.

RESULTS AND CONCLUSIONS

NRBCs were found in 18 of the 20 pregnant wemen at a range of 1 to 200 per 20 ml of venous blood. After hybridization with Y-probe only in one case the signal was detected on 5 of 200 nuclei examined (Tab. 1). NRBCs detected in pregnant women were predominantly of maternal in origin. Pregnancy *per se* seem to induce the appearance that NRBC in the circulation and it cannot therefore be assumed that NRBC isolated from maternal blood are of fetal origin on the basis of morphology alone (5). Discrimination of fetal NRBC must occur for prenatal diagnosis of fetal genetic disorders. The immuno-phenotyping with an antibody specific for fetal haemoglobin simultaneously with FISH is not sufficient proof of their derivation from the fetus haemoglobin, in fact a few cells reacting with antibody against HbF have been observed in non-pregnant women (6). So, additional markers are needed better to identify NRBC of fetal origin.

In conclusion the methods presented in this study show that non-invasive prenatal diagnosis from maternal blood has the potential to became a practical routine procedure but further improvements in methodology are needed in order to apply this new technique to clinical purposes.

Tab. 1: FISH risults using Yspecific probes from venous
blood 20 pregnant women with a male fetus

Subjet N°	Weeks of gestation	N° of NRBCs	Detection of Y signals
1	18	2	-
2	16	1	-
3	17	200	5
4	17	6	-
5	17	12	-
6	18	0	not done
7	18	26	-
8	17	5	-
9	17	7	-
10	16	10	-
11	18	47	-
12	18	13	-
13	18	22	-
14	17	2	-
15	16	1	-
16	16	10	-
17	18	4	-
18	19	0	not done
19	19	32	-
20	19	7	-

REFERENCES

1. Adinolfi M. (1991). On a non-invasive approach to prenatal diagnosis based on the detection of fetal nucleated cells in maternal blood samples. *Prenat.Diagn.*, **11**,799-804
2. Price J.O. et all., (1991). Prenatal diagnosis using fetal cells isolated from maternal blood by multiparameter flow cytometry. *Am.J.Obst.Ginecol.*, **165**,1731-1737
3. Bianchi D.W. et all., (1993). Erythroid-specific antibodies enhance detection of fetal nucleated erythrocytes in maternal blood. *Prenat.Diagn.*, **13**,293-300
4. Ganshirt-Ahlert D. et all., (1993). Detection of fetal trisomies 21 and 18 from maternal blood using triple gradient and magnetic cell sorting. *Am.J.Reprod.Immunol.*, **30**,2-3
5. Slunga-Tallberg A. et all,(1995). Maternal origin of nucleated erythrocytes in peripheral venous blood of pregnant women. *Hum.Genet.*, **96**,53-57
6. Zeng Y. et all., (1993). Prenatal diagnosis from maternal blood: simultaneous immunophenotyping and FISH of fetal nucleated erythrocytes isolated by negative magnetic cell sorting. *J Med Genet* **30**,1051-1056

EARLY PREGNANCY STUDIED BY TRANSVAGINAL COLOR DOPPLER

Asim Kurjak, Sanja Kupešić, Damir Zudenigo, Tomislav Anić, Davorko Đulepa

Department of Obstetrics and Gynecology, Medical School, University of Zagreb, "Sveti Duh" General Hospital, Sveti Duh 64, 10000 Zagreb, Croatia

INTRODUCTION

Remarkable hemodynamic changes occur in the first trimester of pregnancy, the most prominent is the continuous growth and development of the uteroplacental and fetal circulation. Until recently, there has been no reliable tool to obtain noninvasive measurements of maternal, embryonic or fetal blood flow in early pregnancy. The introduction of transvaginal color Doppler has produced significant improvement in the recognition of blood vessels, indicating anatomic location plus direction and velocity of flow. With conventional ultrsound it is often difficult to identify the same vessel reproducibly, and it may be impossible to differentiate small vessels from other soft-tissue areas or fluid-filled structures. Color Doppler overcomes this since flow is displayed over the whole scanning plane as compared with the single line of sight available with pulsed Doppler. Precise investigation of the blood flow changes in maternal and fetal circulation during early pregnancy has become possible due to this technique.

MATERNAL CIRCULATION

The maternal portion of the placental circulation consists of the main uterine arteries and their branches that spread throughout the uterus until they reach the decidual plate of the placenta. The main uterine arteries originate from the iliac arteries, and they give off branches which extend inward for about a third of the myometrium thickness without significant branching. Then they subdivide into an arcuate wreath encircling the uterus. From this network, smaller branches arise, the radial arteries that are directed towards the uterine limen. These arteries become the endometrial spiral arteries as they pass the myometrial-endometrial border (1). After the implantation, spiral arteries become large tortuous channels which is a consequence of the replacement of the normal musculoelastic wall with fibrinoid material and fibrous tissue (2). Such changes enable adequate blood supply to the growing embryo. This process which converts spiral

43

arteries into a low resistance bed is well defined by the 18th week of gestation. These vascular changes have been closely related to the trophoblastic infiltration of the placental bed. It is generally accepted that most of these migrating cells are of the cytotrophoblastic type. There is probably only one continuous trophoblastic wave from the 8-18 weeks period.

All uteroplacental arteries can be clearly identified in the pregnant uterus with their characteristic Doppler signature. The main uterine artery can be visualized at the level of the internal cervical os as it approaches the uterus laterally and curves upward alongside the uterine body. Arcuate arteries may be displayed within the outer third of the myometrium, while radial arteries can be identified at their characteristic anatomical position within myometrium. Spiral arteries may be observed in close proximity of the active trofoblast.

Pulsed Doppler waveform profiles for uterine arteries are characteristic. High peak systolic component of a Doppler sonogram with characteristic notch at the descending slope of the systolic and very low end-diastolic flow is a normal finding in the uterine artery. Doppler sonograms of the arcuate and radial arteries are very similar – moderate peak-systolic and end-diastolic component of blood flow. The present difference is in the values of the peripheral vascular impedance. Impedance values are lower in the radial arteries than in the arcuate arteries. Pulsed Doppler waveform signals obtained from spiral arteries show low impedance to blood flow and a characteristic spiky outline which is indicative of a high turbulence and a tortuous vessel with an irregular wall. The significant differences between uterine arteries in the peripheral impedance values are noticable. During pregnancy, impedance to blood flow decreases from the main uterine to the spiral arteries and with advanced gestational age (3-6). At the same time, an increase of blood flow by means of peak-systolic Doppler shift is observed. A decrease of vascular impedance with gestation is probably a consequence of the dilatation of spiral arteries induced by trophoblast infiltration, hormonal mediated vasodilatation and decrease of maternal blood flow viscosity.

UMBILICAL-PLACENTAL CIRCULATION

Umbilical artery branches into the chorionic arteries and they together form umbilical-placental circulation. Umbilical artery can be located by transvaginal color Doppler sonography very early in pregnancy, even at the 6th week. By the end of the 10th gestational week there is no end-diastolic component of blood flow. Between the 10th and the 14th week, diastolic velocities begin to emerge, but are incomplete and inconsistently present (7). After this, pandiastolic frequencies are consistently present. Visualization of chorionic arteries and intraplacental arterioles can be obtained in significant proportion of the investigated cases. Hsieh and colleagues using a sensitive color flow mapping system, spotted intraplacental arterioles in the upper two thirds of the placenta, beneath the chorionic plate (8). Their results show that resistance to flow in the umbilical artery is the highest at the fetal side, and becomes progressively lower towards the placental side, being the lowest in the fetal arteries within the placenta. There are no significant changes in the umbilical artery blood flow until the 12t[h] gestational week, when significant decrease of vascular impedance is noticed.

The anatomic changes in the villous vasculature, which are characterized by the progressive increase of the number and the surface area occupied by the fetal vessels, must have a key role in the gradual fall in blood flow impedance in the umbilical circulation.

INTERVILLOUS BLOOD FLOW

According to the embryological textbooks, as soon as the blastocyst has implanted, maternal blood enters the future intervillous space bringing nutrients and oxygen to the rapidly growing embryo. This classic concept has been spread by Hustin and Schaaps who performed perfusion experiments using transvaginal sonography, intervillous hysteroscopy and examination of chorionic villous sampling material (9). Using all of these techniques, they were unable to demonstrate a true intervillous blood flow during the first 12 weeks. They suggested that, during this period, the tips of the spiral arteries are obstructed by intravascular trophoblastic plugs and the intervillous space was bathed by a clear fluid, possibly made of filtered plasma and uterine gland secretions. This hypothesis has been supported by the study of perfused hysterectomy specimens showing that, during the first 3 months of gestation, the embryo is totally separated from the maternal circulation by the trophoblastic shell (10). Further support has been supplied by more recent studies using a polarographic oxygen electrode (11). It has been demostrated that between 8 and 10 weeks gestation, placental pO2 levels were significantly lower compared with endometrial pO2 levels, while the levels were similar between 12 and 13 weeks. Recent Doppler studies supported Hustin's theory that intervillous circulation normally becomes established much later in pregnancy than it was previously thought (12).

Only in cases of abnormal early pregnancy has the presence of intervillous blood flow been proven before 12 weeks of pregnancy. Jauniaux and colleagues showed increased blood flow in the intervillous space in 16 out of 23 (70%) of the complicated pregnancies before 12 weeks gestation (13). Their results are consistent with some previous studies showing a higher rate of intervillous flow detection in abnormal early pregnancies (14). Study by Jauniaux showed that, in these cases, the trophoblastic shell was thinner and discontinuous, and that the intervillous space was massively infiltrated by maternal blood. Indeed, this study suggested that one of the functions of trophoblastic plugging of the spiral arteries is to restrict maternal blood flow into the intervillous space in early pregnancy. If this concept is true, the premature entry of maternal blood into the intervillous space could disrupt the maternoembryonic interface, causing the separation of early placenta, which cannot sustain the relatively high pressure from the maternal circulation (15).

However, most of these early color Doppler studies have used less sensitive equipment and have failed to demonstrate continuous blood flow in the intervillous space in the first 12 weeks. After the introduction of the new generation of far more sensitive color Doppler devices in last few years, several authors reported a positive finding of intervillous circulation during first trimester of pregnancy.

In 1995. Kurjak et coauthors (16) presented the first report on a combined Doppler and morphopathological study of intervillous circulation. Using a transvaginal color Doppler, continuous intervillous flow of two types was detected in all examined patients: pulsatile arterial-like and continuous venous-like flow. Parallel histological study has shown that the lumen of spiral arteries was never completely obstructed by the trophoblastic plugs. These data indicate that establishment of the intervillous circulation is a continuous process rather than an abrupt event at the end of the first trimester.

In our recent studies (17,18) of normal and abnormal (missed abortion and anembryonic pregnancy) first-trimester pregnancies the same Doppler features were detected in the intervillous space of all pregnancies; pulsatile arterial-like signals with characteristic spiky outline, and venous-like continuous signals. There was no difference in Doppler parameters between the group with missed abortion and the group of normal pregnancy. However, lower impedance was detected in the group with anembryonic pregnencies.

Valentin performed a combined study of uteroplacental and luteal flow with a patomorphologic analysis (19). Color Doppler measurements revealed positive finding of intervillous cirulation from the 6th week of normal pregnancy onward. The same two types of Doppler signals, the pulsatile and continuous, were detected and measured with a visualization rate of more than 90% from 5 to 11 weeks of gestation. The authors stated that high blood velocities recorded from the subchorionic arteries were not compatible with these arteries being completely occluded by trophoblastic plugs. At the pathomorphologic analysis trophoblast plugging of the spiral arteries was incomplete, allowing passage of red blood cells. The authors concluded that the intervillous circulation was present as early as the first trimester.

In study of Merce (20) similar results were obtained. They were able to detect intervillous flow from 5 weeks 6 days of gestation. It was a slightly undulating venous-like signal with tendency of increasing velocity through the first trimester. They also recorded arterial signals in retrochorionic segments of uteroplacental vasculature. The conclusion was that their results were in accordance with the classic embryological concept of establishment of the intervillous flow from 4th to 7th weeks of gestation.

Definitive proof of the existence of intervillous blood flow in the first trimester of pregnancy is histological study of Meekins and co-workers (21). Using light microscopy, they analyzed placental bed sections from 25 first trimester gravid hysterectomy specimens. Maternal red blood cells were present in the intervillous space in all specimens. Of 232 decidual spiral arteries which were found, 63 per cent contained scattered endovascular trophoblast, 20 per cent had plugs of trophoblast partially occluding the vessel and 17 per cent had plugs totally filling the vessel lumen. Even within plugs of trophoblast red blood cells were easily identified and were seen in continuity entering into the intervillous space giving the impression that the plugs were acting as a sieve to blood flow rather than a total barrier. This mechanism would be compatible with the suggested shielding of the vulnerable uteroplacental interface from the shearing forces of the maternal blood that would be at work if the communication with the maternal circulation and the intervillous space was fully open **(13,15)**. A slowing down of the maternal blood flow may also facilitate the exchange of chemical messages between the fetal and maternal compartments.

FETAL CIRCULATION

Around 21 days after ovulation, corresponding to the end of the 5th week after the last menstrual period, the primitive heart begins to beat. Activity of the embryonic heart has been documented i n u t e r o as early as 36 days post-menstrual age **(22)**. Heart rate increases from 80 to 90 beats/min to 150-170 till the end of the 9th week. Arrhythmias in the first trimester can precede fetal loss, and color Doppler could become the main tool for the detection and screening of such disturbances **(23)**. This technique has also been shown to be helpful in the visualization of normal early fetal cardiac anatomy during the late first and early second trimester of pregnancy. Doppler flow velocities can be measured at the level of the atrioventricular and outflow tracts **(24,25)**. Up to 11-12 weeks of gestation it is not always possible to differentiate between the two atrioventricular valves. An atrioventricular waveform recording at 10 weeks consists of the early diastolic or E-wave component and late diastolic or A-wave component, demonstrating that differentiation between passive diastolic filling and atrial contraction is already feasible at this very early stage of gestation. Of interest is the relatively low peak E-wave velocity compared with the peak A-wave velocity, resulting in an E/A ratio of approximately 0.5, as opposed to E/A ratios ranging between 0.8 and 0.9 in late pregnancy. The clear A-wave dominance of the atrioventricular level reflects the relative stiffness of the cardiac ventricles in early gestation. At 11-12 weeks mean peak E-wave and A-wave velocities of 20.5 +/- 3.2 cm/s and 38.6 +/- 4.7 cm/s have been established. There is a marked rise in peak E-wave velocities and E/A ratios of both the mitral and tricuspid level with advancing gestational age. This suggests a shift of blood flow from late towards early diastole, which may be due to increased ventricular compliance and/or raised ventricular relaxation rate.

Aortic and pulmonary artery flow velocities may also be recorded at the outflow tract level ae early as 10-11 weeks of gestation. At 11-12 weeks, peak and time-averaged flow velocities are lower than observed in late pregnancy, with mean values of 32.1 +/- 5.4 cm/s and 11.2 +/- 2.2 cm/s in the ascending aorta, and 29.6 +/- 5.1 cm/s and 10.8 +/- 2.1 cm/s in the pulmonary artery. In both vessels a gestational age-related rise in peak velocities can be demonstrated during the early second trimester of pregnancy, the highest velocities being reached in the ascending aorta. A difference in left and right cardiac blood flow in favor of the right side was calculated during the first half of the second trimester of pregnancy. The higher peak-systolic velocities in the ascending aorta compared with the pulmonary artery may be a result of a difference in semilunar valve area between the two vessels, as has been suggested on the basis of similar findings in late pregnancy.

Fetal vessels usually analyzed for assessment of fetal well-being are the aorta, carotid arteries and middle cerebral artery. Pulsations from the fetal aorta can be identified as early as the 6th week of gestation.

In the fetal aorta, as in the umbilical artery, there are no significant changes in blood flow until the end of the gestational week. There is then a significant decrease in peripheral vascular impedance. The decrease of impedance is accompanied by an increase of blood flow velocities in all investigated vessels.

EARLY FETAL CEREBRAL CIRCULATION

The intracranial circulation becomes visible as early as the 7th week of gestation. At that time, discrete pulsations of the internal carotid arteries are detectable at the base of the skull. During the 9th and 10th gestational weeks, color patterns representing blood flow can be visualized in the anterolateral quadrant of the skull base. From the 10th gestational week, arterial pulsations can be detected on transverse section, lateral to the mesencephalon and cephalic flexure.

There are few transvaginal color Doppler studies of cerebral blood flow in early pregnancy **(26-8).** In all these studies end-diastolic flow was present earlier in cerebral vessels compared to the fetal aorta and umbilical artery. Moreover, a significant decrease of pulsatility index was observed two weeks earlier in cerebral arteries than in the other parts of the fetal circulation. These results suggest a low vascular impedance at the fetal cerebral level in early gestation, not dependent on changes in the vascular resistance of the fetal trunk or uteroplacental circulation. Cerebral vessels are a separate hemodynamic system that is independent of the other parts of the fetal circulation from the beginning of the pregnancy. This apparently independent and autoregulatory mechanism thus provides an adequate blood supply to the growing fetal brain, protecting it from hypoxia even in early pregnancy.

FETAL CHOROID PLEXUS VASCULARIZATION

The fetal choroid plexus plays a large role in brain development. It is proportionally larger than that of an adult human being and fills more of the space in the ventricles. The choroid plexus and arachnoid membrane act together as barriers between the blood and cerebrospinal fluid. In effect, the choroid plexus is like a "kidney" for the brain **(29)**. It is not a simple excretory organ for creating cerebrospinal fluid, but also provides the fluid with nutrients extracted from the blood. The choroid plexus also has an important role in the cleaning of the cerebrospinal fluid of waste substances that exist in the brain tissues as by-products of metabolic reactions. In early to mid-pregnancy, fetal choroid plexus cells contain significant amounts of glycogen and serve as a storage site.

The choroid plexus of the lateral ventricles receives blood from the anterior and posterior choroidal arteries. A small anterior branch arises from the origin of the middle cerebral artery. The remainder of the blood supply comes from a posterior communicating artery. The choroid vein runs along the whole length of the outer border of the choroid plexus, receiving veins from the hippocampus major, the fornix and corpus callosum. and unites behind the anterior extremity of the choroid plecus with the vein of the corpus striatum.

The vascular network of the choroid plexus vessels is characteristic. Each frond consists of capillaries and other small blood vessels surrounded by a single layer of epithelial cells. One side of each cell, called the basolateral surface, is in contact with blood plasma that filters through the "leaky" wall of the choroid plexus capillaries, which constitute the blood-brain barrier and mediate the diffusion of substances from the blood directly into the interstitial fluid.

In our study of the fetal choroid plexus vascularization **(30)**, choroid plexus vessels can be clearly visualized at 10 weeks and 3 days of gestation . Subtle color and pulsed Doppler signals can be obtained at the inner edge of the lateral ventricle choroid plexus. The pulsed Doppler waveform profile of choroid plexus is characteristic. The systolic component of blood flow within a cardiac cycle is not pronounced, while the slope from the systolic peak until the end of the cycle is very mild. Visualization rate from choroid plexus vessels ranges from 35 to 75% and they are most easily seen at 13 weeks, after that the visualization rate declines. Visualization of the vessels of the choroid plexus increases and decreases as the plexus develops and shrinks. A steady decline of resistance and increment of flow is present in choroid plexus arteries with advanced gestational age. Our results show significant flow velocity differences between the larger cerebral vessels and the smaller, choroidal vessels. The same characteristic has been demonstrated for other organs as well. peripheral vascular indices of the large vessels reflect the resistance in the entire organ, while the same indices of the smaller vessels reflect the resistance in the smaller areas.

EARLY PREGNANCY FAILURE

MISSED ABORTION AND BLIGHTED OVUM

There are some color Doppler studies on the blighted ovum and missed abortion, but results are inconsistent and vary from author to author.

Alfirević and Kurjak (31) analyzed blood flow in uterine and spiral arteries in cases of missed abortions and blighted ova. These arteries showed a slightly lower RI compared with normal pregnancy values, although the difference failed to reach a level of significance. In pregnancies with blighted ovum and missed abortion flow could not be detected in trophoblastic vessels in two out of six and four out of six cases. Jaffe and colleagues (32) reported RI values around and above the cutoff point value of 0.63 in cases of missed abortions and below that value in cases of blighted ova. Although the calculated indices did not differ significantly from those found in normal gestation, they detected blood flow more often in spiral arteries in gestations defined as anembryonic than in those defined as missed abortions (14,33). Although the absence of flow in missed abortions could be a secondary phenomenon, it may indicate that circulatory problems can cause this type of early pregnancy failure. However, the incidence of chromosomal abnormalities was significantly increased in the blighted ova group, indicating that such abnormalities could cause this type of pregnancy failure. Under these circumastances the trophoblast will often develop in the absence of an embryo, and the subplacental circulation is not immediately affected.

Arduini and colleagues found no difference in peripheral vascular impedance between normal pregnancies and those with blighted ova or missed abortions (34).

In the study by Kurjak and colleagues (35), RI was higher in a group of patients with blighted ovum and missed abortion than in a control group. Furthermore, in 31% of blighted ova and 26% of missed abortions no blood flow could be detected in the spiral arteries. It was also found that some blighted ova were richly vascularized and that the intensity of color flow corresponded to the trophoblast activity. Abundant color signals possibly indicate which blighted ova will undergo molar changes.

SUBCHORIONIC HEMATOMA

Subchorionic hematoma is defined sonographically as an echo-free are located between the membranes and the uterine wall. Color flow is necessary to confirm this observation because, occasionally, the echo-free black and white image turns out to be a highly vascularized placental site. Physiologically, this represents a separation of the chorionic plate from the underlying decidua. The precise cause of subchorionic hematoma is unknown. Postulated associative factors include autoimmune reactions, coumarin drugs, or hematologic factor deficiency **(36,37).** In our recent study **(38),** the correlation between the volume of hematoma and blood flow parameters was evaluated, the frequency of spontaneous abortions and preterm deliveries in group with subchorionic hematoma and normal pregnancies was estimated, and the hematoma site with pregnancy outcome was correlated.

More spontaneous abortions occurred in women with subchorionic hematoma compared to control group, while there was no significant difference in the number of preterm deliveries. There was a positive correlation between hematoma volume and RI in the spiral arteries and a negative correlation between hematoma volume and peak systolic velocity, probably as a consequence of the mechanical compression to the spiral arteries caused by the hematoma. When pregnancy continued and hematomas reduced, these indices returned to normal values. The hematoma size did nor affect pregnancy outcome, but the site did. There was no significant difference in the number of spontaneous aboritons between the patients with small hematomas and those with large ones. Most hematomas associated with abortion were found in the corpus or fundus of the uterus, but not in the supracervical area. Since in most cases this is the region of the placental site, it suggests a possible disruption of placental function. Alteration of blood flow in spiral arteries was probably a secondary effect without influence on pregnancy outcome.

CONCLUSION

Transvaginal color Doppler opens new frontiers in the detection and analysis of blood flow in early pregnancy. The extent of this has no parallel with any other breakthrough in the field. It offers not only anatomic information, but in adition allows access to physiologic information regarding uteroplacental and fetoplacental circulation. It minimizes the time for localization of even very small vessels and at the same time it enhances the accuracy and reproducibility. It is our belief that this method will become indispensible in the noninvasive study of early pregnancy in not too distant future.

LITERATURE

1. Ramsey E.M. and Dodder N.W. (1980). Placental vasculature and circulation. (Stuttgart: Georg Thieme)

2. Pijnenborg R., Dixon G., Robertson W.B. and Brosens I. (1980). Trophoblastic invasion of human decidua from 8 to 18 weeks of pregnancy. Placenta, **1**, 3-19

3. Jurković D., Jauniaux E., Kurjak A., Hustin J., Campbell S. and Nicolaides K.H. (1991). Transvaginal color Doppler assessment of uteroplacental circulation in early pregnancy. Obstet. Gynecol.,77, 365-9

4. Kurjak A., Zudenigo D., Funduk-Kurjak B., Shalan H., Predanić M. and Šošić A. (1993). Transvaginal color Doppler in the assessment of the uteroplacental circulation in normal early pregnancy. J. Perinat. Med., **21**, 25-34

5. Kurjak S., Kupešić S., Predanić M. and Salihagić A. (1992). Transvaginal color Doppler assessment of uteroplacental circulation in normal and abnormal early pregnancy. Early. Hum. Dev., **29**, 385-9

6. Kurjak A., Žalud I., Predanić M. and Kupešić S. (1994). Transvaginal color and pulsed Doppler study of uterine blood flow in the first and early second trimester of pregnancy: normal vs. abnormal. J. Ultrasound Med., **13**, 43-7

7. Arduini D. and Rizzo G. (1991). Umbilical artery velocity waveforms in early pregnancy: a transvaginal color Doppler study. J. Clin. Ultrasound, **19**, 335-9

8. Hsieh F.J., Kuo P.L., Ko T.M., Chang F.M. and Chen H.Y. (1991). Doppler velocimetry of intraplacental fetal arteries. Obstet. Gynecol., **77**, 478-82

9. Hustin J. and Schaaps J.P. (1987) Echographic and anatomic studies of the maternotrophoblastic border during the first trimester of pregnancy. Am. J. Obstet. Gynecol., **157**, 162-8

10. Hustin J., Schaaps J.P. and Lambotte K.H. (1991). Anatomical studies of the utero-placental circulation in early pregnancy. Obstet. Gynecol., **77**, 365-9

11. Rodesch F., Simon P., Donner C. and Jauniaux E. (1992). Oxygen measurements in endometrial and trophoblastic tissue during early pregnancy. Obstet. Gynecol., **80**, 283-5

12. Jauniaux E., Jurković D., Campbell S., Kurjak A. and Hustin J. (1991). Investigation of placental circulations by color Doppler ultrasound. Am. J. Obstet. Gynecol., **64**, 486-8

13. Jauniaux E., Zaidi J., Jurković D., Campbell S. and Hustin J. (1994). Comparison of color Doppler features and pathohistological finding in complicated early pregnancy. Hum. Reprod., **9**, 2432-7

14. Jaffe R, Warsof SL. (1992). Color Doppler imaging in the assessment of uteroplacental blood flow in abnormal first trimester intrauterine pregnancies. J Ultrasound Med **(11)**, 41-4

15. Hustin J, Jauniaux E, Schaaps JP. (1990). Histologtical study of the materno-embryonic interface in spontaneous abortion. Placenta, 11, 477-86.

16. Kurjak A., Laurini R., Kupešić S., Kos M., Latin V. and Bulić K. (1995). A combined Doppler and morphological study of intervillous circulation. Book of Abstracts. The Fifth World Congress of Ultrasound in Obstetrics and Gynecology, Kyoto. Ultrasound Obstet Gynecol **6** (Suppl 2)

17. Kurjak A., Kupešić S., Kos M., Latin V. and Zudenigo D. (1996). Early hemodynamics studied by transvaginal color Doppler. Perinat. Neonat. Med., 1, 38-49

18. Kurjak A. and Kupešić S. (1997). Doppler assessment of the intervillous blood flow in normal and abnormal early pregnancy. Obstet. Gynecol., **89**, 252-6

19. Valentin L., Sladkevicius P., Laurini R., Soderberg K. and Marsal K. (1996). Uteroplacental and luteal circulation in normal first trimester pregnancies: Doppler ultrasonographic and morphologic study. Am. J. Obstet. Gynecol., **174**, 768-72

20. Merce L.T., Barco M.J. and Bau S. (1996). Color Doppler sonographic assessment of placental circulation in the first trimester of normal pregnancy. J. Ultrasound Med., **15**, 135-9

21. Meekins JW, Luckas MJM, Pijnenborg R, McFadyen IR (1997). Histological study of decidual spiral arteries and the presence of maternal erythrocytes in the intervillous space during the first trimester of normal pregnancy. Placenta, **18**, 459-64

22. Neiman H.L. (1990). Transvaginal ultrasound embryography. Sem. Ultrasound, CT, NMR., **11**, 22-33

23. Birnholz J.C. (1990). First trimester fetal arrhythmias. Fetal. Diagn. Ther., **8**, (Suppl. 2), 6

24. Rizzo G., Arduini D. and Romanini C. (1991). Fetal cardiac and extracardiac circulation in early gestation. J. Maternal Fetal. Invest., **1**, 73-8

25. Wladiniroff J.W., Huisman T.W.A. and Stewart P.A. (1992). Cardiac Doppler flow velocities in the late first trimester fetus. Am. J. Obstet. Gynecol., **166**, 46-9

26. Wladimiroff J.W., Huisman T.W.A. and Stewart P.A. (1992). Intracerebral, aortic and umbilical artery flow velocity waveforms in the late-first-trimester fetus. Am. J. Obstet. Gynecol., **166**, 36-9

27. Van Zalen-Sprock M.M., Van Vugt J.M.G., Colenbrander G.J. and Geijn H.P. (1994). First-trimester uteroplacental and fetal blood flow velocity waveforms in normally developing fetuses: a longitudinal study. Ultrasound Obstet. Gynecol., **4**, 284-8

28. Kurjak A., Predanić M., Kupešić S., Funduk-Kurjak B., Demarin V. and Salihagić A. (1992). Transvaginal color Doppler study of middle cerebral artery blood flow in early normal and abnormal pregnancy. Ultrasound Obstet. Gynecol., **2**, 424-8

29. Spector J. and Johanson C.E. (1989). The mammalian choroid plexus. Aci. Am., **6**, 48-53

30. Kurjak A., Schulman H., Predanić A., Kupešić S. and Žalud I. (1994). Fetal choroid plexus vascularization assessed by color and pulsed Doppler. J. Ultrasound Med., **13**, 841-4

31. Alfirević Ž. and Kurjak A. (1990). Transvaginal color Doppler ultrasound in normal and abnormal early pregnancy. J. Perinat. Med., **18**, 173-80

32. Jaffe, R. (1991). Uteroplacental blood flow assessment in eartly pregnancy failure. In: Jaffe R. and Warsof, S.L. (eds.) Color Doppler Imaging in Obstetrics and Gynecology (New York: McGraw-Hill)

33. Jaffe R. (1993). Investigation of abnormal first-trimester gestations by color Doppler imaging. J. Clin. Ultrasound, **21**, 521-6

34. Arduini D., Rizzo G. and Romanini C. Doppler ultrasonography in early pregnancy does not predict adverse pregnancy outcome. Ultrasound Obstet. Gynecol., **1**, 180-5

35. Kurjak A., Žalud I., Salihagić A., Crvenković G. and Matijević R. (1991). Transvaginal color Doppler in the assessment of abnormal early pregnancy. J. Perinat. Med., **19**, 155-65

36. Baxi L. and Pearlstone M. (1991). Subchorionic hematomas and the presence of autoantibodies. Am. J. Obstet. Gynecol., **165**, 1423-6

37. Guy G., Baxi L. and Chao C. (1992). An unusual complication in a patient with factor IX deficiency. Obstet. Gynecol., **80**, 502-4

38. Kurjak A., Schulman H., Zudenigo D., Kupešić S., Kos M. and Goldenberg M. (1996). Subchorionic hematomas in early pregnancy: clinical outcome and blood flow patterns. J. Matern. Fetal. Med., **5**, 41-4

Color Doppler assessment of intraplacental circulation in late pregnancy

D. Zoričić, D. Perić

Department of Obstetrics and Gynecology, Pula General Hospital, Zagrebačka 34, 52000 Pula, CROATIA

Summary

Adequate blood flow in an intervillous space which is a final segment of uteroplacental vascular system, is necessary for normal delivery of oxygen and nutrients to growing fetus. Color and spectral Doppler ultrasonography techniques enable noninvasive assessment of intervillous circulation in all three trimesters of pregnancy. Our purpose was to establish reference data representative for normal findings in second half of pregnancy. Cross-sectional study was performed on 70 uncomplicated pregnancies of 22 to 42 completed gestational weeks. Doppler examinations of arterial-like intervillous flow signals were performed using transabdominal route. Color-coded areas were visualized within the placenta in the intrachorionic area, flow velocity waveforms were obtained by pulsed Doppler and pulsatility (PI) and resistance (RI) indices calculated.

Color signals were detected and arterial Doppler flow velocity waveforms recorded within the chorionic area in all women. We noted low-significant increase of Doppler indices of intervillous arterial-like signals ($p < 0,06$) throughout second half of pregnancy from RI $0,26 \pm 0,04$ and PI $0,29 \pm 0,06$ in a group of 22 to 26 gestational weeks to RI $0,30 \pm 0,09$ and PI $0,36 \pm 0,14$ in a group of 37 to 42 weeks. According to our data resistance of blood flow in intervillous space gradually increases during second half of pregnancy. It might be a result of degenerative process in mature placenta. Study of hemodynamic changes within the intervillous space during second half of pregnancy may help in better understanding physiologic and patophysiologic mechanisms of uteroplacental circulation.

Introduction

Scientific interest in the placenta evolved from the recognition of the great metabolic, endocrine and immunological properties of this organ. Placental function includes exchange of metabolic and gaseous products between maternal and fetal blood streams, production of hormones and metabolism. For normal delivery of oxygen and nutritiens to growing fetus adequate blood flow in placenta is necessary. Since the introduction of Doppler ultrasound in perinatal medicine, numerous investigators felt challenged to assess hemodynamical changes in uteroplacental and umbilical arteries[1-4]. Our current interest is focused on intervillous circulation, terminal segment of utero-placental vascular system.

Maternal blood enters the intervillous space in spurts produced by the maternal blood pressure in spiral arteries[5]. Researches which have been recently conducted showed that intervillous circulation begins early in the first trimester[6-9]. During the first half of pregnancy broadening of the spiral arteries diameter due to throphoblastic invasion occurs[10,11]. Spiral arteries convert into uteroplacental arteries, distal part of utero-placental vascular system that supply intervillous space. In the second half of pregnancy only minimal endovascular alterations occur. In contrast to that there are some hyper-tensive pregnancies and pregnancies associated with growth-retarded fetuses where the transformations of spiral arteries are irregular thus causing and inadequate placental perfusion and, probably, serious consequences as hypertension and/or intrauterine growth retardation[12-18].

Color and spectral Doppler ultrasonography techniques enable noninvasive assessment of all segments of uteroplacental circulation. The continuing influx of blood in the intervillous space can be visualized and measured by color and pulsed Doppler from the 6th week of pregnancy to the term as pulsatile, arterial-like signal[6,19-23]. Our purpose was to find out reference data representative for normal findings in second half of pregnancy.

Methods

Doppler examinations were performed on 70 pregnancies of 22 to 42 completed gestational weeks. Only persons with uncomplicated pregnancy were included in the study. We used 3,5 MHz curvilinear probe (Acuson 128 XP/10, Acuson, Mountain View, Calif.). The high-pass filter was set on 125 Hz to exclude low-frequency distorting signals. After localization of placental site by B-mode ultrasonography, color flow imaging was used for visualization of placental site by B-mode ultrasonography. There are three main types of blood flow inside placenta (Figure 1.);

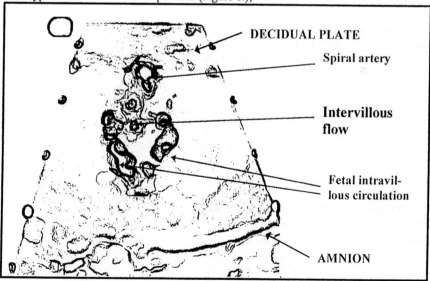

Figure 1. The main types of blood flow in the intraplacental area.

1. Spiral arteries transformed in subchorionic uteroplacental vessels located on the deciduo-myometrial border with irregular and tortuotic appearance.

2. Intervillous flow located in intrachorionic space which represents final segment of uteroplacental perfusion.

3. Fetal intravillous vessels.

After localization of vessel with color Doppler, arterial blood flow velocity waveforms in intervillous space was obtained by placing the Doppler gate in interchorionic area, 1-2 cm above dicicluo-myomatrial border. In the same manner 3 color coded areas of intervillous space were assessed. Distinction between the intervillous circulation and fetal intravillous space was made by heart rate analysis because frequencies in intravillous vessels are higher and fetal blood flow vaweforms have typical patterns similar to umbilical arteries. Finally, intravillous fetal vessels begin from amnion and lie in opposite direction of maternal intervillous flow that begin from decidual part of placenta.

Intervillous flow signals were described using resistance (RI) and pulsatility (PI) indices. The patients were divided in groups according to the gestational age in the following manner: 22-26, 27-31, 32-36, 37-42 weeks. Statistical significance between the groups was calculated using Student t-test.

Results

Color was detected and maternal bloodflow waveforms recorded from intervillous area in all women. Signals obtained from distal part of uteroplacental circulation are characterized by low velocities and arterial-like pattern with little variation between systole and diastole (Figure 2). Results of Doppler measurements are presented in table 1. We noted low significant increase of Doppler indices of intervillous flow (Figure 3. and 4.) from RI $0,26 \pm 0,05$ and PI $0,29 \pm 0,06$ in a group of 22 to 26 gestational weeks to RI $0,30 \pm 0,09$ and PI $0,36 \pm 0,14$ in a group of 37 to 42 weeks (p<0,06).

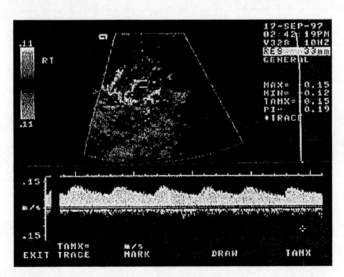

Figure 2. Pulsatile signals obtained from the intervillous space.

Table I. *Pulsatility index (PI) and resistance index (RI) obtained from the intervillous space in second half of pregnancy. Data are expressed as mean ± SD.*

GESTATIONAL AGE GROUP	PI	RI
22-26	0,29± 0,07	0,26 ± 0,05
27-32	0,30 ± 0,12	0,27 ± 0,07
33-36	0,34± 0,11	0,29 ± 0,07
37-42	0,36 ± 0,1	0,30 ± 0,09

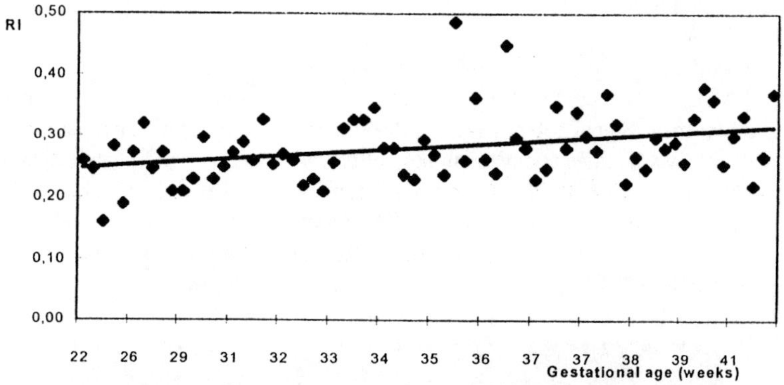

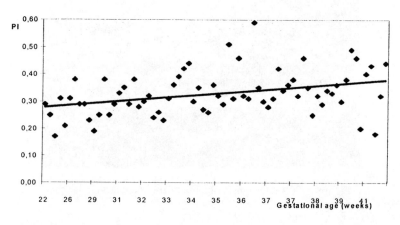

Figure 3. Resistence index of intervillous flow during second half of pregnancy.

Figure 4. Pulsatility index of intervillous flow during second half of pregnancy.

Comment

Our study has confirmed the practicality of obtaining satisfactory Doppler blood flow signals from the intervillous circulation in second half of pregnancy. According to our data with advancing gestation there was progressive elevation of Doppler indices. Contrary to that, according to research conducted by Kurjak impedance to blood flow within the intervillous space significantly decreased towards the midpregnancy, and then remained stable without significant change till the term. The regulatory mechanisms of the blood circulation trough the intervillous spaces are still unknown. One can speculate that process of aging of placenta could be responsible for decrement of blood flow velocity and changes in Doppler indices. At present we need prospective studies with a larger number of patients to confirm or exclude that hypothesis.

A decision about the time of preterm birth if fetal distress occurs means balancing between consequences of preterm delivery and risk of intrauterine deterioration due to placental insufficiency. So, it is particularly important to know as many parameters of placental function as possible. Doppler velocimetry of umbilical and uterine arteries is no longer a research tool limited to an investigational setting but rather a common component of prenatal units dealing with high-risk pregnancies. Also, by use of color Doppler equipment we have a possiblity to measure blood flow in small intraplacental vessels on distal part of uteroplacental circulation. Today there are still some limitation to the clinical use of these measurements. First, ishemic-hemorrhagic damage of the placenta may be related to obstruction of one or few uteroplacental arteries, but others may have normal function. Second, and the main problem is in standardization of measurements because Doppler finding strongly depends on localization of caliper (signals from the spiral arteries and intervillous flow are similar). Finally, if endovascular lesion of distal part of uteroplacental circulation exists and blood flow decreased at that point, we will probably not see it by color Doppler. In this situation we could see another vessel that probably represents the best functioning part of that placenta.

Dispute of that it is obviously that using color Doppler technique we have possibility to noninvasive assess placental circulation in vivo. This may help in better understanding physiolgic and patophysiologic mechanisms of uteroplacental circulation and intervillous space.

References

1. Alfirević Z, Neilson JP. The current status of Dopplere sonography in obstetrics. Curr Opin Obstet Gynecol 1996;8:114-8.
2. Hitschold T, Weiss E, Beck T, Hunterfering H, Berle P. Low target birth weight or growth retardation? Umbilical Doppler flow velocity waveforms and histometric analysis of fetoplacental vascular tree. Am J Obstet Gynecol 1993;168:1260-4.
3. Coppens M, Loquet P, Kollen M, De Neubourg F, Buytaert P. Longitudinal evaluation of uteroplacental and umbilical blood flow changes in normal early pregnancy. Ultrasound Obstet Gynecol 1996;7:114-121.
4. Merce LT, Barco MJ, Bau S. Color Doppler sonographic assessment of placental circulation in the first trimester of normal pregnancy. J Ultrasound Med 1996;15:135-142.
5. Gruenwald P. Maternal blood supply to conceptus. Eur J Obstet Gynecol Reprod Biol 1975;5:23-34.
6. Kurjak A, Dudenhausen JW, Hafner T, Kupešic S, Latin V, Kos M. Intervillous circulation in all three trimestrers of normal pregnancy assessed by color Doppler. J Perinat Med 1997;25:373-380.

7. Kurjak A, Kupešić S, Hafner T, Kos M, Kostović-Knežević L, Grbeša D. Conflicting data on intervillous circulation in early pregnancy. J Perinat Med 1997;25:373-380.

8. Jaffe R, Jauniaux E, Hustin J. Maternal circulation in the first-trimester human placenta-myth or reality? Am J Obstet Gynecol 1997;176:695-705.

9. Simpson NA, Nimrod C, De Vermette R, Fournier J. Determination of intervillous flow in early pregnancy. Placenta 1997;18:287-293.

10. Meekins JW, Luckas MJ, Pijnenbort G, McFadyen IR. Histological study of decidual spiral arteries and the presence of maternal erythrocytes in the intervillous space during the first trimester of normal human pregnancy. Placenta 1997;18:459-464.

11. Lin S, Shmizu I, Suehara N, Nakayama M, Aono T. Uterine artery Doppler velocimetry in relation to trophoblast migration into the myometrium of the placental bed. Obstet Gynecol 1995:85:760-5.

12. Abitbol MM, LaGamma EF, Demeter E, Cipollina CM. Umbilical Flow in the normal and pre-eclamptic placenta. A study in vitro. Acta Obstet Gynecol Scand 1987;66:689-694.

13. Jacques SM, Qureshi F. Chronic intervillositis of the placenta. Arch Pathol Lab Med 1993;117:1032-1035.

14. Zelop CM, Richardson DK, Heffner LJ. Outcomes of severely abnormal umbilical artery doppler velocimetry in structurally normal singleton fetuses. Obstet Gynecol 1996;87:434-8.

15. Macara L, Kingdom JC, Kaufmann P, Kohnen G, Hair J, More IA, Lyall F, Greer IA. Structural analysis of placental terminal villi from growth-restricted pregnancies with abnormal umbilical artery Doppler waveforms. Placenta 1996;17:37-48

16. Jauniaux E, Zaidi J, Jurković D, Campbell S, Hustin J. Comparison of colour Doppler features and pathological findings in complicated early pregnancy. Hum Reprod 1994;9:2432-2437.

17. Harrington K, Carpenter RG, Nguyen M, Campbell S. Changes observed in Doppler studies of the fetal circulation in pregnancies complicated by pre-eclampsia or the delivery of a small-for-gestational-age baby. I. Cross-sectional analysis. Ultrasound Obstet Gynecol 1995;6:19-28.

18. Iwata M, Matsuzaki N, Shimizu I, Mitsuda N, Nakayama M. Prenatal detection of ischemic changes in the placenta of growth-retarded fetus by Doppler flow velocimetry of the maternal uterine artery. Obstet Gynecol 1993;82:494-9.

19. Kurjak A, Zalud I, Salihagić A, Crvenković G, Matijević R. Transvaginal color Doppler in the assessment of abnormal early pregnancy. J Perinat Med 1991;155-165.

20. Hoogland HJ. The ultrasound display of intervillous circulation. Placenta 1987;537-544.

21. Clavero JA, Negueruela J, Ortiz L, De los Heros JA, Modrego SP. Blood flow in the intervillous space and fetal blood flow. I. Normal values in human pregnancies at term. Am J Obstet Gynecol 1973;116:340-346.

22. Clavero JA, Ortiz L, De los Heros JA, Negueruela J. Blood flow in the intervillous space and fetal blood flow. II. Relation to placental histology and histometry in cases with and without high fetal risk. Am J Obstet Gynecol 1973;116:1157-1162.

23. Burchell RC. Arterial blood flow into the human intervillous space. Am J Obstet Gynecol 1967;98:303-311.

DOPPLER ULTRASOUND IN PERINATAL MEDICINE:

MEASUREMENTS AND ARTIFACTS

Ivica Zalud, MD, PhD

Gary Eglinton, MD

Division of Maternal-Fetal Medicine, Department of OB/GYN
Georgetown University, School of Medicine

Washington, DC, USA

INTRODUCTION

Doppler ultrasound has been in use for many years. The primary long-standing applications include monitoring of the fetal heart rate during labor and delivery and evaluating blood flow in the carotid artery. Applications that have developed largely in the last decade have extended its use to virtually all-medical specialties including obstetrics and gynecology, cardiology, neurology, radiology, pediatrics, and surgery. Flow can be detected even in vessels that are too small to image. Doppler ultrasound can determine the presence or absence of flow, flow direction, and flow character.

Doppler methods are unique among clinical techniques in ultrasound in that they have the potential to offer information related to the function of an organ beside its morphology. For intelligent and successful application of the technique to medical diagnosis, an understanding of Doppler physics, its possibilities and limitations is necessary. In obstetrics and gynecology, Doppler ultrasound has been used to investigate fetal and maternal hemodynamics during pregnancy, and pelvic vessels in nonpregnant women. Color flow has been found to be useful in elucidating complex cardiac malformations of the fetus, in directing spectral Doppler interrogation of fetal cerebral, renal and other circulations, in diagnosing ectopic pregnancy and in assessing pelvic tumor vascularity. It should be recognized, however, that the instrumental setting and characteristics significantly influence the information generated by Doppler color flow mapping. The reliability of the method, thus, depends on the appropriate use of the device by the operator who should have a clear understanding of the basic principles of Doppler ultrasound and its implementation[1-6].

BASIC PRINCIPLES

Doppler color flow imaging is based on multigated sampling of multiple scan lines using bursts of short pulses of ultrasound. For each emitted pulse of ultrasound along a single scan line, many range gated samples are obtained by opening the receiving gate sequentially to the echo signals arriving from various depths along the scan line. The time needed for the return journey of the echo is used to determine the spatial origin of the returning echoes. In reality, many samples are collected and the consecutive sampling of the signals along the scan line are timed according to the depth of the sampling location.

Each returning echo is referenced to its range gate, which identifies it with the spatial location of its origin and is electronically stored by using delay circuitry. After all the echoes from the first pulse are received, a second pulse in phase with the first pulse is sent along the same scan line. Appropriate timing of the pulse repetition is a critical consideration for pulsed Doppler, since the transmission of a pulse before the return of the echoes from the previous pulse will cause range ambiguity. In two-dimensional Doppler imaging, range ambiguity is not permissible. The backscattered echo signals of the second pulse are collected from range locations identical to those of the first pulse and are referenced to their respective range gates. In order to determine the mean Doppler shift, each echo signal from each pulse sampled from a given range gate is compared with that from the previous pulse sampled from the same gate. As an enormous amount of samples are collected, the comprehensive spectral processing techniques can not be implemented in Doppler color flow mapping. Instead, autocorrelation technique is utilized to obtain mean Doppler phase shift.

Each scan line is repeatedly sampled using multiple pulses. The signals from the identical range gates are collected and compared to obtain mean Doppler shifts that are averaged for each gate. The number of pulses per scan line is called the ensemble length. There are several reasons for this repeated sampling of a single scan line. The most important is the fact that blood flow is a continuously changing phenomenon and the duration of each pulse in Doppler color flow mapping is too short (<2 msec) to provide an acceptable mean value. As the number of pulses per scan line is increased, the quality of flow information improves in terms of reliability and completeness. Another distinct advantage of increasing the samples is greater Doppler sensitivity to detect low velocity circulations. This may be useful in gynecological applications, specifically in detecting ovarian, uterine or tumor blood flow where it is more important to detect flow than to be concerned with the temporal resolution. Moreover, as the samples are repeated and averaged against a constant background of noise, the signal to noise ratio improves. Multiple sampling also contributes toward stabilization of the high pass filter. Once sampling of a scan line is completed, the next scan line is interrogated in the same manner as described above. Multiple scan lines sweeping across the imaging field complete the color map.

Multigated sampling of multiple scan lines of the color flow imaging field generates an enormous amount of data. Color flow mapping requires real time processing and display of this data. The demands of processing such a vast flow of information can not be met by the currently available comprehensive spectral analytic techniques such as Fast Fourier Transform. This is usually achieved by autocorrelation technique that generates mean Doppler shift information, rather than the comprehensive power spectral data generated by full spectral processing.

It is important to note that the autocorrelation method does not estimate the peak frequency shift.

INSTRUMENTATION

The instrumentation for Doppler ultrasound consists of multiplex systems that combine multiple ultrasound modalities providing a comprehensive array of sophisticated diagnostic tools. It is not surprising that the technology employed in these devices is highly complex, especially in the Doppler mode. In addition, commercially available devices not only demonstrate a fair degree of diversity in the engineering implementation of the Doppler technology, they also differ in the organization and the choice of system controls they offer to the operator.

The basic components of a Doppler signal processing system consist of the following :

(a) A transducer for transmitting the ultrasound beam and receiving the echoes for both imaging and Doppler analysis.

(b) The receiver which receives and amplifies the incoming signals from the transducer for further processing for gray scale tissue imaging and for color Doppler.

(c) The echo information for tissue imaging is processed and converted to digital format and is stored in the digital scan converter for subsequent integration with color flow.

(d) Backscattered echoes for Doppler processing are first converted from analog (electrical voltage variations) data to numeric or digital data.

(e) The digitized signals are then subjected to filtering to remove noise generated by stationery and slow moving tissue structures; the filter is known as the moving target indicator.

(f) The filtered data is then analyzed by the autocorrelator to determine the Doppler phase shift. The autocorrelator output consists of 3 types of information: Doppler mean frequency shift, variance and Doppler amplitude (power or energy). These are fed to the digital scan converter where it is integrated with the tissue image information.

(g) Finally, the Doppler related data is color encoded by the color processor and the combined gray scale tissue image and the Doppler color map is sent to the video display via digital to analog conversion.

The above description is only a general outline; the actual implementation of color Doppler sonography involves highly complex technology and proprietary engineering innovations, information that is not accessible in the public domain.

There are various types of transducers used for Doppler ultrasound. Of these, electronic array systems are used in most devices for color flow imaging. Mechanical transducers do not offer an optimal platform for Doppler color flow implementation as simultaneous tissue imaging and Doppler interrogation, and other advanced features such as beam steering can not be performed with these transducers. With these devices, one must freeze the tissue image before using the Doppler mode. These limitations preclude their use in obstetrical Doppler sonography.

Doppler ultrasound has been implemented using linear sequenced array, convex sequenced array, linear phased array and annular phased array transducers. The scan lines are perpendicular along the length of the transducer face producing a rectangular field. Although this configuration provides the optimal imaging approach, it not optimal for Doppler imaging of vessels or flow channels located across the beam path. This can be mitigated by the hybrid sequenced and phased systems in which Doppler beam can be steered independent of the direction of the imaging beam, producing a more favorable angle of insonation. As all scan lines are parallel to one another, they incur the same angle with a given flow axis. However, beam steering reduces the effective aperture and increases the beam thickness, and may compromise the sensitivity and lateral resolution. These transducers are advantageous in peripheral vascular imaging. However, they are not particularly useful for obstetrical and gynecological applications.

A modification of the linear sequence design, the convex sequenced array offers distinct advantages over the previous design for obstetrical scanning because of its smaller footprint while offering a wider field of imaging at depth. Furthermore, the wider field of view is achieved without the grating lobe problem of the linear phased array. The angle of Doppler insonation is better achieved in the convex than in the linear array despite some of the disadvantages of the former as previously discussed.

The linear phased array offers a sector shaped field of image and is very useful in cardiologic applications. These transducers, however, are not optimal for fetal imaging applications. They do not provide the wide angle of view at depth and may produce from side lobe problem resulting in spurious flow depiction. Annular array transducers are seldom used for Doppler obstetrical applications.

QUALITY DOPPLER IMAGING
Transducer Frequency
The operating frequency of the transducer is an important contributor for the functional efficacy of the system. A higher carrier frequency results in a better spatial resolution of the image, but reduces the depth of penetration. The Doppler mode is more vulnerable to depth limitation than gray scale tissue imaging. For most obstetrical applications, a two to four MHz frequency provides adequate penetration and resolution, and is usually preferred. For transvaginal applications, a higher frequency (five to twelve MHz) is used as penetration is not a problem. Currently, piezzo electric elements capable of resonating at more than one frequency are available so that a single transducer may operate at multiple frequencies. This offers a unique advantage for color flow mapping as a lower frequency may be used for the combined tissue imaging and color Doppler mode while one may default to a higher frequency for tissue imaging to ensure a higher gray scale resolution.

Pulse Repetition Frequency (PRF)
Doppler color flow imaging is based on pulsed Doppler insonation. The magnitude of the frequency shift in color flow Doppler is, therefore, dependent on

the PRF of the transmitted ultrasound. The PRF is adjustable and should be optimized for specific applications. As the PRF is changed, the range of Doppler shifts for a given PRF is shown in the color bar. The displayed range is a qualitative approximation and can not be used as quantitative information. The PRF setting should be manipulated to accommodate a changing velocity pattern. A low PRF in the presence of a high velocity flow will result in aliasing of the displayed frequencies. A high PRF, on the other hand, reduces the sensitivity so that a low velocity flow may not be identified. The location of the baseline can be changed in order to depict optimally the entire range of frequencies encountered in a target vessel in the appropriate direction. The PRF is inter-related to the frame rate and also affects the depth of imaging. All these factors should be taken into consideration for increasing the efficiency of Doppler imaging.

Doppler Gain
The gain control deals with signal amplification. Most Doppler devices offer separate gain controls for pulse echo imaging, spectral Doppler and Doppler color mapping functions. The greater the gain, the more sensitive the Doppler. Appropriate color gain adjustment is essential for generating reliable hemodynamic information. A higher gain setting improves the sensitivity of color Doppler for identifying low velocity flow states. However, increased gain also amplifies the noise component of the signal. This causes display of misleading information that includes appearance of random color speckles in the color window, overflow of color outside vascular areas, and semblance of mosaic patterns. The latter falsely suggests the presence of turbulence when the flow is actually nonturbulent. The optimal gain setting should, therefore, be tailored to the specific examination situation. As a practical guideline, the gain should be initially increased until random color speckles start to appear; the gain then should be turned down until the speckles disappear. Further manipulation should take into account other attributes of the color image and the characteristics of the flow.

High Pass Filter (Wall Filter)
A high pass filter eliminates high amplitude low frequency Doppler shift signals generated by the movement of vascular wall, cardiac structures or the surrounding tissues. Such signals, because of their high power content, obfuscate Doppler signals generated by blood flow. This filter is called high pass because it allows higher frequencies to pass through for further processing. High pass filters are an essential part of signal processing in spectral Doppler ultrasound. They are also an integral part of Doppler color flow mapping. The technique, however, is relatively more complex in this application, as an immense amount of Doppler data needs to be processed in real time. A filter that simply eliminates low frequency signals will also remove low velocity blood flow signals with consequent loss of important hemodynamic information. In obstetrical and gynecological application, low speed flow is encountered in ovarian and tumor vessels, placental circulation, and fetal splanchnic vessels. The filters can be implemented at various levels of high pass threshold. The thresholds are defined in

terms of either frequency values or predesignated levels optimized for specific applications. The threshold may change automatically as the PRF is increased. In many devices, a minimum level of filter operates at all times.

For proper use of high pass filter, the circumstances of its application should be taken into account. As a rule of thumb, a low level filter should be used for imaging ovarian, pelvic tumor, fetal splanchnic, intrauterine and placental vessels; a medium level is useful in imaging umbilical or fetal venous flow; and a high level is recommended for fetal intra cardiac flow, or pelvic vessels such as the internal iliac or the uterine arteries. Although the exact algorithm of filtering is proprietary and varies according to the vendor, the current generation of high pass filters is sophisticated and use multivariate techniques capable of discriminating between low velocity blood flow and wall motion. Introduction of such filtering techniques has led to the recent resurgence of interest in Doppler amplitude mode (also known as power Doppler or energy Doppler) in color flow mapping, which may be helpful in identifying slow flow circulations.

Power Doppler

Doppler signal amplitude implies the intensity of the signal and is also referred as power or energy Doppler. Doppler flow signals have three dimensions: (a) frequency, which is proportional to the speed of red cell movement; (b) amplitude or intensity of the signal, which is proportional to the number of red cells scattering the transmitted ultrasound beam; and (c) time, during which the above two parameters change. Whereas the frequency information and its temporal changes form the basis for clinical application of Doppler technique, the amplitude data remains largely unutilized. However, amplitude reflects the scattering power and, therefore, may prove useful in clinical application. In Doppler color flow processing, the autocorrelator measures the amplitude from the phase analysis of the returning echoes. Although it was theoretically possible to produce two dimensional Doppler color flow mapping based on the intensity of the Doppler signal, it is only recently that the systems have seriously attempted to resolve the technical challenge of producing an amplitude based map that would be independent of Doppler shifted frequency.

The energy or power Doppler display, however, does not indicate directionality of flow in relation to the transducer. In contrast to the frequency mode which, as apparent from the Doppler equation, is angle dependent, the amplitude mode is virtually unaffected by the angle of insonation. Power or energy Doppler imaging is also affected by gain. A higher gain results in an increased sensitivity for detecting slow velocity circulations but also results in the extension of color flow areas beyond the vascular margin, and the depiction of tissue or wall movements. Other factors, that interdependently or independently affect the power or energy mode display, include the transmitted acoustic power, color sensitivity, preponderance of gray scale (write priority) and persistence. The actual implementation of these controls and the resultant changes in the amplitude color maps vary from device to device

Amplitude mapping may be helpful in identifying blood flows which are of low volume or of low velocity. Doppler mean frequency shift based on color mapping may not be sensitive enough to detect such a flow system. Examples of such potential uses in obstetrics include demonstration of splanchnic flow in fetal lungs and placenta. In gynecological practice, amplitude may optimize our ability to detect flow in pelvic organs such the ovaries, especially in postmenopausal women. However, the extent of its clinical utility is still being explored. Very recently, spatially three-dimensional reconstruction of the vascular channels has been accomplished utilizing the Doppler amplitude mode. This feature may have potentially promising clinical applications.

DOPPLER MEASURENTS

Because of inherent difficulties in evaluating blood flow, or even taking depicted velocities as accurate, the blood flow velocity waveform has commonly been interpreted to distinguish patterns associated with high and low resistance in the distal vascular tree. Three indices are in common use, the systolic/diastolic ratio (S/D ratio), the pulsatility index (PI, also called the impedance index), and the resistance index (RI, also called the Pourcelot ratio).

The S/D ratio is the simplest and can be calculated by hand, but it is irrelevant when diastolic velocities are absent, and the ratio becomes infinite. Common practice has grouped values above 8.0 into a single category "extremely high". The PI requires computer-assisted calculation of mean velocity, which still may be subject to very large experimental error. In a normal pregnancy, neither the S/D ratio nor PI is normally distributed across all gestational ages. The RI is moderately complicated but has the appeal of approaching 1.00 when diastolic velocities are abnormally low and does, therefore, reflect the relative impairment of flow by high resistance. These indices are ratios, independent of the angle between the ultrasound beam and the insonated blood vessel, and therefore not dependent on absolute measurement of true velocity.

The indices were derived initially by their statistically demonstrated association with adverse clinical findings. They are commonly regarded as "resistance indices," reflecting the belief that they indicate the degree of downstream resistance. However, the RI must not be considered independent of changes in physiologic variables such as heart rate, cardiac contractility, blood pressure, and the many other determinants of flow.

The three indices are highly correlated, with coefficients in excess of 0.9 being reported[2,3]. Such is the degree of correlation that it is unlikely one index provides an advantage over another. There are intrinsic errors in all that have been quantified and lie between 10 and 20%. There may be advantages to the RI or PI where flow is markedly abnormal or in early pregnancy, when a very low end-diastolic velocity can be a normal finding. Given the many modifications and adaptations proposed in the literature, use of particular index becomes a matter of personal choice.

LIMITATIONS

Inspite of the impressive technological innovations of the Doppler ultrasound that revolutionized noninvasive diagnosis, there are important limitations of the method which need to be considered. These limitations are inherent in the physical principle and the engineering implementation of the method. They are also responsible for various artifacts that one may encounter during the use of this technique. An understanding of these limitations and artifacts is essential for the appropriate use and interpretation of Doppler color flow mapping. Several artifacts are encountered in Doppler ultrasound[7-12]. These are incorrect presentations of Doppler flow information. The most common of these is aliasing. However, others occur, including range ambiguity, spectrum mirror image, location mirror image, speckle, and electromagnetic interference.

Aliasing

Aliasing is the most common artifact encountered in Doppler ultrasound. There is an upper limit to Doppler shift that can be detected by pulsed instruments. If the Doppler shift frequency exceeds one half the pulse repetition frequency (normally in the 1 to 30 kHz range), aliasing occurs and improper Doppler shift information (improper direction and improper value) results. An analogous optical form of aliasing occurs in motion pictures when wagon wheels appear to rotate at various speeds and in reverse direction. Higher pulse repetition frequencies permit higher Doppler shifts to be detected but also increase the chance of the range ambiguity artifact. Continuous-wave Doppler instruments do not have this limitation but neither do they provide depth selectivity.

Aliasing in a color flow system is exposed in a spatial two-dimensional plane in which the aliased flow is shown in reversed color surrounded by nonaliased flow. This pattern mimics the color flow appearance of separate streams in differing directions. The two patterns are, however, clearly distinguishable. In an aliased flow, the higher velocity generates a higher Doppler shifted frequency that is depicted with greater brightness. The higher the frequency shifts, the brighter the color. The brightest level in the color calibration bar (the uppermost for the flow toward the transducer and lowermost for the flow away from the transducer) represents the Nyquist limit. As the velocity and, therefore, the frequency shift exceeds this limit, the color wraps around the calibration bar and appears at the other end as the most luminous color of the opposite direction. For example, a flow toward the transducer with an increasing velocity is depicted with an increasingly bright red color changing to yellow. As the Nyquist limit is reached, the color flow shows brightest yellow in the color bar and as the limit is exceeded, flow is shown in the brightest blue. Thus in an aliased flow, bright or pale color of one direction is juxtaposed against bright color of the opposite direction. In contrast, in genuine flow separation the distinct flow streams are depicted in the directionally appropriate colors that are separated by a dark margin. It should be noted that the hue that demarcates an aliased flow would depend on the choice of the color-mapping scheme.

In demonstrating aliasing, an apparent contradiction may be seen between the spectral Doppler and the Doppler color flow interrogations. Doppler color flow mapping may show nonaliased flow pattern when aliasing is observed with the spectral Doppler waveform. This is explained by the fact that the mean frequency is less than the peak frequency and Doppler color flow depiction is based on the use of mean frequency, so that Nyquist limit is not reached as readily as with the peak frequency depiction by the spectral Doppler.

Aliasing can be eliminated by increasing pulse repetition frequency, increasing Doppler angle (which decreases the Doppler shift for a given flow), or by baseline shifting. The latter is an electronic "cut and paste" technique that moves the misplaced aliasing peaks over to their proper location. It is a successful technique as long as there are no legitimate Doppler shifts in the region of the aliasing. If there are, they will get moved over to an inappropriate location along with the aliasing peaks. Other approaches to eliminating aliasing include changing to a lower frequency Doppler transducer or changing to a continuous-wave instrument. Aliasing occurs with the pulsed system because it is a sampling system. If samples are taken often enough, the correct result is achieved. Sufficient sampling yields the correct result. Insufficient sampling yields an incorrect result.

Range ambiguity

In an attempt to solve the aliasing problem by increasing pulse repetition frequency, the range ambiguity problem can be encountered. This occurs when a pulse is emitted before all the echoes from the previous pulse have been received. When this happens, early echoes from the last pulse are simultaneously received with late echoes from the previous pulse. This causes difficulty with the ranging process. The instrument is unable to determine whether an echo is an early one (superficial) from the last pulse or a late one (deep) from the previous pulse. To avoid this difficulty it simply assumes that all echoes are derived from the last pulse and that these echoes have originated from some depth. As long as all echoes are received before the next pulse is sent out, this will be true. However, with high pulse repetition frequencies, this may not be the case. Doppler flow information may, therefore, come from locations other than the assumed one (the gate location). In effect, multiple gates or sample volumes are operating at different depths. Instruments often increase pulse repetition frequency (to avoid aliasing) into the range where range ambiguity occurs. Multiple sample gates are shown on the display to indicate this condition. Range ambiguity in color-flow Doppler, as in sonography, places echoes (color Doppler shifts in this case) that have come from deep locations after a subsequent pulse was emitted in shallow locations where they do not belong. In practice, however, most Doppler color flow devices prevent this problem by automatically reducing the depth when the pulse repetition frequency is increased to the threshold of range ambiguity.

Temporal ambiguity

Temporal ambiguity occurs when Doppler color flow mapping fails to depict hemodynamic events with temporal accuracy. Specifically, such a situation arises when the frame rate for color flow is too slow relative to the circulatory dynamics. As discussed earlier, the basic unit of color flow depiction is a single frame which when completed shows the average mean frequency shifts color coded and superimposed on the gray scale tissue image. The flow dynamics are, therefore, summarized for the duration of one frame. As we have noted above, the frame rate is inversely proportional to the number of scan lines and the number of samples per scan line. The slower the frame rates the better the color image quality in terms of both spatial resolution and Doppler sensitivity. Herein lies the paradox as a slower rate means longer duration of a frame. As the frame duration increases, there is a progressive loss of the ability to recognize discrete hemodynamic events.

Angle of insonation

Angle dependency of the Doppler shifted frequencies is also a critical factor in blood flow analysis. In sector scanning, multiple scan lines spread out from the transducer in a fan-like manner. When the sector scanner is used to interrogate a circulatory system in which the direction of flow is across these scan lines in a color window, the angle of insonation between the flow axis and the ultrasound beam changes. The angle is smallest when the flow stream enters in the sector field and progressively rises to $90°$ as the flow approaches the center of the field. Concurrently, the Doppler shifted frequencies progressively decline and may become undetectable at the center of the color field.

A sector scanner may also create apparently contradictory directional information in a vessel traversing across the color field. As the flow approaches the midline of the field, the flow is depicted in color encoding for flow toward the transducer which usually is red; as the flow moves away, it will be encoded blue. Thus, the same vessel will show bi-directional flow. This paradox actually highlights the basic concept of representation of flow directionality by any Doppler system.

Mirror imaging

The mirror image artifact can also occur with Doppler systems. This means that an image of a vessel and a source of Doppler shifted echoes can be duplicated on the opposite side of a strong reflector (such as a bone). The duplicated vessel containing flow could be misinterpreted as an additional vessel. It will have a spectrum similar to that for the real vessel. A mirror image of a Doppler spectrum can appear on the opposite side of the baseline when, indeed, flow is unidirectional and should appear only on one side of the baseline. This is an electronic duplication of the spectral information. It can occur when receiver gain is set too high (causing overloading in the receiver and cross talk between the two flow channels) or with low gain (where the receiver has difficulty determining the sign of the Doppler shift). It can also occur when Doppler angle is near 90 degrees. Here the duplication is usually legitimate. This is because beams are focused and not cylindrical in shape. Thus, portions of the beam can experience flow toward while other portions can experience flow away.

Other artifacts

Doppler spectra have a speckle quality to them similar to that observed in sonography. Speckle is a result of interference effects of scattered sound from the distribution of scatters (erythrocytes) in the blood. Because the ultrasound pulse encounters several scatters at any point in its travel, several echoes are generated simultaneously. These may arrive at the transducer in such a way that they re-enforce (constructive interference) or partially or totally cancel (destructive interference) each other. This results in a displayed dot pattern that does not directly represent individual scatters but rather represents an interference pattern of the scatter distribution scanned. This phenomenon is called acoustic speckle. Occasionally, a spectral trace can show a straight line adjacent to and parallel to the baseline, often on both sides. Apparently, this is due to 60 Hz interference from power lines or power supply. It can make determination of low or absent diastolic flow difficult. Electromagnetic interference from power lines and nearby equipment can also cloud the spectral display with lines or "snow".

CONCLUSIONS

Doppler ultrasound has ushered in a new era in diagnostic sonographic imaging. The application of this technique in obstetrical and gynecological imaging has proved very useful. However, a prerequisite for optimal utilization of this technique is an in depth knowledge of the principles and limitations of this technique. Furthermore, it is important to appreciate that the appearance of Doppler images is influenced by the operational setting of the equipment that must be taken into account for any reliable interpretation. Finally, there are newer modalities of flow imaging which present exciting possibilities for the future of noninvasive hemodynamic investigation in clinical practice.

Doppler imaging is unique among clinical techniques in that way that Doppler has the potential to offer information related to the function of an organ beside its morphology. Due to its sensitivity to measurement artifacts, the ultrasonic Doppler technique has not yet become a clinically useful tool for blood perfusion measurements. One of these measurement artifacts is caused by ultrasonic wave interference in combination with the small changes of structures inside the ultrasonic field. These changes are a result of variations in blood pressure, small movements in muscles, and involuntary movements of the transducer. The changes alter the ultrasonic interference pattern, causing fluctuations in the measured perfusion value. The need to develop clinical methods for the noninvasive monitoring of regional blood perfusion, i.e., the blood flow through the very fine capillaries in body tissue, has long been felt. Hitherto existing methods exhibit limitations, such as insufficient measurement depth and poor time- or space-resolution, which restrict the measurements that can be performed. Unexpectedly large variations in the recorded perfusion values lead to further investigation of the method, both in vitro using a specially designed flow phantom and in vivo.

Aliasing is the most common artifact in Doppler measurements. Recognizing these artifacts is important to avoid image misinterpretations and, when possible, to overcome them by modifying either techniques or unit settings, or both. It must be kept in mind that an accurate analysis of unit settings during scanning, and the meticulous evaluation of the obtained Doppler images are of the utmost importance for the proper use of this valuable but difficult diagnostic modality. Doppler ultrasound has potential for both false positive and false negative results. Misdiagnosis is far more dangerous than any effect that might result from the ultrasound exposure. Therefore, diagnostic ultrasound should be performed only by persons with sufficient training and education. One of the major reasons for so many conflicting and controversial results in the literature originates from technique complexity and inadequate education in Doppler physics and technique. Standardization in Doppler technique would significantly help to properly evaluate all clinical potential in Doppler ultrasound in obstetrics and gynecology.

LITERATURE

1. Omoto, R., Kasai, C. (1987). Physics and instrumentation of Doppler color mapping. Echocardiography 4:467-471
2. Taylor, K.J.W. and Holland, S. (1990). Doppler ultrasound. Part I: Basic principles, instrumentation, and pitfalls. Radiology, 174, 297-307
3. Burns, P.N. (1993). Principles of Doppler and color flow. Radiol Med, 85, 3-16
4. Maulik, D. (1997). Sonographic color flow mapping: Basic principles. In: Maulik D: Doppler ultrasound in obstetrics and gynecology. Springer, New York, 68-87
5. Kremkau, F.W. (1992). Doppler color imaging: Principles and instrumentation. Clin. Diagn. Ultrasound, 27, 7-60
6. Jaffe, R. (1992). Color Doppler imaging: A new interpretation of the Doppler effect. In Jaffe, R. and Warsof, S.L. (eds.). Color Doppler imaging in obstetrics and gynecology. McGraw-Hill, New York, 17-34
7. Mitchell, D.G. (1990). Color Doppler imaging: principles, limitations, and artifacts. Radiology, 177, 1-10
8. Zalud, I., Breyer, B., Kurjak, A. (1998). Accuracy, precision and artifacts of Doppler measurements in gynecology. In Kurjak A, Fleischer AC: Doppler ultrasound in gynecology. Parthenon Publishing, London - New York, 1-17
9. Derchi, L.E., Giannoni, M., Crespi, G., Pretolesi, F. and Oliva, L. (1992). Artifacts in echo-Doppler and color-Doppler. Radiol. Medica, 83, 340-352
10. Winkler, P., Helmke, K. and Mahl, M. (1990). Major pitfalls in Doppler investigations. Part II: Low flow velocity and colour Doppler application. Ped. Radiology, 20, 304-310
11. Suchet, I.B. (1994). Colour-flow Doppler artifacts in anechoic soft-tissue masses of infants. Can Assoc Radiol J, 45, 201-203
12. Pozniak, M.A., Zagzebski, J.A. and Scanlan, K.A. (1992). Spectral and color Doppler artifacts. Radiographics, 12, 35-44

Three-dimensional imaging in human reproduction in normal and pathological conditions: a new approach by high resolution electron microscopy after maceration techniques and vascular casts

[1]PM MOTTA, [1]S CORRER AND [1-2]E VIZZA

[1]Department of Anatomy, University of Rome "La Sapienza, via Borelli 50, 00161 Rome, Italy;

[2]Department of Gynaecology "San Carlo di Nancy-IDI Sanità" Hospital, via Aurelia 275, 00165 Rome, Italy.

SUMMARY.

This study updates important morphodynamic features related to human female reproductive organs such as ovary, tube and uterus at different stages (reproductive and postmenopausal ages) including relevant pathological conditions.

All these organs and their fine structure have been systematically analysed by parallel and integrated observations by high resolution transmission and scanning electron microscopy (TEM and SEM). Furthermore, methods of chemical maceration (2N-NaOH and 6N-NaOH) of selected tissues as well as vascular corrosion casts preparations have been largely used. This systematic study provided clear three-dimensional dynamic pictures (*real three-dimensional microanatomy*) easy to integrate and correlate with parallel physiopathological and clinical events as seen by different clinical methods (endoscopy, histopathology).

INTRODUCTION.

Till recently, the study of the micro-anatomical modifications of the sexual organs during sexual life and menopause was mainly based on bidimensional techniques such as the observations under light microscopy (LM) of sections alone. In the last three decades the development of scanning electron microscopy (SEM) resolution, and more recently, of maceration techniques as well as *vascular corrosion casts* methods in anatomy and cell biology (1, 2), made possible a three-dimensional (3-D) evaluation of the microanatomy of the female reproductive organs during the various phases of the reproductive life (3). The combination of TEM and SEM allowed the visualization of the 3-D microanatomy of the

73

inner uterine structures such as glands, interglandular stroma and vessels including the sub-epithelial capillary network (3, 4). Furthermore, the 3-D organization of smooth muscle cells of myometrium and myosalpinx (5), the extracellular fibrillar matrix skeleton of the endometrium, myometrium (3-5) and myosalpinx (1) including some pathological forms such as the myoma (6) could be easily revisited by these techniques. Therefore, an innovative approach to the study of the real 3-D microanatomy of the uterus, fallopian tube and ovary - in a sense complementary to the actual microendoscopic view obtainable by hysteroscopy and laparoscopy - is rapidly merging (2, 5). Finally, the artificial addition of key colours to different cells, tissues and their cell components emphasizes the morphodynamics and aids comprehension of the fine details in various structures of the human body (7, 8).

MATERIAL AND METHOD.

For this study were used biopsies of ovary, endometrium and falloppian tube at different phases of the female cycle and in menopause. The material was obtained during laparoscopic or hysteroscopic procedures with the consent of the patients. All the samples were fixed by immersion in 2.5% glutaraldehyde in PBS. *Maceration of the extracellular matrix for studying the cellular spatial organization.* The samples were incubated in an aqueous solution of 6N NaOH at 60 °C for 10-15 min, rinsed in tap water for 20 min., conductive stained, critical point dried with CO_2 and finally sputtered with platinum (9). *Maceration of cells for studying the collagen fibrillar architecture.* The samples incubated with an aqueous solution of 2N NaOH at room temperature for 7 days and rinsed in distilled water for 10-15 days were conductive stained, critical point dryed with CO_2 and sputtered with platinum (10). *Vascular corrosion cast.* Casting medium (methyl methacrilate) was injected into the vascular system and maceration of the tissues from the replicas was obtained by immersing the resin-injected tissues into 20% KOH at 60 °C (11). Then, the casts were dissected, dried, mounted on stubs and sputtered with gold. Observations were made with a Hitachi S4000 SEM at 7kV.

RESULTS and DISCUSSION.

Due to a rapid development in imaging technologies - which integrate high resolution SEM and TEM with computerised analysis - nowadays real 3-D microanatomical images of tissues and cells components clearly revealed new fundamental insights in great details. When these methods are applied to study the cycling organs of the woman's reproductive organs original unexpected microtopographical dynamic views are disclosed which can be easily coupled with concurrent biochemical and physiopathological data. These pictures compared to parallel cycling normal organs and relevant pathological cases offer the unique opportunity to

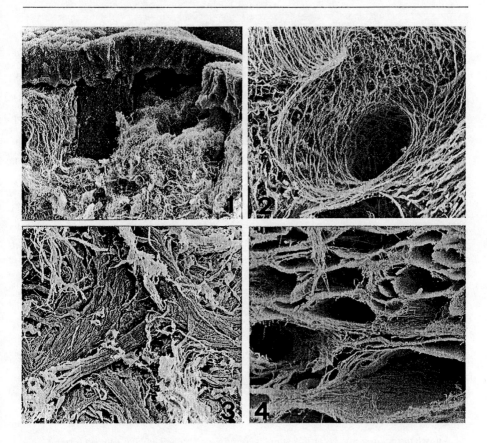

CAPTIONS. **Fig.1**. Endometrium, early proliferative phase. Endometrial glands and their extracellular fibrillar matrix baskets. SEM 1000X. **Fig. 2**. Endometrium, secretive phase. Extracellular fibrillar basket of an endometrial gland. Note the convolute shape of the basket. SEM 1200X. **Fig. 3**. Myosalpinx. The muscular network of the muscle cells in the human myosalpinx as seen after maceration of the extracellular matrix (6N NaOH). SEM 900X. **Fig. 4**. The honeycomb arrangement of the extracelluar matrix around the smooth muscle bundles of the myosalpinx after maceration of the cells (2N NaOH). SEM 1300X.

clearly evaluate the real significance of basic physiopathological cellular events in reproduction. In addition, the recent development of selective maceration techniques for SEM (12) opened a new era in the study of the microanatomy of cell and tissues. In fact, these techniques made possible, for example, direct visualisation by SEM of the real 3D organisation of the fibrillar component of the extracellular matrix (EM). These approaches consist in the chemical digestion of cells (2N NaOH maceration) preserving the fibrillar component of the EM (mainly collagen fibres). The present study shows as the SEM observations combined with alkali macerated and corrosion casted samples allows a new 3-D view of the female genital organs in a sense very close to that visible at micro-endoscopic level or under a dissecting stereo-microscope (3). In fact, for example, by this technique it is possible to investigate the fine interaction among epithelial cells and EM of endometrial glands and their dynamic changes during the cycle (figs. 1 and 2), or the morphofunctional interaction of the smooth muscle cells of the myosalpinx and the EM of the fallopian tube (figs. 3 and 4).

Such a *new microanatomy* allowing a more precise clinical evidence of various dynamics in female physio-pathology, can be considered as a sort of *micro-operative anatomy* complementary to the microendoscopy. In addition, this microanatomic view is likely to help much the gynaecologist in the selection of the most appropriate therapy to improve the health and the quality of the woman's life.

Acknowledgements: Funds for this study were provided by M.U.R.S.T. 1995-97, Italy.
REFERENCES.

1. **Motta PM, Murakami T, Fujita T.** (eds) *Scanning Electron Microscopy of Vascular Casts: Methods and Applications.* Kluwer Academic Publishers. Boston, Dordrecht, London, pp.231-44, 1992

2. **Motta PM, Vizza E, Correr S.** The microanatomy of the uterus by coloured high resolution scanning electron microscopy. In: *Hysteroscopy Update.* Phillips J, Hunt R, Loffer FD (eds.) AAGLPC, pp 3-7 1997

3. **Goranova V, Vizza E, Motta PM.** Collagen fibrillar network in estrous and hCG-stimulated rabbit uterus: a SEM study after NaOH maceration. Arch Histol Cytol 56, 231-41, 1993

4. **Motta PM, Vizza E.** The three-dimensional arrangement of the human myosalpinx. In: *New Horizons in Reproductive Medicine.* Coutifaris G, Mastroianni L (eds.) Parthenon, New York, London 1997

5. **Vizza E, Heyn R, Magos AL et al.** Smooth muscle cells and extracellular fibrillar matrix

of human myometrium and myosalpinx studied by SEM after alkali maceration. In: *Recent Advances in Microscopy of Cells, Tissues and Organs.* P.M. Motta (ed.). A. Delfino Publisher. Rome 1997

6. **Vizza E, Mazzon I, Sbiroli C et al.** Microanatomia 3D del mioma uterino e del miometrio. Studio comparativo al microscopio elettronico a scansione dopo macerazione con alcali. Proceedings of the 37th Congress of the Italian Society of Obstetrics and Gynaecology, Florence, Vol. 32, pp 728-31, 1996

7. **Ewing WA.** *Inside Information. Imaging the Human Body.* Thames and Hudson Publisher U.K. 1996

8. **Motta PM, Nottola SAR.** Colored Scanning Electron Microscopic Pictures in Teaching Anatomy (P.M. Motta ed.) *Cells and Tissues: A Three-Dimensional Approach by Modern Techniques in Microscopy* pp 629-34, Alan R. Liss. New York 1989

9. **Vizza E, Muglia U, Macchiarelli G, et al.** Three-dimensional architecture of the human myosalpinx isthmus. SEM after NaOH digestion and ultrasonic macrodissection. Cell Tissue Res 226: 219-21, 1991

10. **Vizza E, Correr S, Goranova V, et al.** The collagen skeleton of the human umbilical cord at term. A scanning electron microscopic study after 2N-NaOH maceration. *Reproduction Fertility and Development* 8: 1-10, 1996

11. **Ohtani O.** Three - dimensional organization of the connective tissue fibers of the human pancreas: A scanning electron microscopic study of NaOH treated tissue. Arch. Histol. Jap. 50: 557-566, 1987

COLOR DOPPLER IN CONGENITAL DEFECTS

Kurjak A, Kupesic S

Department of Obstetrics and Gynecology, Medical School University of Zagreb,

Sveti Duh Hospital, Zagreb, Croatia

The use of color Doppler ultrasound offers a novel approach for the investigation of human uteroplacental and fetal circulations. Using this modality our understanding of the integrity of the materno-fetal circulation has tremendeously improved, allowing precise assessment of the circulatory modifications in cases of abnormal pregnancy. There is an obvious benefit from this technique in performing invasive procedures in prenatal diagnosis, particularly in identification and differentiation of the umbilical arteries and vein during the funiculocenthesis.

This chapter attempts to demonstrate the role of color Doppler in the diagnosis of fetal malformations, and evaluation of the chromosomal defects.

1. COLOR DOPPLER IN THE DIAGNOSIS OF FETAL MALFORMATIONS

A. Malformations of the cephalic pole

During the 7th gestational week it is already possible to observe early cerebral circulation, which is potentially helpful in the evaluation of cranial malformations and/or the degree of their effect on the central nervous system.

Anencephaly can be diagnosed very early, from the 8th week onwards (1-4). In these cases color Doppler studies reveal normal or even increased blood flow in carotid arteries, while the cerebral blood flow is absent.

In patients with **exencephaly**, blood flow is detected arising from the circle of Willis by an aberrant route (5). In normal pregnancies the pulsed Doppler waveform analysis indicates permanent diastolic flow and significantly lower impedance to flow than in other fetal vessels. In exencephalocoele vascular structures are clearly detected within the herniated cerebral mass and show an abnormal Doppler feature: absence of diastolic flow. This fact permits a differential diagnosis from cystic hygroma.

Cystic hygroma Is produced by a blockade of the lymphatic drainage at the level of the outlet of the jugular vein. Therefore, it is at first associated with the appearance of a bursa in the lateral aspect of the neck, which later due to its extension occupies the posterior portion, giving rise to a septated aspect, or simply a cystic image (5). In many cases, when it progresses it is accompanied by ascites, generalized edema and anasarca.

The cystic hygroma is accompanied by a frequency of chromosomopathies of between 40 and 90%: Turner's syndrome being the most common followed by trisomy 21 and mosaicisms (5). The presence of cystic hygroma, detectable during the first trimester of pregnancy obliges one to carry out an amniocentesis or chorial biopsy (6-22).

It is clearly shown that the malformation may disappear during gestation, even at the end of the first trimester (6,9,10,14,18). Cystic hygromas never manifest vascular flow in the tumor mass. However, blood flow signals from cerebral vessels are easily obtainable.

Numerous cystic formations (such as cysts of arachnoid fossae, agenesis of the corpus callosum, Dandy-Walker sy etc) may affect the cerebral mass. In these cases color Doppler accurately differentiates between cystic and vascular origin.

It has already been reported (23-26) that aneurism of the vein of Galen demonstrates a turbulent blood flow that permits a differential diagnosis from an arachnoid cyst. Commonly, this finding is associated with other malformations of the central nervous system.

Choroid plexus cysts are very common, and occur as a consequence of vascular dilatations with an accumulation of cerebrospinal liquor, so that they do not show any blood flow alterations. Today they are considered completely physiological and they tend to disappear spontaneously towards the 24th-26th week (5). However, there has been a lot of discussion about their significance as indirect signs of chromosomal malformations (27-29).

Based on our experience, choroid plexus cysts do not demonstrate increased flow and do not alter blood flow in other cerebral vessels.

Hydrocephaly and hydranencephaly are among the most common malformations of the central nervous system. Their origin is associated with obstruction or stenosis of the cerebral aqueduct. In general, they tend to be bilateral, although they may appear unilateral due to obliteration of the foramen of Monro.

In hydrocephaly and hydranencephaly a progressive compression of the vessels takes place, increasing the resistance to blood flow. This causes hypoxia and progressive degeneration of the cerebral parenchyma (30). In cases of unilateral hydrocephaly, a marked difference in the cerebral flow between the affected and the contralateral hemispheres has been observed (28).

It is clearly assumed that the increase in cerebral flow resistance is a reflection of the increase in intracranial pressure, and therefore its finding in these lesions, particularly in the beginning, involves a worse prognosis.

Color Doppler has a very limited application in detection of the **neural tube defects** since they do not modify the embryonic and fetal circulations.

B. Malformations of the thorax

Color Doppler may assist in detection of the malformations of the thorax. In pulmonary sequestration, color Doppler permits the identification of the aberrant origin of the systemic vascularization of the pulmonary parenchyma, allowing it to be differentiated from an adenomatoid cystic malformation. Similarly, color Doppler improves the diagnosis of all intra- or extra-cardiac malformations that are accompanied by an anomalous venous return (inferior or superior vena cava, portal vein, etc.) that can be located early on with this technique (30,31).

This method has significantly increased our diagnostic capacity in prenatal diagnosis of congenital cardiopathies. Starting from the 8th week of gestation it becomes possible to detect heart action and to obtain the cardiac frequency of an embryo. It was clearly demonstrated by De Vore (32) that sudden decrease of the fetal cardiac frequency is one of the most harmful prognostic factors in the first trimester of pregnancy. Knowledge of the normal embryonic and fetal cardiovascular anatomy is significantly increased allowing rapid identification of

major cardiac defects.

Color Doppler is very useful in the first phase of the echocardiographic examination since it provides rapid identification of the great vessels, such as the aorta and the pulmonary artery, allowing for immediate orientation by the examiner (31).

In a normal fetus, color Doppler allows evaluation of the cardiovascular hemodynamics with great simplicity (33). Venous circulation is easily observed by identifying blood flow in the superior vena cava and inferior to the right atrium, as well as blood flow through the foramen ovale to the left atrium. It is also easy to define both afferent and efferent vessels of both ventricles. The aortic arch is also identified without difficulty and the presence of an "aliasing" phenomenon in the region of the ductus often facilitates the identification of this structure (31). In the same manner, it is possible to clearly observe the turbulent flow of the pulmonary artery and its branches. The fact that color Doppler completely opacifies these vessels greatly facilitates the measurement of their diameters.

In fetuses with **congenital cardiopathies**, the additional information provided by color Doppler facilitates the identification and documentation of a certain number of anomalies, especially septi, valvular regurgitation and complex lesions. According to Coppel and colleagues (34) 20% of cardiopathies can be diagnosed in utero only with the use of color Doppler. Therefore, this technique is considered essential in these cases. In 47% of cardiopathies, the contribution of color Doppler is considered useful but not essential, and in 24%, color Doppler does not provide any additional diagnostic information than that provided by conventional echocardiography.

In general, color Doppler is essential to determine the course and direction of blood flow in the great vessels, is helpful but not essential in identifying the tiny "jets" in areas of regurgitation from the atrioventricular valves, and, finally, it is not essential in diagnosing the majority of anatomic congenital cardiopathies which are generally readily identified with two dimensional ultrasond (31,34). Color Doppler may be very useful in evaluation of the cardiac flow in patients with generalized non-immune hydrops.

C. Abdominal wall defects

Color Doppler permits the confirmation of structural pathologies that are difficult to diagnose early in pregnancy. The primitive gut is morphologically formed in the 6th week. The interstinal tract and liver grow more rapidly than the abdominal wall, and therefore the abdominal cavity becomes temporarily too small to contain the bowel, so they are displaced into the umbilical cord. Towards the 8th week, this physiological migration (35-37) is clearly visible using transvaginal ultrasound.

During the 10th week these organs return to their normal intra-abdominal position, due to the more rapid growth of the abdominal wall. During this process the midgut undergoes 270° of rotation, which occurs in two stages: the first stage of 90° when the midgut is herniated, and the second of 180° after the return to the intra-abdominal location. The definitive intra-abdominal location is completely established in the 11th week.

Due to this physiological herniation, it is difficult to diagnose abdominal wall defects before the 11th week, although with experience they may be suspected.

Such defects, which occur in one out of 5000 living newborns (5), include a very common group formed by omphalocoeles and gastroschisis, and an exceptional second group that includes ectopia cordis, cloaca and bladder extrophy, the limb-body wall complex and Cantrell's pentalogy.

Apart from gastroschisis, 70% of these defects are accompanied by chromosomal abnormalities and by other severe organ malformations. Therefore, there is an obvious importance of an early diagnosis which can be carried out using transvaginal ultrasound coupled with color flow imaging. Using this technique one can observe the displacement of the entire hepatic vascular map into the interior of the defect in the case of gastroschisis, or the vascular absence in the omphalocele and visualization of the mesenteric vessels at the base of the defect.

D. Malformations of the genito-urinary tract

Renal and urinary tract anomalies represent 40-50% of all malformations diagnosed with sonography (38). Although the kidneys are formed in the 10th week (39) and the existence of urine production is known from the 12th week on (38), it is difficult to diagnose these anomalies prior to the 16th week (5).

Color Doppler has been used to confirm the diagnosis of renal genesis, poly- micro and macrocystic kidneys and obstructive uropathies (5,31,40-43). In cases of renal agenesis, the existence of normal flow in the aorta and umbilical cord has been observed (40), with no visualization of the renal arteries. In renal ectopias the displaced renal vessels have been observed with normal velocimetric indices (41,42).

In cases of multicystic renal dysplasia Bonilla et al. (5) observed renal flow with normal indices which, as the gestation advanced and the lesion progressed, became highly pathological. The abnormal kidney tissue changes the vessels' diameter increasing the resistance to flow (expressed through RI and PI. These alterations initially have few consequences on the fetal systemic circulation but affects the function of the renal parenchyma, increasing the oligohydramnios and furthering the hemodynamic consequences. Color Doppler serves to establish a neonatal prognosis (43) as well as to determine whether one or both kidneys are involved.

E. Other abdominal tumors

Transvaginal color Doppler may be used for identification of the intra-abdominal cystic lesions (44) as well. They are easily identified by their lack of blood flow using this modality. In cases of vascularized cystic tumors one can differentiate their origin due to location and vascular relationship with kidneys, ovaries or interstines. In cases with obstructive uropathy color Doppler can detect local circulatory changes and may be used for follow-up of the functional changes produced by the lesion. Furthermore, it may facilitate the visualization of minor lesions such as pyelectasia, which is a well know phenotypic marker of chromosomal defects.

F. Other malformations

In contrast to cystic hygroma, non-immune edema produces a loosening of the neck and back skin, and is not accompanied by chromosomopathies. The origin of this state is very variable (45,38): in 52% is caused by cardiopathy, sometimes is associated with nephropathy, placental and cord anomalies, sacrococcygeal teratomas etc. In severe cases complicated by anemia, hypopoteinemia and cardiac insufficiency color Doppler measurements show significant alterations.

Doppler features of some vascular hepatic tumors such as cavernous hemangiomas (46) or hemangioendotheliomas (47,48,49) were reported as well. Sacrococcygeal teratomas are highly vascularized tumors characterized with numerous arteriovenous shunts, polyhydramnios, hypertrophic placenta and congestive cardiac insufficiency (50,51,52). Terefore, color Doppler seems to be useful in detection and follow-up of the hemodynamic changes in pregnancies complicated by sacrococcygeal teratoma.

This method allows us to study the kinetic patterns of different fluids, such as amniotic fluid or fetal urine. Abnormal movements of these fluids may lead an ultrasonographer to definition of some anomalies that are difficult to be detected such as cleft lip and palate, pharyngeal anomalies, etc.

2) COLOR DOPPLER IN DIAGNOSIS OF INDIRECT SIGNS OF CHROMOSOMAL DEFECTS

A single umbilical artery is a sign commonly associated with chromosomal defects, perinatal complications, intrauterine growth retardation and existence of fetal malformations. Since the incidence of this sign is around 1% in singleton pregnancies, and 4.6% in twin gestations, one should be aware of the importance of the early and safe detection of this entity by color and pulsed Doppler (31).

Pseudocysts of the umbilical cord display focal degeneration of the Wharton's jelly without involving embryonic vestigial structures of the omphalomesenteric or alantoid canals. Since these structures are associated with trisomies 18 and 13, their visualization by color Doppler indicates further cytogenetic evaluation.

Cord angiomyxomas are vascular tumors in a close contact with one or more umbilical vessels from which they arise. Due to infiltration of the cord by the angiomatous tissue and progressive shortening of the cord, a cesarean section is recommended.

Shortening of the length of the umbilical cord is associated with several chromosomal defects and congenital malformations (53). Color Doppler allows precise measurement of the umbilical cord, and exact "tracing" from the placenta insertion to the fetal insertion.

Increased resistance of the umbilical artery blood flow, without simultaneous alteration of the uterine flow is a warning signal, commonly described in patients with chromosomal defects and perinatal complications (54). Umbilical vein pulsations are an omnious sign indicating alterations in cardiac function. They are associated with severe growth retardation, end-diastolic velocities in the umbilical artery and abnormal fetal heart rates.

Although color Doppler improves the imaging of some markers of aneuploidy such as nuchal translucency, intestinal hyperechogenicity or visualization of the pyelectasis, it does not increase the sensitivity of ultrasound in detection of the fetuses with chromosomal defects.

However, the use of color Doppler may significantly improve the identification of the heart defects. Since between 16 and 20% of fetuses with congenital heart defects are carriers of chromosomal anomalies (55,56) and between 50 and 52% of the chromosomal defects indicate complex heart defects, there is an obvious need for early and proper recognition of heart defects.

The results of ultrasound examinations in the study carried out by DeVore and Alfi (55) are clearly very different depending on whether conventional echography is done in real time or whether color Doppler is added. In the first case only 12% of trisomy 21 cases would have been suspected, the percentage increased to 47% using color Doppler ($p<0.05$ and $R=6.1$). The differences are even more significant if all chromosomal abnormalities are grouped together: 7% sensitivity in real time as compared to 43% with color Doppler ($p<0.004$ and $R=9.7$).

Carrera (31) clearly stated that in pregnant women aged 35 or over, echographic examination using color Doppler considerably alters the thoretical risk of trisomy 21. If we accept that the potential risk of this trisomy is 1/270 at the age of 35 and 1/134 for any chromosomal anomaly, these indices are only reached at the age of 42 if a color Doppler examination is performed to exclude anomalies. Beyond that age, the risk of trisomy 21 or any other anomaly increases as it usually does beyond the age of 35. Therefore, if the color Doppler study is normal, no cytogenetic study needs to be carried out until after the age of 42.

CONCLUSIONS

Since the introduction of diagnostic ultrasound to obstetrics, there has been a dramatic increase in the quantity and quality of the information that can be obtained regarding fetal malformations. Color Doppler imaging has opened new fields in the investigation of the physiology and pathophysiology of pregnancy. Apart from investigations during the first trimester of pregnancy (57-59), analysis of the early cerebral flow (60,61), fetomaternal circulation in patients with threatened abortions (62) and studies on intervillous circulation (63) our group conducted a prospective study on fetuses with congenital defects. Part of these results are demonstrated and illustrated in this chapter indicating that color Doppler provides information that can contribute to the improved diagnosis of structural abnormalities of the fetus.

REFERENCES:

1. Rottem, S., Bronshtein, M., Thaler, I. And Brandes, J.M. (1989). First trimester transvaginal sonography diagnosis of fetal anomalies. *Lancet*, **1**, 444-5

2. Benacerraf, B.R. (1988). First-trimester diagnosis of fetal abnormalities. A report of three cases. *J. Reprod. Med.*, **33**, 777-80

3. Goldstein, R.D., Filly, R.A. and Cullen, P.W. (1989). Sonography of anencephaly: pitfalls in early diagnosis. *J. Clin. Ultrasound*, **17**, 397-402

4. Johnson, A., Losure, T.A. and Neiner, S. (1985). Early diagnosis of fetal anencephaly. *J. Clin. Ultrasound*, **13**, 503-5

5. Bonilla-Musoles, F., Ballester, M.J. and Raga, F. (1994). Transvaginal color Doppler in early embryonic malformations. In Kurjak, A. (ed.) *An atlas of transvaginal color Doppler: The current state of the art*, pp.105-23, (London-Casterton-New York: The Parthenon Publishing Group)

6. Gustavii, B. and Edvall, H. (1984). First trimester diagnosis of cystic nuchal hygroma. *Acta Obstet. Gynecol. Scand.*, **63**, 377-8

7. Van Salen-Sprock, M.M., Van Vugt, J.M.G., Van der Harten, H.J. and Van Geign, H.P. (1992). Cephalocele and cystic hygroma: diagnosis and differentiation in the first trimester of pregnancy with transvaginal sonography: report of two cases. *Ultrasound Obstet. Gynecol.*, **2**, 289-92

8. Bronshtein, M., Rotterm, S., Yoffe, N. and Blumenfeld, Z. (1989). First-semester and early second-trimester diagnosis of nuchal cystic hygroma by transvaginal sonography: diverse prognosis of the septated from the non septated lesion. *Am. J. Obstet. Gynecol.*, **161**, 78-84

9. Mostello, D.J., Bofinger, M.K. and Siddigi, T.A. (1989). Spontaneous resolution of fetal cystic hygroma and hydrops in Turner syndrome. *Obstet. Gynecol.*, **73**, 862-5

10. Rodis, J.F., Vintzileos, A.M., Campbell, W.A. and Nochimson, D.I. (1988). Spontaneous resolution of fetal cystic hygroma in Down's syndrome. *Obstet. Gynecol.*, **71**, 976-7

11. Rahmani, M.R., Fong, K.W. and Connor, T.P. (1986). The varied sonographic appearance of cystic hygromas in utero. *J. Ultrasound Med.*, **5**, 165-8

12. Fisk, N., Vaugghan, J., Smidt, M. and Wigglesworth, J. (1991). Transvaginal ultrasound recognition of nuchal edema in the first-trimester diagnosis of achondrogenesis. *J. Clin. Ultrasound*, **19**, 586-90

13. Ville, Y., Lalondrelle, C., Doumerc, S., Daffos, F., Frydman, F., Oury, J.F. and Dumez, Y. (1992). First trimester diagnosis of nuchal anomalies: significance and fetal outcome. *Ultrasound Obstet. Gynecol.*, **2**, 314-16

14. Cullen, M.T., Gabrielli, S., Green, J.J., Rizzo, N., Mahorney, M.J., Salafia, C., Whethan, J. and Hobbins, J.C. (1990). Diagnosis and significance of cystic hygroma in the first trimester. *Prenat. Diagn.*, **10**, 643-51

15. Nicolaides, K.H., Azar, G., Byrne, D., Mansur, C. and Marks, K. (1992). Fetal nuchal translucency: ultrasound screening for chromosomal defects in first trimester of pregnancy. *Br. Med. J.*, **304**, 867-9

16. Schulman, L.P., Emerson, D.S., Myers, C.M., Philips, O.P. and Elias, S. (1991). Longitudinal evaluation of 11 fetuses with cystic hygromata detected in the first trimester. *Am. J. Obstet. Gynecol.*, **164**, 351-2

17. Podobnik, M., Singer, Z., Podobnik-Sarkanji, S. and Bulic, M. (1992). First-trimester diagnosis of cystic hygromata by transvaginal sonography. *Ultrasound Obstet. Gynecol.*, **2**, 124-5

18.Van Zalen-Spock, M.M., Van Vugt, J.M.G. and Gein, H.P. (1992). First trimester diagnosis of cystic hygroma, course and outcome. *Am. J. Obstet. Gynecol.*, **167**, 94-8

19.Rebarber, A. and Mohon, R. (1992). Prenatal diagnosis of cystic adenomatoid malformation of one fetus in a twin pregnancy: an unusual presentation. *J. Ultrasound Med.*, **11**, 305-8

20.Shulman, L.P., Emerson, D.S., Felker, R.E., Philips, G.P., Simpson, J.L. and Elias, S. (1992). High frequency of cytogenetic abnormalities in fetuses with cystic hygroma diagnosed in the first trimester. *Obstet. Gynecol.*, **80**, 80-2

21.Reuss, A., Pijpers, L., Van Swaij, E., Jahoda, M.G. and Wladimiroff, J.W. (1987). First-trimester diagnosis of recurrence of cystic hygroma using a vaginal ultrasound transducer. *Eur. J. Obstet. Gynecol. Reprod. Biol.*, **26**, 271-3

22.Cullen, M.T., Gabrielli, S. and Green, J.J. (1990). Diagnosis of significance of cystic hygroma in the first trimester. *Prenat. Diagn.*, **10**, 643-51

23.Johnson, W., Berry, J.M., Einzig, S. and Bass, J.L. (1988). Doppler findings in nonimmune hydrops fetalis and cerebral arteriovenous malformation. *Am. Heart J.*, **115**, 1138-40

24.Hirsch, J.H., Cyr, D., Eberhardt, H. and Zunkel, D. (1983). Ultrasonographic diagnosis of an aneurysm of the vein of Galen *in utero* by duplex scanning. *J. Ultrasound Med.*, **2**, 231-3

25.Rizzo, G., Arduini, D., Colosimo, C., Boccolini, M.R. and Mansuco, S. (1987). Abnormal fetal cerebral blood flow velocity waveforms as a sign of an aneurysm of the vein of Galen. *Fetal Ther.*, **2**, 70-5

26.Hata, T., Hata, K. and Senoh, D. (1988). Antenatal Doppler color flow mapping of arteriovenous malformation of the vein of Galen. J. Cardiovasc. *Ultrasonogr.*, **7**, 301-3

27. Bonilla-Musoles, F. (1991). In Salvat (ed.). *Tratado de Endosonografia en Obstetricia y Ginecologia*, 2nd edn. (Barcelona)

28. Bronshtein, M. and Ben-Shlomo, I. (1991). Choroid plexus dysmorphism detected by transvaginal sonography: the earliest sign of fetal hydrocephalus. *J. Clin. Ultrasound*, **19**, 547-53

29. Rotmensch, S., Luo, J.S., Nores, J.A., Dimaio, M.S. and Hobbins, J.C. (1992). Bilateral choroid plexus cyst in trisomy 21. *Am. J. Obstet. Gynecol.*, **166**, 591-2

30. Jaffe, R. and Warsof, S.R. (1992). *Color Doppler imaging in Obstetrics and Gynecology.* (NY: McGraw-Hill)

31. Carrera, J.M., Devesa, R., Torrents, M., Mortera, C., Comas, C. and Munoz, A. (1996) Color Doppler in prenatal diagnosis. In Chervenak, F.A. and Kurjak, A. (eds) *Current Perspectives on The Fetus as a Patient*, pp 39-48 (NY-London: The Parthenon Publishing Group)

32. De Vore, G.R. (1992). The use of color Doppler imaging to examine the fetal heart. Normal and pathologic anatomy. In Jaffe, R. (ed). *Color Doppler Imaging in Obstetrics and Gynecology*, pp. 121-54

33. Mortera, C., Carrera, J.M. and Torrents, M. (1992). Doppler pulsado codificado en color. Mapa Doppler color de la circulacion fetal. In Carrera, J.M. (ed). *Doppler en Obstetricia*, pp. 185-98. (Barcelona: Salvat-Masson)

34. Copel, J.A., Morotti, R., Hobbins, J.C. and Kleinman, C.H.S. (1991). The antenatal diagnosis of congenital heart disease using fetal echocardiography: is color flow mapping necessary? *Obstet. Gynecol.*, **78**, 1-8.

35. Cyr, D.R., Mack, L.A. and Schoenecker, S.A. (1986). Bowel migration in the normal fetus: US detection. *Radiology*, **161**, 119-23

36. Schmidt, W., Yarkoni, S., Crelin, E.S. and Hobbins, J. (1987). Sonographic visualization of physiologic anterior abdominal wall hernia in the first trimester. *Obstet. Gynecol.*, **69**, 911-15

37. Timor-Tritsch, I.E., Warren, W.B., Peisner, D.B. and Pirrone, E. (1989). First-trimester midgut herniation: a high frequency transvaginal sonographic study. *Am. J. Obstet. Gynecol.*, **161**, 831-3

38. Merz, E. (1991). *Ultrasound in Gynecology and Obstetrics.* (Stuttgart: Thieme Verlag)

39. Bronshtein, M., Kushnir, O., Ben-Rafael, Z., Shalev, E., Nebel, L., Mashiach, S. and Shalev, J. (1990). Transvaginal sonographic measurement of fetal kidneys in the first trimester of pregnancy. *J. Clin. Ultrasound*, **18**, 299-301

40. Jaffe, R. and Warsof, S.R. (1992). *Color Doppler Imaging in Obstetrics and Gynecology.* (NY: McGraw-Hill)

41. Campbell, S. and Vyas, S. (1988). Color flow mapping in measurement of flow velocity in fetal renal arteries. Presented at the *First International Meeting, Fetal and Neonatal Color Flow Mapping,* Dubrovnik, Croatia

42. Hecker, K., Spernol, R. and Szalay, S. (1989). Doppler blood flow velocity waveforms in the fetal renal artery. *Arch. Gynecol. Obstet.*, **246**, 133-7

43. Kaminopetros, P., Dukes, E.H. and Nicolaides, K.H. (1991). Fetal renal artery blood velocimetry in multicystic kidney disease. *Ultrasound Obstet. Gynecol.*, **1**, 410-12

44. Zimmer, E.Z. and Bronshtein, M. (1991). Fetal intra-abdominal cysts detected in the first and early second trimester by transvaginal sonography. *J. Clin. Ultrasound*, **19**, 564-7

45. Bonilla-Musoles, F. (1983). *Diagnostico Prenatal de las Malformaciones Fetales.* (Barcelona: Jims)

46. Rizzo, G. and Arduini, D. (1992). Prenatal diagnosis of an intraabdominal ectasia of the umbilical vein with color Doppler ultrasonography. *Ultrasound Obstet. Gynecol.*, **2**, 55-7

47. Diakoumakis, E.E., Weinberg, B., Seife, B., Beck, A.R. and Guttenberg, M.E. (1986). Infantile hemangioendothelioma of the liver. *J. Clin. Ultrasound*, **14**, 137-9

48. Nakamoto, S.K., Dreilinger, A. and Dattel, B. (1983). The sonographic appearance of hepatic hemangioma in-utero. *J. Ultrasound Med.*, **2**, 239-41

49. Platt, L.D., De Vore, G.R., Brenner, P., Siassi, B., Ralls, P.W. and Mikity, V.G. (1983). Antenatal diagnosis of a fetal liver mass. *J. Ultrasound Med.*, **2**, 521-2

50. Gergely, R.Z., Eden, R., Schifrin, B.S. and Wade, M.E. (1989). Antenatal diagnosis of congenital sacral teratoma. *J. Reprod. Med.*, **24**, 229-31

51. Kohler, H.G. (1976). Sacrococcygeal teratoma and nonimmunological hydrops fetalis. *Br. Med. J.*, **2**, 422-4

52. Alter, D.N., Reed, K.L., Marx, G.R. and Anderson, C.F. (1988). Prenatal diagnosis of congestive heart failure in a fetus with a sacrococcygeal teratoma. *Obstet. Gynecol.*, **71**, 978-81

53. Szabo, J., Gellen, J. and Szemere, G. (1992). Nuchal edema as an ultrasonic sign of trisomy 21 during the first trimester of pregnancy. *Orv. Hetil.*, **133**, 3167-8

54. Carrera, J.M. and Mortera, C. (1991). Estudio Doppler de los Defectos Congenitos. Presented at *I Congreso Mundial de Obstetricia y Ginecologia*, January, London

55. DeVore, G.R. and Alfi, O. (1995). The use of color Doppler ultrasound to identify fetuses at increased risk for trisomy 21: an alternative for high-risk patients who decline genetic amniocentesis. *Obstet. Gynecol.*, **85**, 378-86

56. Allan, L.D., Sharland, G.K., Chita, S.K., Lockhart, S. and Maxwell, D.J. (1991). Chromosomal anomalies in fetal congenital heart disease. *Ultrasound Obstet. Gynecol.*, **1**, 8-11

57. Kupesic, S. (1996). The first three weeks assessed by transvaginal color Doppler. *J. Perinat. Med.*, **24**, 301-17

58. Kurjak, A., Zudenigo, D., Predanic, M. and Kupesic, S. (1994). Recent advances in the Doppler study of early fetomaternal circulation. *J. Perinat. Med.*, **22**, 419-23

59. Kurjak, A., Zalud, I., Predanic, M. and Kupesic, S. (1994). Transvaginal color and pulsed Doppler study of uterine blood flow in the first and early second trimester of pregnancy: normal vs. abnormal. *J. Ultrasound Med.*, **13**, 43-7

60. Kurjak, A., Schulman, H., Predanic, M., Kupesic, S. and Zalud, I. (1994). Fetal choroid plexus vascularization assessed by color and pulsed Doppler. *J. Ultrasound Med.*, **13**, 841-4

61. Kupesic, S., Kurjak, A. and Babic, M.M. (1997). New data on early cerebral circulation. *Prenatal Neonatal Med.*, **2**, 48-55

62. Kurjak, A., Schulman, H., Zudenigo, D., Kupesic, S., Kos, M. and Goldenberg, M. (1996). Subchorionic hematomas in early pregnancy: clinical outcome and blood flow patterns. *J. Matern. Fetal. Med.*, **5**, 41-4

63. Kurjak, A. and Kupesic, S. (1997). Doppler assessment of the intervillous blood flow in normal and abnormal early pregnancy. *Obstet. Gynecol.*, **89**, 252-6

Correlation between antepartum cCTG and

umbilical cord gas-analysis at birth

M. Anceschi, G. Vozzi, A. Silvestri, S. Modesto,

E. Marchiani, J. Piazze and E.V. Cosmi

2nd Institute of Obst. & Gyn., «La Sapienza University «- Rome, Italy

Abstract

Objective: To correlate computerized cardiotocography (cCTG) parameters to umbilical cord blood gas analysis (UBGA) values, in order to assess its predictivity for fetal well-being.

Study design: Antepartum cCTG was performed in 207 pregnant women and cCTG parameters were correlated to umbilical cord blood (arterial and venous) gas analysis (UBGA) values. cCTG was performed by means of an Oxford-Sonicaid Team Fetal Monitor connected to a System 8002 software, and the UBGA by an AVL Compact 2 analyzer. For statistical analysis, Pearson product moment correlation and unpaired t-tests were performed. When normality criteria were not satisfied, a Mann-Whitney signed rank test was run. UBGA parameters were considered as dependent variables.

Results: The mean gestational age at cCTG was 37.4 ± 2.9 (26.5-43.7) wks and at delivery was 37.7 ± 2.8 (28-43.7) wks. Venous values were found as follows: pH=7.24 ± 0.5, range=7.17-7.49, PO2=28.1 ± 16.6, range=10.2-46, BE=-5.5 ± 4.1, range=-25.4/7.8; on the other hand arterial values were: pH=7.20 ± 0.06, range=7.40-7.09, PO2=17.4 ± 9.7, range=4.3-49, BE=-6.16 ± 3.8, range=-22.3/6.6. The following parameters of cCTG correlated positively with gestational age: acc>10 ($p<0.001$), acc>15 ($p<0.001$), decel>20 ($p<0.006$), HV (min) and HV (msec) ($p<0.0003$), LV (min) (0.0006), STV (msec) ($p<0.01$) and peaks of uterine contraction (60 min) ($p<0.0002$). Birth weight was positively correlated with STV (msec) ($P<0.009$), while Apgar score at 1 min. and 5 min. were positively correlated with HV (msec) ($P<0.03$ and $P<0.01$, respectively) and arterial BE ($P<0.02$ and $P=0.02$, respectively).

Conclusion: cCTG parameters such as Acc>10, Acc>15, Decel>20, HV (min), HV (msec), LV (min), STV (msec) and peaks, increase with gestational age which may reflect the increase of fetal activity and the maturation of CNS. HV (msec) seems to be the most reliable predictor of fetal well-being . (Supported by CNR)

INTRODUCTION
Antepartum computerized CTG (cCTG) was introduced with the aim of providing a more objective and reproducible mean of fetal heart rate (FHR) reporting. Computerized analysis of the FHR tracing has been validated by comparing computer FHR analysis results with umbilical cord blood gas analysis at cesarean birth. Several authors have found correlations between heart rate variation as determined by cCTG and umbilical vein and artery blood gases at birth (1-4). In our study we evaluated the correlation of FHR indices, as determined by cCTG, with umbilical blood gas analysis at birth to establish their ability in detecting fetal acidemia at birth.

MATERIALS AND METHODS
We excluded twin pregnancies and fetal malformations for this study. All pregnants recruited underwent cesarean section. Antepartum cCTG was performed within 4 hours from delivery by the System 8002 (Oxford Sonicaid, UK), the duration of traces was at least 40 minutes. The following cCTG parameters were considered: Fetal Heart Rate (FHR) in beats/min (bpm), number of accelerations, defined as the changes of the heart rate greater than 10 and 15 bpm above the baseline for at least 15 seconds; number of decelerations, defined as changes of the heart rate greater than 20 bpm under the baseline for at least 15 seconds; episodes of high (HV) and low (LV) variation measured in minutes (min) and milliseconds (msec) and identified when in 5 of 6 consecutives minutes the mean minute range is more than 32 or less than 30 milliseconds, respectively; short-term variation (STV) measured in milliseconds and defined as variation of FHR in 1/16 minutes (3.75 seconds) epochs; peaks of contractions (per hour); fetal movements (FM) (per hour). The system has been described elsewhere (5-9). Immediately after delivery, a segment of 10 to 15 cm of umbilical cord was doubly clamped before the first neonatal breath. To collect cord blood samples for artery and vein we used 1 ml plastic syringe flushed with 1.000 units/ml of heparine. UBGA was performed within 5 minutes from collection with an UBGA system AVL compact 2 analyser. The following UBGA parameters were considered: pH, PO2 and BE.

For statistical analysis, Pearson product moment correlation and unpaired t-test were performed. When normality criteria were not satisfied, a Mann-Whitney signed rank test was run. UBGA parameters were considered as dependent variables.

RESULTS

The average gestational age at cCTG was 37.4$\pm$2.9 (26.5-43.7) wks and at delivery it was 37.7$\pm$2.8 (28-43.7) wks.

Venous values were found as follows: pH=7.24$\pm$0.5, range=7.17-7.49, PO2=28.1$\pm$16.6, range=10.2-46, BE=5.5$\pm$4.1, range=-25.4/7.8; on the other hand arterial values were: pH=7.20$\pm$0.06, range=7.40-7.09, PO2=17.4$\pm$9.7, range=4.3-49, BE=-6.16$\pm$3.8, range=-22.3/6.6.

Regarding cCTG parameters, we found positive correlations between gestational age and acc>10 ($p<0.001$), acc>15 ($p<0.001$), decel>20 ($p<0.006$), HV (min) and HV (msec) ($p<0.0003$), LV (min) (0.0006), STV (msec) ($p<0.01$) and peaks of uterine contraction (60 min) ($p<0.0002$).

Birth weight was positively correlated with STV (msec) ($p<0.009$), while Apgar score at 1 min and 5 min were positively correlated with HV (msec) ($p<0.03$) and $p<0.01$, respectively) and arterial BE ($p<0.02$ and $p=0.02$, respectively). Table 1 summarizes correlations between variables.

CONCLUSIONS

Our data shows that computerized FHR indices can potentially be used individually or collectively as independent variables to predict umbilical blood pH at birth. Several investigators have examined the correlation between fetal pH and computer FHR indices. Ribbert et al (3) performed funipuncture in 25 severely small for gestational age (SGA) fetuses and found a significant correlation between long-term variation and umbilical vein pH (r=0.69). Guzman et al (10) found a significant correlation betwee long-term variation and umbilical artery pH at birth. Nevertheless, not all authors agree with these findings (1,2,11). The NST has been widely used during the last years as a primary fetal surveillance procedure, with uncertain results because of the subjective evaluation of CTG traces

Tab. 1. Correlations between cCTG parameters and UBGA values.

		FHR	Acc>10	Acc>15	Decel>20	HV (min)	HV (msec)	LV (min)	FM (60')
V	pH	NS	$P<0.007$ $r=-0.22$	$P<0.001$ $r=-0.27$	NS	$P<0.02$ $r=-0.19$	NS	NS	NS
E	PO$_2$	NS	$P<0.02$ $r=0.19$	NS	NS	NS	NS	NS	NS
I	PCO$_2$	NS	NS	NS	NS	NS	NS	NS	NS
N	BE	NS	NS	NS	NS	NS	NS	NS	NS
	BB	NS	NS	NS	NS	NS	$P<0.01$ $r=0.24$	NS	$P<0.02$ $r=0.22$
	HCO$_3$	$P<0.04$ $r=0.16$	NS	NS	NS	NS	NS	$P<0.05$ $r=0.16$	NS
	SatO$_2$ %	NS	$P<0.04$ $r=0.23$	NS	NS	NS	NS	NS	NS
A	pH	NS	NS	NS	NS	NS	$P<0.02$ $r=0.18$	NS	NS
R	PO$_2$	NS	NS	NS	NS	NS	NS	NS	$P<0.03$ $r=-0.17$
T	PCO$_2$	NS	NS	NS	NS	NS	NS	NS	NS
E	BE	NS	NS	NS	NS	NS	NS	NS	NS
R	BB	NS	NS	NS	$P<0.03$ $r=-0.17$	NS	$P<0.03$ $r=0.18$	NS	NS
Y	HCO$_3$	NS	NS	NS	NS	NS	NS	NS	NS
	SatO$_2$ %	NS	NS	NS	NS	NS	NS	NS	$P<0.01$ $r=-0.19$

NS: Not Significant

and the poor reproducibility of the method (12-13). An important role may be played in this regard by computerized analysis of FHR. A computer system gives the objectivity, precision and reproducibility of analysed traces. We have examined, according to others studies (3,10), the relationship between the parameters of the computerized analysis of the FHR and the fetal acid-base status which is considered the more objective criterion to detect perinatal asphyxia.

The data showed in this study confirm that cCTG parameters increase with gestational age which may reflect the increase of fetal activity and the maturation of CNS; in particular episodes of high variation (measured in minutes and milliseconds) may be predictive for fetal acidosis and allow the identification of fetuses at risk.

REFERENCES
1. Bekedam DJ, Visser GH, Mulder EJH, Poelmann-Weesjes G. Heart rate variation and movement incidents in growth retarded fetuses: The significance of antenatal late heart rate decelerations. *Am J Obstet Gynecol* 1987; 157: 126-33.

2. Smith JH, Anand KJ, Cotes PM, Dawes GS, Harkness RA, Howlett TA, et al. Antenatal fetal heart rate variation in relation to the respiratory and metabolic status of the compromise human fetus. *Br J Obstet Gynaecol* 1988; 95: 980-9.

3. Ribbert LS, Snijders RJ, Nicolaides KH, Visser JH. Relation of fetal blood gases and data from computer assisted analysis of fetal heart rate patterns in small for gestation fetuses. *Br J Obstet Gynecol* 1991; 98: 820-3.

4. Snijders RJ MSc, Ribbert LS, Visser GH, Mulder EJ. Numeric analysis or fetal heart rate variation in intrauterine growth retarded fetuses: a longitudinal study. *Am J Obstet Gynecol* 1992; 166: 22-7.

5. Dawes GS, Visser JH, Goodman JD, Redman CW. Numerical analysis of the human fetal heart rate: the quality of ultrasound records. *Am J Obstet Gynecol* 1981; 141: 43-52.

6. Visser JH, Dawes GS, Redman CW. Numerical analysis of the normal human antenatal fetal heart rate. *Br J Obstet Gynecol* 1981; 88: 792-802.

7. Dawes GS, Houghton CR, Redman CW. Baseline in human fetal heart rate records. *Br J Obstet Gynecol* 1982; 89: 270-5.

8. Street P, Dawes GS, Moulden M, Redman CW. Short term variation in abnormal antenatal fetal heart rate records. *Am J Obstet Gynecol* 1991; 165: 515-23.

9. Guzman ER, Conley M, Stewart R, Ivan J, Pitter M, Kappy K. Phenytoin and magnesium sulfate effects on fetal heart rate tracings assessed by computer analysis. *Obstet Gynecol* 1993; 82: 375-9.

10. Edwin R, Guzman ER, Vintzileos AM, Martins M, Benito C, Houlihan C, Hanley M. The efficacy of individual computer heart rate indices in detecting acidemia at birth in growth-restricted fetuses. *Obstet Gynecol* 1996; 87: 969-74.

11. Henson GL, Dawes GS, Redman CW. Antenatal fetal heart rate variability in relation to the fetal acid-base status at cesarean section. *Br J Obstet Gynecol* 1983; 90: 516-21.

12. Trimbos I.B. et al: Observer variability in assessment of antepartum cardiotocogram. *Br J Obstet Gynaecol* 1978; 85: 900-906.

13. Borgatta L. et al: Realiability and riproducibility of non stress test readings. *Am J Obstet Gynecol* 1988; 159: 554.

Maternal-fetal cytomegalovirus infection

G. Nigro, M. Mazzocco, M.A. Porcaro, M.M. Anceschi, R. La Torre, A. Krzysztofiak, F. D'Orio, U. Bartmann, O. Capuano, O. Bederti, D. Di Ruzza, C. D'Emilio, and E.V. Cosmi

2nd Institute of Obstetrics/Gynecology and Pediatric Institute of "La Sapienza" University, Viale Regina Elena 324, 00161 Rome, Italy.

Microbiology
Cytomegalovirus (CMV) is a large (150-200 nm), enveloped DNA virus which shows several biologic and epidemiologic properties of the herpesvirus family, including the persistence in human cells with alternance of latent periods and viral activity. There are no distinct serotypes of CMV but numerous different strains, which are genetically homologous though not identical, and reinfection of a CMV-seropositive individual is possible in spite of pre-existing and cross-reacting antibodies (1,2).

Epidemiology
CMV infection is usually transmitted by direct human-to-human contact, being infected persons capable of excreting CMV in urine, saliva, semen, cervical secretions and breast milk. CMV is the most common and serious congenital infection being associated with important neurologic sequelae, although the majority of infants are asymptomatic at birth. Approximately 0.5 to 2.5% of infants show viruria in the neonatal period. Intrapartum and immediately postnatal (through the breast milk or other sources) transmission account for an additional 10 to 15% of infants acquiring CMV infection in the first 4 to 8 weeks of life. In low-birth-weight infants, blood transfusions are an important source of infection (1-3).
In pregnancy, active infection, as shown by CMV DNAemia, is detected in 3 to 6% of women, viruria is present in 3% to 12%, and cervical viral shedding increases as gestation advances: 0 to 5% in the first trimester, 6% to 10% in the second trimester and 11% to 28% in the third trimester. The low viral shedding in the first trimester, during which organogenesis occurs, is correlated with a low rate of fetal abnormalities. Viral shedding is better correlated with intrapartum than prenatal transmission (4).
Primary CMV infection occurs in 0.7% to 4.1% of pregnancies with an annual seroconversion rate in women of childbearing age of about 2% in higher socioeconomic groups and about 6% in lower groups. The annual rate of primary infection in pregnancy appeared to be correlated with socioeconomic status, being higher in women of low income than those of mid-to-upper income (6.8% versus 2.5%), in spite of a higher seropositivity rate (64.5% versus 23.4%) (5). The presence of young children attending daycare centers, young maternal age and mid-to-upper income are significant risk factors for primary infection during pregnancy. The role of sexual transmission in

primary CMV infection is unclear and varies with the populations: young age, lower socioeconomic status, number of sexual partners and other sexually transmitted diseases are risk factors for sexual CMV transmission. Saliva is a significant source of viral transmission in this setting (2).

Pathogenesis

Infection with CMV is differentiated in primary or recurrent, including reactivation of a pre-existing viral strain or reinfection by an exogenous strain. CMV is transmitted to the fetus following viremia and placentitis during a primary maternal infection, while recurrent infections could also be transmitted after CMV reactivation in the cervix. Neuropathologic processes include meningoencephalitis, periventricular calcifications, microcephaly, polymicrogiria and other migrational alterations. Meningoencephalitis is characterized by the presence of meningeal and perivascular inflammatory cells, necrotic neuronal cells (particularly in the periventricular areas) often associated with calcifications, enlarged neuronal and glial cells containing intranuclear CMV inclusions, and glial proliferation. Viral predilection for the periventricular area may relate to the proximity to the cerebrospinal fluid (CSF) pathway, through which CMV probably spreads, and to the actively proliferating subependymal germinal matrix cells, which are particularly vulnerable to CMV (6). Microcephaly relates to encephaloclastic viral effects and possible neuro-proliferative troubles consequent to the CMV prediletion for actively proliferating cells. Alterations in neuronal migration include polymicrogyria, which occurs in approximately 65% of reported cases and may involve both cerebral and cerebellar cortex, lissencephaly, pachygiria, and neuronal heterotopias (7). These manifestations show that the teratogenic effects of CMV may also occur in the second trimester of pregnancy, when neuronal migration takes place (8). In fact, CMV is the only congenitally transmitted pathogen causing alterated gyral development, the pathogenesis of which include both teratogenic and encephaloclastic mechanisms. Porencephaly, hydranencephaly, hydrocephalus, cerebellar hypoplasia, and diffuse cerebral calcifications are less frequent neurologic manifestations of congenital CMV infection. Schizencephaly has also been recently reported to be consequent to fetal CMV infection (9).

Clinical manifestations

In pregnancy, approximately 10% of women with primary infection may have a mononucleosis-like syndrome including persistent fever as a prominent clinical feature; the remaining patients generally are asymptomatic. Congenital CMV infection may occur in approximately 40% of infants born to mothers with primary infection; of these, 10 to 12% are symptomatic at birth. Symptomatic congenital CMV infection predominantly include signs of reticuloendothelial involvement (hepatosplenomegaly, jaundice, thrombocytopenia). Although fatal cirrhosis can occur, liver abnormalities generally disappear completely, sometimes after several months. Pneumonia and a purpuric rash may also be present. Intrauterine growth retardation (IUGR) is frequent and about one third of infected infants have a gestational age lower than 38 weeks. Approximately 25% of infants show inguinal hernia (10).

Neurologic syndrome, including seizures, microcephaly and often periventricular calcifications, is the most serious consequence of congenital CMV infection and occurs in 30 to 50% of the symptomatic infants (9). Approximately 20% of these also develop sensorineural hearing loss. The majority of patients have CSF signs of encephalitis (e.g., pleocytosis, elevated protein concentration); diabetes insipidus may also occur. Neuroimaging studies show a variety of neurologic abnormalities, ranging from lissencephaly to multicystic encephalomalacia. The clinical course is generally slow, but progressive encephaloclastic disease or hearing loss may occur (11). In fact, viruria still persists in about 50% of patients at 5 years of age.

Diagnosis
Prenatal diagnosis of CMV infection may be obtained by viral isolation or CMV DNA detection with polymerase chain reaction in the amniotic fluid which, however, does not predict an adverse fetal outcome. Fetal CMV infection should be closely monitored for evidence of growth retardation, ventriculomegaly, intracranial calcifications or microcephaly. Congenital CMV infection is diagnosed by viral isolation or CMV DNA detection from urine or blood. Neurologic involvement is clearly demonstrated by viral presence in the CSF, but this is only occasionally possible.
CMV infection can also be diagnosed by detecting specific IgM antibodies in cord or neonatal blood specimens, but false positive or negative results may occur. CMV-specific IgA antibodies appeared to be an useful complementary tool for serodiagnosis of congenital or perinatally-acquired CMV infection (1,2).
Periventricular calcifications as well as precise definition of the cerebral damage can be obtained by computerized tography (CT) scanning which is more sensitive than radiography, magnetic resonance imaging (MRI) or ultrasonography. Cranial ultrasound scans can also demonstrate abnormalities consisting of periventricular cysts, ventriculomegaly, periventricular echolucencies due to leukomalacia and thalamic echodensities representing arteries. MRI is very useful in revealing altered neuronal migration, parenchymal loss, delayed myelination and cerebellar hypoplasia. In symptomatic as well as asymptomatic infants, testing of brain stem auditory evoked potentials could reveal abnormalities (6).

Prognosis
In children with symptomatic congenital CMV infection, the outcome is closely related to the severity of neurologic syndrome. In fact, approximately 95% of the infants with microcephaly, periventricular calcifications or chorioretinitis may have major neurologic sequelae such as mental retardation, seizures, deafness, spasticity. Children with microcephaly without calcifications may not have mental retardation. Among children with asymptomatic congenital infections, approximately 10% have been reported to develop bilateral hearing loss which may not be diagnosed until serious language impairment occurs. However, hearing loss may not be detectable before the first year of life, being related to a direct and progressive lesion of the cochlear cells and of the neurons of the eighth cranial nerve (1-3,6,10,11).

Prevention
A subunit vaccine consisting of recombinant-derived CMV glycoprotein B (UL55) combined with an adjuvant derived from saponin, QS-21, appeared to be potentially useful for the immunoprophylaxis of CMV disease (12). However, a suitable CMV vaccine, particularly for women in the childbearing age, has not yet been developed. Appropriate hygienic measures (e.g., handwashing, avoidance of contact with oral secretions) can prevent CMV transmission. Prevention of maternal-fetal transmission may be probably obtained by giving hyperimmune immunoglobulins to women with primary infections, but data are lacking probably due to the difficulty in detecting these infections. For prevention of transfusion-acquired CMV infections, fewer units, red blood cells or CMV-seronegative blood should be used (1,2).

Therapy

In pregnancy, CMV-specific immunoglobulins could be used for therapy of fetal infection following primary infection, because of their high content in neutralizing CMV IgG antibodies. We recently obtained encouraging results both for prevention and treatment of fetal infection, but the number of cases is too low to draw definitive conclusions.

Antiviral therapy for infants with severe CMV disease can be attempted with ganciclovir or foscarnet, which are capable of inhibiting CMV replication by inactivating its DNA polymerase with different mechanisms. Clinical benefit (e.g., reversal of hepatosplenomegaly, improvement in tone) has been associated with a ganciclovir regimen based on an initial course with a high dosage and a long maintenance course, to inhibit as long as possible CMV replication (13).

References

1.Naraqi S. Cytomegaloviruses. In: Belshe RB. Textbook of human virology. Second Edition. Mosby Year Book, St Louis. 1991.

2.Ho M. Cytomegalovirus: biology and infection. Plenum Press, New York. 1991.

3.Stagno S, Pass RF, Sworsky ME, et al. Congenital and perinatal cytomegalovirus infection. Semin Perinatol 1983;7:31.

4. Raynor, B.D. (1993). Cytomegalovirus infection in pregnancy. Semin. Perinatol., 17, 394-402.

5.Berge, P., Stagno, S., Federer, W., et al. (1990). Impact of asymptomatic congenital cytomegalovirus infection on size at birth and gestational duration. Pediatr. Infect. Dis. J., 9, 170-5

6.Volpe JJ. Viral, protozoan, and related intracranial infections. In: Neurology of the newborn. Third Edition. WB Saunders Co., Philadelphia. 1995.

7.Hayward JC, Titelbaum DS, Clancy RR, Zimmermann RA. Lissencephaly-pachygyria associated with congenital cytomegalovirus infection. J Child Neurol 1991;6:109.

8.Baskar JF, Furnari B, Huang ES. Demonstration of developmental anomalies in mouse fetuses by transfer of murine cyomegalovirus DNA-injected eggs to surrogate mothers. J Infect Dis 1993;167:1288.

9. Iannetti P, Nigro G, Spalice A, Faiella A, Boncinelli E. Cytomegalovirus infection and schizencephaly: Case reports. Ann Neurol 1998;43:123-7.

10.Boppana SB, Pass RF, Britt WJ, Stagno S, Alford CA. Symptomatic congenital cytomegalovirus infection: neonatal morbidity and mortality. Pediatr J Infect Dis 1992;11:93.

11.Williamson WD, Demmler GJ, Percy AK, Catlin FI. Progressive hearing loss in infants with asymptomatic congenital cytomegalovirus infection. Pediatrics 1992;90:862.

12.Britt W, fay J, Seals J, Kensil C. Formulation of an immunogenic human cytomegalovirus vaccine: responses in mice. J Infect Dis 1995;171:18.

13. Nigro G, Scholz H, Bartmann U. Ganciclovir therapyfor symptomatic congenital cytomegalovirus infection in infants: a two-regimen experience. J Pediatr 1984;124:318.

Prognosis of birth term: new developments

Klimek R., Frączek A. and Klimek M.

OB/GYN Chairs, Jagiellonian University, Cracow, Poland

INTRODUCTION

In the beginning of this century great physicists changed the world and conquered the space, because for them time stopped to be absolute and self-contained event. Only obstetrics retained the concept of one, absolute time measured from the date of the last menstrual period and when it showed to be inadequate in its nineteenth-century Newtonian form. The rescue came from ultrasonography, which - although examining structures (events always in time and space) - enriches them with the calendar scale of pregnancy duration being them "only right one, because it is absolute". Yet even the term pregnancy itself became complex towards the end of its advanced phase, as it was preceded with the epithets of pre-, at- and post-term. Unfortunately it comes useful only in the court of law as an excuse for iatrogenic failures [1,2]

In practice the number of the instrumental labours is on the rise, while there is no change in the number of the premature infants, for whom obstetricians (deprived of the understanding of arithmetics) shorten the pregnancy if they decide it lasts longer than 287 or 294 days or - which is worse - they do not prevent its pathologic termination even by several weeks if biologically premature labour begins in $37^0/_7$-$^6/_7$ week! This cannot be resolved by absolute calendar scale but only by the ability to determine the developmental age.

The foetus, which so far has been only a statistical object, now turned out to be an individual patient. In spite of that the scales of all ultrasonographic devices which have been used to date are based on the absolute time, which dominated the nineteenth-century science. When used, they made it possible to determine the statistical birth-term with an accuracy of ± 3 weeks, which resulted in an increase in the number of caesarean sections and instrumental deliveries ever since ultrasonographic pregnancy dating was generally introduced. Thus, ultrasonographic biometry became an example of backwardness in perinatology, as it uses nonsensical indicators of foetal development in the last few weeks of pregnancy duration. These indicators are equal for all children at the same postmenstrual calendar age, although they refer to foetuses which differ by even several weeks in their gestational age. [6,7]

Out of all foetuses at the gestational calendar age of $37^0/_7$-$37^6/_7$ weeks, only a few percentage will be born within that week, 15% - in a week's time, but more than a half will be born only in three weeks' time at the earliest, including 20% at the age of $\geq 41^0/_7$ weeks. Only computer technology enables a prospective determination of the calendar week in which the foetus will reach full maturity, which makes it possible to prevent premature births even up to 42nd week, as well as inducing births in case of their postmaturity already from 38th week on [3-5].

Modern birth-term prognosis - although with much delay - made use of the achievements of quantum mechanics, which changed nearly all branches of knowledge. Quantization of maturity based on the gestational increase rate of spatial parameters of the foetus makes it possible to determine the inherently related duration of pregnancy up until the time of examination of the mother and the time-spatial values of the newborn, including its birth-date with an accuracy of ±3 days. So far any attempts at determining the maturity of the foetus were based solely on weight, height and postmenstrual foetal age. By virtue of quantisation of full maturity (equivalent to 39±3 points on Ballard-Klimek scale), M. Klimek introduced a computer-aided method of determining the degree of foetal maturity based on the measurement of the increase rate of biophysical and enzymatic parameters of individual foetuses [3].

RESULTS

Table I shows the characteristics of 374 observed pregnancies with natural delivery (group A) - 306 cases and caesarean section (group B) - 68 cases. Gestational age was predicted with accuracy of 1.2 day (t=1.15, Not Significant). Also the mean weight of newborns was predicted with great accuracy of 24g (t=0.95, NS) as well as their maturity. Mode of delivery did not change the accuracy of predicted parameters, but according to the clinical knowledge the actual values of age, weight and maturity were statistically lower in case of caesarean section.

CONCLUSIONS

The data obtained from these examinations enable to predict the birth-term with the accuracy of several days instead of weeks. Therefore, it is unethical to take the range of the expected birth-term - whether it is five or six weeks - as justification of obstetrical actions or desistance, because the delivery took place "at term". This is a fraud from the professional point of view, since everybody knows that they were born on a given day, while every obstetrician is able to prove that the commencing delivery and its prodromes occur during just two or three days of profound transformations from pregnancy to labour. Therefore the delivery date has to be estimated with accuracy of ± 3 days.

There is clinically important difference between developmental biological gestational age (in quantum theory called "imaginary time") and calendar gestational one, although both are expressed in days or weeks. For example, at the calendar gestational $36^{6/7}$ weeks only 2-3% of all newborn are mature while at the calendar gestational age $\geq 39^{6/7}$ weeks at least 50% of fetuses are still maturing. So, it is an often unintentional deviation from truth to interpret all deliveries beyond $36^{6/7}$ weeks as occurring "at term". The same error is done even with some deliveries beyond $41^{6/7}$ weeks, but under the notion "post term" birth.

Improper scales found in ultrasonographic equipment obstruct the use of this wonderful apparatus in birth prognosis and first of all lead to unnecessary blood loss by thousands of women undergoing instrumental deliveries in the most industrialized countries of the world. If such births cause only an average of more 100 ml blood loss during each delivery then their sum total of useless loss must call to mind the tragedy of I.F. Semmelweis. Therein lies the essence of an author's personal responsibility in various existing birth scales. However, it is most important to entrust this task to the editors of textbooks and obstetrical journals, whose authors still publish data mistaking the notion of pregnancy weeks and birth week as well as attaching greater importance to the beginning of pregnancy rather than to its more important goal which is, of course, its successful conclusion.

Table 1. Characteristics (mean±SD, t, p) of observed pregnancies with natural birth (group A) and caesarean section (group B)

	Total	A	B	A/B t, p
N	374	306	68	
Mother				
age (years)	26.3±5.5	25.9±5.1	28.0±6.4	2.92,
	16-48	16-43	19-48	0.01
gravity	2.1±1.3	2.0±1.3	2.2±1.4	1.13,
	1-8	1-8	1-7	NS
parity	2.1±1.3	2.0±1.3	2.2±1.4	1.13,
	1-8	1-8	1-7	NS
Birth week				
<37	36 (9.6)	20 (6.5)	6 (8.8)	
37	31 (8.3)	30 (9.8)	4 (5.9)	
38	48 (12.8)	41 (13.4)	6 (8.8)	χ^2=2.53,
				NS
39-40	147 (39.4)	120 (39.2)	35 (51.5)	
41	40 (10.7)	34 (11.1)	6 (8.8)	
42	39 (10.4)	32 (10.5)	7 (10.3)	
>42	33 (8.8)	29 (9.5)	4 (5.9)	
Newborn	374	306	68	
Gestation age				
actual (days)	277.3±12.7	278.4±12.1	272.3±14.2	3.64,
	215-302	215-302	231-291	<0.001
predicted (days)	278.5±17.4	278.2±17.1	280.1±18.9	0.81,
	226-355	226-327	235-355	NS
Actual weight (g)	3338±496	3380±337	3152±477	4.64,
	1300-4600	1950-4600	1300±4600	<0.001
Predicted weight	3314±274	3299±288	3380±182	2.22,
	2048-4250	2048-3250	2561±3515	0.05
Apgar scores	9.5±1.0	9.5±0.9	9.1±1.4	2.96,
	3-10	5-10	3-10	0.001
actual B-K	39.9±2.1	39.2±1.7	38.2±2.3	4.09,
	25-45	26-41	25-45	<0.001
predicted B-K	39.2±1.6	39.2±1.7	39.5±1.2	1.38,
	26-49	32-48	26-49	NS

REFERENCES
1. Cosmi E.V., Klimek R. Philosophy of birth: natural process or artificial obstetrical procedure? *Int J Gynecol Obstet* 1993; 41: 231.
2. Klimek M., Frączek A. New charts of fast, regular, and slow fetal growth. *Arch Obstet. Ginecol* 1995; 2: 35.
3. Klimek M. A critical evaluation of fetal weight assessment in late pregnancy. *Int J Prenatal and Perinat Psychol and Med* 1995; 7: 17.
4. Klimek M. Fetometria ultra-sonica computadorizada na prenhez avancada. *Ginecol Obstet Atual*, Junho, Ano IV, 1995; 6: 85.
5. Klimek M. Medical prognosis versus statistical prediction of birth. In: Klimek R., Fedor-Freybergh P., Janus L., Walas-Skolicka E.: A time to be born, DREAM Publishing, Cracow 1996; 9-33.
6. Klimek R. Monitoring of pregnancy and prediction of birth-date. The Parthenon Publishing Group, New York-London 1994.
7. Klimek R., Fedor-Freybergh P., Janus L., Walas-Skolicka E. A time to be born. DREAM Publishing, Cracow 1996.

CARNITINE IN PERINATAL MEDICINE REVISITED

Carrapato MRG
Paediatric Department, Maria Pia Children's Hospital, Oporto, Portugal

INTRODUCTION

Carnitine is a quarternary compound (β-hydroxy-γ-trimethylammonium butyrate) first identified in 1927 (1) and for nearly 30 years was almost ignored until it was found to be essential for life in the meal worm *tenebrio mollitor* and hence the designation of vitamin Br (2) for which it became known. A few more years elapsed before the discovery of its role in the transferral of activated long-chain fatty acids across the inner mitrochondrial membrane for β-oxidation and energy release (3,4,5,6). For a long time this was the sole function ascribed to carnitine. In recent years other and perhaps more important aspects have been uncovered, namely that it may act as an acyl sink in order to maintain adequate cellular levels of free CoA (7,8) and also as a modulator of physicochemical properties of cell membranes (9,10,11,12). In addition, carnitine may also provide an essential contribution to the metabolism of medium-chain fatty acids in skeletal and cardiac muscle (13,14,15), in regulating ketogenesis (17,18,19,20) in non-shivering thermogenesis (21,22,23,24) and in branched-chain amino acids metabolism and disorders (25,26,27,28).

In Perinatal Medicine, especially in the neonatal period, many of these carnitine-dependent functions may be of paramount importance both in health and disease.

CARNITINE SYNTHESIS AND AVAILABILITY

Carnitine is synthesised from the essential amino acids lysine and methionine (29,30,31,32) through a complex pathway involving several enzymes and co-factors as well as the presence of ferrous ions and a number of vitamins: ascorbate, niacine and pyrodoxine (33). A more detailed account of these biosynthetic processes is beyond the scope of this review and can be found elsewhere (34,35,36). It is noteworthy, however, to point out that the last enzyme in the carnitine pathway, γ-butyrobetaine hydroxylase, necessary for the conversion of γ-butyrobetaine to carnitine is only found in the liver and kidney, perhaps the testis and possibly the brain (37,38). Furthermore the activity of γ-butyrobetaine hydroxylase is age-dependent with only about 12% of the adult activity present in the first week of life, rising to 30% by the third year of life and reaching adult levels by adolescence (37,39). This is probably one reason why the neonate is unable to synthesise carnitine (40,41); the other might be due to the anabolic status of the newborn limiting protein degradation and therefore available substrates of carnitine precursors. However, even in the adult in health, and in spite of a fully-competent pathway system, the main source of carnitine is of dietary origin. Carnitine is found in high concentrations in animal products especially in red meats and milk (42,43,44). Plants with very few exceptions (avocado pears) contain no carnitine or only very small amounts (45). Vegetarians may have an unbalanced carnitine status, especially if compromised by disease, namely liver or kidney (46,47,48,49) or by the increasing metabolic demands of, for instance, pregnancy (50,51,52).

CARNITINE DEFICIENCY

Carnitine deficiency is defined as a carnitine concentration in plasma and tissues that is below the requirements for the normal function of the organism (53). An abnormal ratio of acylcarnitine to free carnitine (greater than 0.4) is considered *carnitine insufficiency* (53) indicating that more carnitine is necessary to counterbalance the excessive production of acyl carnitines.

Although plasma levels are commonly used to diagnose carnitine deficiency, this may not always reflect the tissue carnitine concentration. Another important point in clinical practice is that tissue carnitine levels may have to be substantially reduced often below 20%, before the biological effects become clinically significant (54).

Primary carnitine deficiencies, systemic or myopathic, have been identified as autosomal recessive inherited disorders (55,56,57,58). Their prevalence remains low especially as some of the early cases were quite likely to be carnitine insufficiency states rather than true carnitine deficiencies (53,55,58).

The pathogenesis of primary systemic deficiency has been variously ascribed to either defective biosynthesis, increased degradation or, most probably, to an abnormal transport affecting uptake or release of carnitine from tissues (58,59,60,61,62). As a result of the intracellular carnitine deficiency the inner mitochondrial membrane becomes impermeable to the transferral of activated long-chain fatty acids impairing not just β-oxidation and energy release but also affecting the shuttling of intra mitochondrial CoA with the consequent accumulation of acyl-CoA esters and impairment of the intermediary metabolisms requiring free CoA – Krebs Cycle, pyruvate oxidation, amino acids oxidation, etc. (54,63).

The clinical presentations of primary systemic carnitine include an acute non-ketotic hypoglycaemic encephalopathy with hepatomegaly, raised liver enzymes and hyperammonaemia (younger children), a progressive cardiomyopathy (most common) or very rarely, an isolated myopathy (53,57,59,61,64,65,66,67,68). All these forms may coexist in the same family (59,60,67).

High doses of oral carnitine, 100-200 mg/kg/day, will correct the metabolic disturbance of hypoketonaemia, will greatly improve myocardial function and to a lesser extent, the myopathy (59,60,65,67,68,73).

The primary myopathic form (low muscle carnitine levels with normal plasma levels) points to an altered muscle carnitine transport and recent evidence suggests the possibility of a developmental defect in the muscle-specific carnitine carrier (69,70). However, short-chain acyl CoA dehydrogenase deficiency has been documented in cultured fibroblasts of one patient with the myopathic form and therefore other fatty acid oxidation defects, either generalised or tissue specific, could also be responsible for this entity (71,72,73,74,75). Moreover, the clinical response to carnitine supplementation is greatly variable from near normalisation of muscle strength to no improvement and carnitine stores are rarely completely restored (73,76,77).

Secondary carnitine deficiencies with reduced levels of plasma or tissues, are associated with genetically determined inborn errors of metabolism, acquired medical conditions or iatrogenically induced (54,58,78,79,80,81,82,83,84). The most representative causes of secondary carnitine deficiency are metabolic inherited defects of impaired oxidation of acyl-CoA intermediates in the mitrochondria, namely fatty acid oxidation disorders and amino acids oxidation defects (80,83,84,85). The intramitrochondrial block in fatty acid or amino acids oxidation leads to the accumulation of acyl-CoA which is subsequently transferred out of the cell, leading to an increasing ratio of acyl to free carnitine. The postulated mechanism of carnitine deficiency in these disorders results from an imbalance between the urinary excretion of the accumulated acyl carnitines and the dietary intake and endogenous synthesis (80,83). Carnitine supplementation in long-chain fatty acids oxidation defects and organic acidurias remains controversial because whilst correcting the existing carnitine deficiency, restoring CoA levels and removing toxic intermediates, on the other hand may also promote the accumulation of long-chain esters leading to cardiac arrythmias and cell membrane disfunction (86).
Iatrogenic factors have also been implicated as contributors to carnitine deficiency namely patients on haemodialysis due to the loss into the dialysate fluids (47,48,49,58) and amongst several drugs considerable attention has been focused on valproic acid, a branched-chain fatty acid used in the treatment of epilepsy, migraine, behavioural disorders, etc (87,88,89,90,91). Although not all patients on valproate will develop carnitine deficiency, the carnitine status should be assessed and replaced especially in high risk cases (89,90,91).
Acquired medical conditions especially liver and kidney, may adversely affect carnitine homeostasis leading to secondary carnitine deficiency (46,47,78,79,80,84,85). In recent years there has been an increasing body of evidence that human immunodeficiency virus (HIV)/AIDS patients may be carnitine deficient either directly from the cytokine dysregulation upon the fatty acid metabolism or indirectly from HIV complications of malnutrition, opportunistic infections, reduced nutritional intake, drug toxicity, mainly Zidovudine or a combination of several different inter-related factors (92,93,94,95,96,97,98,99,100). Carnitine therapy in these patients has not been systematically assessed given the multifactorial basis of the carnitine deficiency and the absence of control studies; nevertheless, from the available data and the low carnitine toxicity, carnitine replacement may play a significant role in the overall care of these patients (93,94,101,102,103).

CARNITINE STATUS IN PREGNANCY, LACTATION AND NEONATES AND POSSIBLE CLINICAL IMPLICATIONS

Reduced body stores and increasing demands may lead to carnitine deficiency in pregnancy (50,51,52,81,104). The falling levels of total carnitine observed with increasing gestational age could argueably be only the result of the concommitant increase in plasma volume. Against this possibility is the fact that the reduction in total carnitine is mainly caused by a fall in free carnitine (50,81,104) and that the red blood cell content of carnitine increases with advancing gestation (52). The elevated ratio of acylcarnitine to free carnitine towards the end of pregnancy, often in the range of secondary carnitine deficiencies, can either be the result of the conversion of free carnitine to acylcarnitine to meet the physiological demands of fatty acid oxidation of late gestation and delivery (105) or conversely, represent a true secondary carnitine deficiency (52). Thus, carnitine supplementation may be necessary in certain high risk pregnancies – diabetics, underlying and complicating liver and kidney disorders or even simple vegetarians.

Data from animal studies and a limited number of clinical trials have appeared (and been overlooked?) on the possibility of carnitine supplementation, alone or together with antenatal steroids, in the prevention of respiratory insufficiency of prematurity, presumably due to its effects on the dipalmitoylphosphatidylcholine (DPPC) content of surfactant (106,107,108,109). Should these observations be confirmed it would render carnitine an interesting and useful tool in perinatal medicine.

The neonate, in contrast to the fetus, the older child and the adult, switches from mainly carbohydrates to fatty acids and ketone bodies for its immediate energy requirements (110,111,112,113,114). Fat is a major content in the diet of the newborn.

Traditionally, for many years, infant formulae for pre-terms have been substantially enriched with medium-chain fatty acids. The proposed arguments in favour for these high concentrations of MCFA in formulae being: readily-abosorbed by the intestine; completely metabolised by the liver into ketone bodies and CO_2; improved nitrogen retention and growth and especially to be metabolised independently of carnitine. This is true, but only partially. In fact, although carnitine may not be necessary for the oxidation of MCFA in the liver (and even this is debatable in the neonate, especially pre-terms under stress), carnitine will be required for their oxidation in skeletal and cardiac muscle (14,15,16,115,116,117,118). At such high proportions of MCFA, up to 50% of the whole fat content in some formulae, it is unlikely that they would be completely converted to ketogenesis in the liver and therefore the incompletely oxidised MCFAs would lead to the accumulation of dicarboxylic acids, the removal of which is carnitine dependent (117,118). Further arguments against the incorporation of unphysiological MCFA in formulae would be the limited availability of long and very long chain polyunsaturated fatty acids (including essential fatty acids) for cell membrane synthesis and differentiation especially of brain, retina, vascular and reproductive organs (119,120,121,122,123,124,125,126).

Carnitine plays a major role in many of these functions of fat metabolism but may also be an essential co-factor in the regulation of non-shivering thermogenesis (21,22,23,24), in gluconeogenesis (127,128,129,130,131,132) and in branched-chain amino acids metabolism (25,26,27,28).

We have demonstrated some years ago that the newborn is unable to synthesise carnitine (40,41) an observation corroborated by other authors (133, 134, 135, 136,

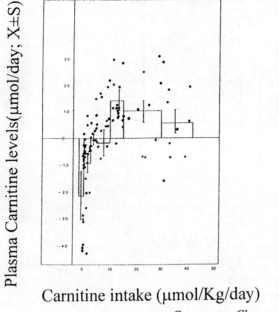

Carnitine intake (μmol/Kg/day)

Carrapato; Cheeseman; Gamsu

Figure 1   Carnitine homeostasis in the newborn

137,138) presumably due to the immaturity of the γ-butyrobetaine hydroxylase, the last converting enzyme in the pathway of carnitine and an age-dependent enzyme (37,38).

From our studies we have also shown that the daily requirements of carnitine to maintain homeostasis to be in the region of 10μmol/kg/day (Fig.1)(41).

The daily carnitine needs of the newborn are met from the exogenous supply of either milk formula or from breast milk.

Cows milk formula contains various amounts of carnitine (41,44) but until the mid eighties many soya bean preparations and highly purified casein and protein hydrolysates in use for the newborn contained no, or extremely low levels of carnitine (Table 1)(41). Recently many of these dietary products have been supplemented with carnitine.

Breast milk contains various amounts of carnitine, the highest being found in the colostrum of mothers delivering very pre term infants (Fig.2)(41). Whether milk banks, often the result of donations of mothers in advanced stages of lactation, will contain enough carnitine for these very immature babies remains open to question.

Solutions for parenteral nutrition, unless otherwise supplemented, contain no carnitine and neonates fed this diet develop increasingly low levels of plasma (Fig.3)(41) and tissue carnitine content (133,134,137,138). Again it is debatable whether the low levels of carnitine observed in these babies will have any significant immediate (metabolic) effects in the newborn or in the long term (developmental) consequences – in other words, is carnitine an essential or a conditional nutrient for the neonate (139)?

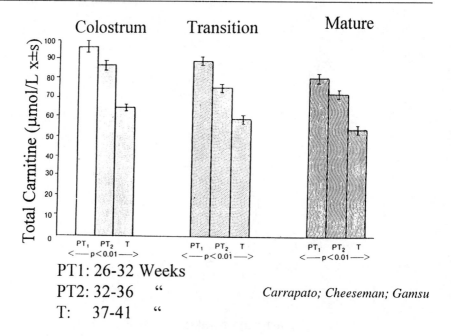

Figure 2   Carnitine content in the diet of the newborn

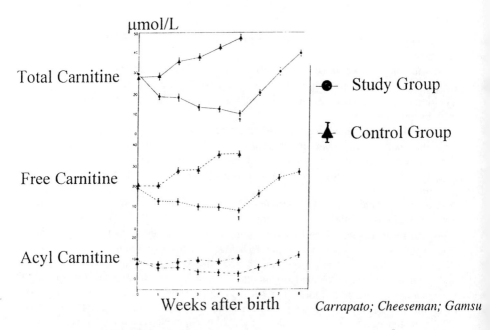

Figure 3   Carnitine 'deficiency' in neonates

Table 1   Carnitine content in the diet of the newborn

	TOTAL CARNITINE	FREE CARNITINE	ACYL CARNITINE	%
Prosobee	-	-	-	-
Pregestamil	-	-	-	-
Pepti-Junior	-	-	-	-
Al 110	-	-	-	-
Galactamin	-	-	-	-
Intralipid	-	-	-	-
Vamin	-	-	-	-
Comm.Chicken	49.24 ± 2.74	45.66 ± 2.92	3.53 ± 0.14	7.25 ± 0.77
Osterprem	70.23 ± 5.86	63.58 ± 6.52	7.27 ± 0.67	9.05 ± 1.63
Lactogen	91.39 ± 3.64	47.43 ± 1.92	43.95 ± 1.72	48.09 ± 0.03
Cow & Gate Plus	98.78 ± 1.74	64.19 ± 0.97	34.59 ± 2.72	35.00 ± 2.12
Pellargon	98.97 ± 5.54	51.33 ± 2.09	47.63 ± 3.45	48.11 ± 0.79
Aptamil	113.43 ± 2.55	102.43 ± 0.12	11.02 ± 2.42	9.69 ± 1.92
Premium	125.91 ± 2.79	96.84 ± 4.50	28.91 ± 1.93	22.95 ± 2.05
Nan	132.66 ± 0.18	65.64 ± 0.35	67.01 ± 0.54	50.51 ± 0.33
Nenatal	157.64 ± 3.75	155.88 ± 3.93	1.77 ± 0.17	1.15 ± 0.10
Osterfeed	168.76 ± 0.29	131.82 ± 6.59	39.43 ± 9.84	23.37 ± 5.05
Prematalac	173.41 ± 6.30	162.08 ± 4.60	11.30 ± 4.60	6.45 ± 2.33
Pre-Aptamil	178.28 ± 7.25	163.78 ± 11.30	14.49 ± 3.38	8.18 ± 2.27
SMA Gold	179.72 ± 6.40	153.10 ± 2.70	26.63 ± 8.50	14.72 ± 4.77

- Undetected

Carrapato; Cheeseman; Gamsu

REFERENCES

1. Tomita M, Sendju Y: Uber die Oxyaminoverxbindungen, Welche die Biuretreaktionzeigen. III Spaltung der γ-amino-β-oxybuttersaure in die optisch-aktiven komponenten Hoppe-Seyler's Z.   *Psyiol Chem 1927;169:263*

2. Carter HE, Bhattacharya PK, Weidman KR, Fraenkel G: Chemical Studies on vitamin B_T: isolation and characterisation as carnitine.   *Arch Biochem Biophys 1952;38:405*

3. Fritz IB: The effects of muscle extract on the oxidation of palmitic acid by liver slices and homogenates. *Acta Physiol Scand 1955;34:367*

4. Fritz IB: Carnitine and its role in fatty acid metabolism.   *Adv Lipid Res 1963; 1:285*

5. Fritz IB, McEwen B: Effects of carnitine on fatty acid oxidation by muscle. *Science 1959;129:334*

6. Fritz IB, Yue KTN: Long chain carnitine acyltransferase and the role of acylcarnitine derivatives in the catalytic increase of fatty acid oxidation induced by carnitine.   *J Lipid Res 1963;4:279*

7. Bieber LL, Emaus R, Valkner K, et al: Possible functions of short chain and medium chain carnitine acyltransferases. *Fed Proc 1982;41:2858*

8. Roe CR, Hoppel CL, Stacey T, et al: Metabolic response to carnitine in methylmalonic aciduria. *Arch Dis Child 1983;58:916*

9. Fritz IB, Burdzy K: Novel action of carnitine : inhibition of aggregation of dispersed cells elicited by clusterin in vitro. *J Cell Physiol 1989;140:18*

10. Criddel DN, Dewar GH, Wathey WB, et al: The effects of novel vasodilator long-chain carnitine esters in the isolated perfused heart of the rat. *Br J Pharmacol 1990;99:477*

11. Arduini A, Mancinelli G, Ramsey RR: Palmitoyl-L-carnitine, a metabolic intermediate of the fatty acid incorporation pathway in erithrocyte membrane phospholipids. *Biochem Biophys Res Commun 1990;173:212*

12. Arduini A, Mancinelli G, Radatti GL, et al: Role of carnitine and carnitine palmitoyl transferase as integral components of the pathway for membrane phospholipids fatty acid turnover in intact human erithrocytes. *J Biol Chem 1992;267:12673*

13. Otto DA: Relationship of the ATP/ADP ratio to the site of octanoate activation *J Bio Chem 1984;259:5490*

14. Rossle C, Carpentier YA, Richelle M, et al: Medium chain triglycerides induce alterations in carnitine metabolism. *Am J Physiol Endocrinol Metab 1990; 258:E944*

15. Rebouche CJ, Panagides DD, Nelson SE: Role of carnitine in utilisation of dietary medium-chain triglycerides by term infants. *Am J Clin Nut 1990; 52:820*

16. McGuire BS, Carroll JE, Chancey VF, et al: Mitochondrial enzymes responsible for oxidising medium-chain fatty acids in developing rat skeletal muscles, heart and liver. *J Nut Biochem 1990;1:410*

17. Robles-Valdes C, McGarry JD, Foster DW: Maternal-fetal carnitine relationship and neonatal ketosis in the rat. *J Biol Chem 1976;251:19*

18. McGarry JD: New perspective in the regulation of ketogenesis. *Diabetes 1979; 28:517*

19. McGarry JD, Foster DW: Regulation of hepatic fatty acid oxidation and ketone body production. *Am Rev Biochem 1980;49:395*

20. McGarry JD, Robles-Valdes, Foster DW: Role of carnitine in hepatic ketogenesis. *Proc Nat Acad Sci USA 1975;72:4385*

21. Hahn P, Novak M: The development of brown and white adipose tissue. *J Lipid Res 1975;16:79*

22. Hahn P, Skala J: Carnitine and brown adipose tissue metabolism in the rat during development. *Biochem J 1972;127:107*

23. Hittelman KJ, Lindberg O, Cannon B: Oxidative phosphorylation and compartmentation of fatty acid metabolism in brown fat mitochondria. *Eur J Biochem 1969; 11:183*

24. Hull D: Brown adipose tissue. *Br Med Bull 1966;22:92*

25. May ME, Aftring RP, Buse MG: mechanism of the stimulation of branched-chain oxoacid oxidation in liver by carnitine. *J Biol Chem 1980;225:517*

26. Paul HS, Adibi SA: Effect of carnitine on branched-chain amino acids oxidation by liver and skeletal muscle. *Am J Physiol 1978;2:34*

27. Van Hinsbergh VWM, Veerkaamp J, Cordwener JHG: Effect of carnitine and branched-chain acylcarnitine on the 2-oxo acid dehydrogenase activity in intact mitrochondria of rat muscle. *Int J Biochem 1980;12:559*

28. Borum PR: Expanding our tunnel vision to see carnitine's horizon. *Nutrition 1988; 4:251*

29. Horn DW, Broquist HP: Role of lysine and Σ-N-Trimethyllysine in carnitine biosynthesis. I Studies in Neurospora Crassa. *J Biol chem 1975;248:2170*

30. Horn DW, Tanphaichitr V, Broquist HP: Role of lysine in carnitine biosynthesis in Neurospora Crassa. *J Biol Chem 1971;246:4373*

31. Bremer J: Biosynthesis of carnitine in vivo. *Biochem Biophys Acta 1961; 48:622*

32. Hulse JD, Ellis SR, Henderson LM: Carnitine biosynthesis. *J Biol Chem 1978; 253:1654*

33. Rebouche CJ: Ascorbic acid and carnitine biosynthesis. *Am J Clin Nut 1991; 54:1147S*

34. Rebouche CJ: Carnitine function and requirements during the lifecycle. *FASEB J 1992;6:3379*

35. Siliprandi N, Sartorelli L, Ciman M, et al: Carnitine : metabolism and clinical chemistry. *Clin Chim Acta 1989;183:3*

36. Bieber LL: Carnitine. *Ann Rev Biochem 1988;57:261*

37. Rebouche CJ, Engel AG: Tissue distribution of carnitine biosynthetic enzymes in man. *Biochem Biophys Acta 1980;630:22*

38. Englard : Hydroxylation of γ-butyrobetaine to carnitine in human and monkey tissues. *FEBS Lett 1979;102:297*

39. Olson AL, Rebouche CJ: γ-butyrobetaine hydroxylase activity is not rate limiting for carnitine biosynthesis in the human infant. *J Nut 1987;117:1024*

40. Gamsu HR, Cheeseman P, Carrapato MRG: Carnitine synthesis in the newborn. *Proc Br Paed Assoc 1986; G34*

41. Carrapato MRG: Carnitine in neonatal metabolism: *MD Thesis, Oporto Med School 1987*

42. Marquis NR, Fritz IB: The distribution of carnitine, acylcarnitine and carnitine acyltransferase in rat tissues. *J Biochem 1965;240:2193*

43. Sandor A, Pecsuvac K, Kerner J, et al: On carnitine content of the human breast milk. *Pediatr Res 1982;16:89*

44. Borum PR, York CM, Broquist HP: Carnitine content of liquid formulae and special diets. *Am J Clin Nut 1979;32:2272*

45. Panter RA, Mudd JB: Carnitine levels in some higher plants. *FEBS Lett 1969;5:169*

46. Rudman D, Sewell CW, Ansley JD: Deficiency of carnitine in cachetic cirrhotic patients. *J Clin Invest 1977;60:716*

47. Bartel LL, Hussey JL, Shrago E: Perturbation of serum carnitine levels in human adults by chronic renal disease and dialysis therapy. *Am J Clin Nut 1981;34:1314*

48. Battistella PA, Angelini C, Vergani L, et al: Carnitine deficiency in use during hemodialysis. *Lancet 1978;1:939*

49. Bohmer T, Bergrem H, Eiklid K: Carnitine deficiency induced during intermittent hemodialysis for renal failure. *Lancet 1978;1:126*

50. Hahn P, Skala JP, Seccombe DW: Carnitine content of blood and amniotic fluid. *Pediatr Res 1977;11:818*

51.   Scholte HR, Stinis JT, Jennekens FGI: Low carnitine levels in serum of pregnant women.   *N Engl J Med 1979; 299*

52.   Shoderbeck M, Auer B, Legenstein E, et al: Pregnancy-related changes of carnitine and acylcarnitine concentrations of plasma and erythrocytes. *J Perinat Med 1995;23:477*

53.   Angelini C, Vergani L, Martinuzzi A: Clinical and biochemical aspects of carnitine deficiency and insufficiency : transport defects and inborn errors of β-oxidation. *Crit Rev Clin Lab Sci 1992;29:217*

54.   Stanley CA: New genetic defects in mitrochondrial fatty acid oxidation and carnitine deficiency. *Adv Pediatr 1987;34:59*

55.   Engel AG, Angelini C: Carnitine deficiency in human skeletal muscle with associated lipid storage myopathy : a new syndrome. *Science 1973;179:899*

56.   Engel AG: Possible causes and defects of carnitine deficiency in man.   *In Carnitine biosynthesis, metabolism and functions.   Edited by RA Frenkel, J D McGarry, New York Academic Press 1980; 271*

57.   Karpati G, Carpenter S, Engel AG: The syndrome of systemic carnitine deficiency. *Neurology 1975;25:16*

58.   DeVivo DC, Tein I: Primary and secondary disorders of carnitine metabolism. *Int Pediatr 1990;5:134*

59.   Stanley CA, De Leeuw S, Coats PM, et al: Chronic cardiomyopathy and weakness or acute coma in children with a defect in carnitine uptake.   *Ann Neurol 1991;30:709*

60.   Tein I, DeVivo DC, Bierman F, et al: Impaired skin fibroblasts carnitine uptake in primary systemic deficiency manifested by childhood carnitine – responsive cardiomyopathy. *Pediatr Res.1990,28:247*

61.   Treem WR, Stanley CA, Finegold DN, et al: Primary carnitine deficiency due to a failure of carnitine transport in kidney, muscle and fibroblasts. *N Engl J Med 1988;319:1331*

62.   Erikson BO, Lindstedt S, Nordin: Hereditary defects in carnitine membrane transport is expressed in skin fibroblasts. *Eur J Pediatr 1988;147:662*

63.   Brass EP: Overview of coenzyme A metabolism and its role in cellular toxicity. *Chem Biol Int 1994;90:203*

64.   Waber LJ, Valle D, Neill C: Carnitine deficiency presenting as familial cardiomyopathy : a treatable defect in carnitine transport.   *J Pediatr 1982;101:700*

65.   Chapoy PR, Angelini C, Brown WJ et al: Systemic carnitine deficiency. A treatable, inherited lipid storage disease presenting as Reye's Syndrome. *N Engl J Med 1980;303:1389*

66.   Tripp ME, Catcher ML, Peters HA: Systemic carnitine deficiency presenting as familial endocardial fibroelastosis. *N Engl J Med 1981;305:385*

67.   Garavaglia B, Uziel G, Dworzak F, et al: Primary carnitine deficiency : heterozygote and intrafamilial variation. *Neurology 1991;41:1691*

68.   Engel AG: Carnitine deficiency syndromes and lipid storage myopathy. *In Engel AG, Bunker BQ (eds): Myology: basic and clinical. New York McGraw—Hill 1986;1663*

69.   Martinuzzi A, Vergani MR, Angelini C: L-carnitine uptake in differentiating human cultured muscle. *Biochim Biophys Acta 1991;1095:217*

70. Mesmer OT, Lo TCY: Hexose transport properties of myoblasts isolated from a patient with suspected muscle carnitine deficiency. *Biochem Cell Biol 1990;68:1372*

71. Coats PM, Hale D, Finochiaro G, et al: Genetic deficiency of short-chain acyl CoA dehydrogenase in cultured fibroblasts from a patient with muscle carnitine deficiency and severe skeletal muscle weakness. *J Clin Invest 1988;81:171*

72. DiDonato S: Disorders of lipid metabolism affecting skeletal muscle: carnitine deficiency syndromes, defects in the catabolic pathway and Chanarin disease. *In Engel AG, Franzini-Armstrong CL (eds) Myology: Basic and Clinical 2nd ed. New York, McGraw-Hill 1994;1587*

73. Carrol JE. Brooke M, DeVivo DC, et al: Carnitine deficiency: lack of response to carnitine therapy. *Neurology 1980;30:618*

74. Angelini C, Govoni E, Bragaglia MM et al: Carnitine deficiency : acute postpartum crisis. *Ann Neurol 1978;4:558*

75. DiDonato S, Cornelio F, Storchi G, et al: Hepatic ketogenesis and muscle carnitine deficiency. *Neurology 1979;29:780*

76. Hart ZH, Chang C, DiMauro S et al: Muscle carnitine deficiency and fatal cardiomyopathy. *Neurology 1978;28:147*

77. Trevisan CO, Reichman H, DiVivo DC, et al: β-oxidation enzymes in normal human muscle and in muscle from a patient with an unusual form of myopathic carnitine deficiency. *Muscle Nerve 1985;8:672*

78. Mori T, Tsuchiyama A, Nagai K, et al: A case of carbamoylphosphate synthetase-1 deficiency associated with secondary carnitine deficiency – L-carnitine treatment of CPS-1 deficiency. *Eur J Pediatr 1990;149:272*

79. Voit T, Kramer H, Thomas C, et al: Myopathy in Williams-Beuren Syndrome. *Eur J Pediatr 1991;150:521*

80. Chalmers RA, Roe CR, Stacey E, et al: Urinary excretion of L-carnitine and acyl carnitines by patients with disorders of organic acid metabolism : evidence for secondary insufficiency of L-carnitine. *Pediatr Res 1984;18:1325*

81. Tanphaichitr V, Lelahagul P: Carnitine metabolism and human carnitine deficiency. *Nutrition 1993;9:246*

82. Winter SC, Szabo-Aczel S, Curry CJR, et al: Plasma carnitine deficiency. *Am J Dis Child 1987;141:660*

83. Rebouche CJ: Carnitine metabolism and function in humans. *Ann Ver Nut 1986;6:41*

84. Bohles H, Evangeliou A, Bervoets K, et al: Carnitine esters in metabolic diseases. *Eur J Pediatr 1994;153(Suppl 1):57*

85. Stanley CA, Berry GT, Bennet MJ, et al: Renal handling of carnitine in secondary carnitine deficiency disorders. *Pediatr Res 1993;34:89*

86. Corr PB, Gross RW, Sabel BE: Amphipatic metabolytes and membrane disfunction in ischemic myocardium. *Circ Res 1988;55:135*

87. Coulter DL: Carnitine, valproate and toxicity. *J Child Neurol 1990;6:7*

88. Shapira Y, Gutman A: Muscle carnitine deficiency in patients using valproic acid. *J Pediatr 1991;118:646*

89. Matsuda I, Ohtani Y, Ninomiya N: Renal handling of carnitine in children with hyperammonemia associated with valproate therapy. *J Pediatr 1986;109:131*

90. Bratton SL, Garden AL, Bohan TP, et al: A childhood with valproic acid associated carnitine deficiency and carnitine responsive cardiac disfunction. *J Child Neurol 1992;7:413*

91. Chabrol B, Mancini J, Chretien D, et al: Valproate-induced hepatic failure in a case of cytochrome C oxidase deficiency. *Eur J Pediatr 1994:153:133*

92. Simone CD, Tzantzoglous S, Jrillo E, et al: L-carnitine deficiency in AIDS patients. *AIDS 1992;6:203*

93. DeSimone C, Famularo G, Tzantzoglous S, et al: Carnitine depletion in peripheral blood mononuclear cells from patients with AIDS : effects of oral L-carnitine. *AIDS 1994;8:655*

94. DeSimone C, Tzantzoglous S, Famularo G, et al: High dose L-carnitine improves immunologic and metabolic parameters in AIDS patients. *Immunopharmacol Immunotoxicol 1993;15:1*

95. Tomaka FL, Cimoch PJ, Reiter WM, et al: Prevalence of nutritional deficiencies in patients with HIV-1 infection. *Abstract N° PB0898 Int Conf AIDS. 1994;10:221*

96. DeSimone C, Tzantzoglous S, Jrillo E, et al: L-carnitine deficiency in AIDS patients. *AIDS 1992;6:203*

97. Bogden JD, Baker H, Frank O, et al: Micronutrient status and human immunodeficiency virus (HIV) infection. *Ann NY Acad Sci 1990;587:189*

98. Walter EB, Drucker RP, McKinney RE, et al: Myopathy in human immunodeficiency virus in infected children receiving long-term zidovudine therapy. *J Pediatr 1991;119:152*

99. Arnaudo E, Dalakas M, DiMauro S, et al: Depletion of muscle mitrochondrial DNA in AIDS patients with zidovudine-induced myopathies. *Lancet 1991;337:508*

100. Dalakas M, Leon-Monzon ME, Bernardini I, et al: Zidovudine-induced mitochondrial myopathy is associated with muscle carnitine deficiency and lipid storage. *Ann Neuro 1994;35:482*

101. Semino-Mora MC, Leon-Monzon ME, Dalakas M: Effect of L-carnitine on the zidovudine-induced destruction of human myotubes. Part I L-carnitine prevents the myotoxicity of AZT in vitro. *LAB INVEST 1994;71:102*

102. Semino-Mora MC, Leon-Monzon ME, Dalakas M: Effect of L-carnitine on the zidovudine-induced destruction of human myotubes Part II Treatment with L-carnitine improves the AZT-induced changes and prevents further destruction. *LAB INVEST 1994;71:773*

103. Fauci A: Multifactorial nature of human immunodeficiency virus disease : implications for therapy. *Science 1993;262:1011*

104. Novak M, Monkus EF, Chung D, et al: Carnitine in perinatal metabolism of lipids. Relationship between maternal and fetal plasma levels of carnitine and acylcarnitine. *Pediatrics 1981;67:95*

105. Kashyap MC, Sivasambo R, Sothy SP: Carbohydrates and lipid metabolism during human labour. *Metabolism 1976;25:865*

106. Lohninger A, Krieglsteiner P, Nikiforov A, et al: Comparison of the effects of betamethasone and L-carnitine on depalmitoyl phosphatidylcholine content and phosphatidylcholine species composition in fetal rat lungs. *Pediatr Res 1984;18:1246*

107. Czeszynska MB: Evaluation of fetal lung maturation in rabbits after giving carnitine and carnitine with betamethasone to pregnant rabbits. *Ann Acad Med Stetin 1993;39:185*

108. Lohninger A, Laschan C, Auer B: Animal experiment and clinical studies of the significance of carnitine for energy metabolism in pregnant patients and the fetus during the pre- and perinatal period. *Wien Klin Wochenschr 1996;108:33*

109. Lohninger A, B"ock P, Dadak C, et al: Effect of carnitine on fetal rat lung dipalmitoyl phosphatidylcholine content and lung morphology. *J Clin Chem Clin Biochem 1990;28:313*

110. Melichar V, Novak M: Energy metabolism in human fetus and newborn. Utilisation of nutrients during postnatal development. *Hahn P, Koldovsky O (Eds) 121 Pergamon Press, Oxford 1966*

111. Novak M, Melichar V, Hahn P, et al: Release of free fatty acids from adipose tissue obtained from newborn infants. *J Lipid Res 1965;6:91*

112. Warshaw JB: Fatty acid metabolism during development. *Sem Perinat 1979;3:131*

113. Warshaw JB, Maniscalco WM: Perinatal adaptations in carbohydrate and lipid metabolism. *In Stern's Intensive Care of the Newborn 1978;2:251*

114. Warshaw JB, Terry ML: Cellular energy metabolism during fetal development. VI Fatty acid oxidation by the developing brain. *Dev Biol 1976;52:161*

115. Groot PHE, Hulsmann WC: The activation and oxidation of octanoate and palmitate by rat skeletal muscle mitochondria. *Biochim Biophys Acta 1973;316:124*

116. Reichmann H, Maltese WA, DeVivo DC: Enzymes of fatty acid β-oxidation in developing brain. *J Neurochem 1988;51:339*

117. Sulkers EJ, Lafeber HN, Sauer PJJ: Quantification of oxidation of medium chain triglycerides in pre-term infants. *Pediatri Res 1989;26:294*

118. Borum PR: Medium chain triglycerides in formulae for pre-term neonates : implications for hepatic and extra hepatic metabolism. *J Pediatr 1992;120:S139*

119. Clark KJ, Makrides M, Neumann MA: Determination of the optimal ratio of linoleic acid to α-linolenic acid in infant formulas. *J Pediatr 1992;120:S151*

120. Bazan HEP, Bazan NG, Feeney-Burns L, et al: Lipids in human lipofusin-enriched subcellular fractions of two age populations : comparison with rod outer segments and neural retina. *Invest Ophthalmol Vis Sci 1990; 31:1433*

121. Martinez M, Ballabriga A, Gil-Gibernau JJ: Lipids of the developing human retina: 1 Total fatty acids, plasmalogens and fatty acid composition of ethanolamine and choline phosphoglycerides. *J Neurosci Res 1988;20:484*

122. Holman RT, Johnson SB, Hatch TF: A case of human linolenic acid deficiency involving neurological abnormalities. *Am J Clin Nut 1982; 35:617*

123. Uauy RD, Birch DJ, Birch EE, et al: Effect of dietary omega-3 fatty acids on retinal function of very low birthweight neonates. *Pediatr Res 1990;28:485*

124. Carlson SE, Rhodes BG, Rao VS, et al: Effects of fish oil supplementation on the n-3 fatty acid content of red blood cell membranes in pre-term infants. *Pediatr Res1987; 21:507*

125. Innis SM, Foote KD, MacKinnon MJ, et al: Plasma and red cell fatty acids of low birthweight infants fed their mother's expressed breast milk or pre-term infant formula. *Am J Clin Nut 1990;51:994*

126. Neuringer M, Connor WE: n-3 fatty acids in the brain and retina : evidence for their essentiality. *Nutr Rev 1986;44:285*

127. Exton JH: Gluconeogenesis. *Metabolism 1972;21:945*

128. Ferré P, Satabin P, Manoubi LEL, et al: Relationship between ketogenesis and gluconeogenesis in isolated hepatocytes from newborn rats. *Biochem J 1981;200:429*

129. Pilkis SJ, Park CR, Claus TH: Hormonal control of hepatic gluconeogenesis. *In* vitamins and hormones. *Munzo PL, Diezfalusy E, Glover J (Eds) 1978;36:383 NY Academic*

130. Williamson JR, Browning ET, Scholtz R, et al: Inhibition of fatty acid stimulation of neoglycogenesis by (+)-decanolylcarnitine in perfused rat liver. *Diabetes 1968;17:194*

131. Williamson JR, Rostand SG, Peterson MJ: Control factors affecting gluconeogenesis in perfused liver. *J Biol Chem 1970;245:3242*

132. Benmiloud M, Freinkel N: Stimulation of glucogenesis by carnitine in vivo. *Metabolism 1967;16:458*

133. Schiff D, Chan G, Seccombe D, et al: Plasma carnitine levels during intravenous feeding of the newborn. *J Pediatr 1979;95:1043*

134. Schmidt-Sommerfeld E, Penn D, Wolf H: Carnitine blood concentrations and fat utilisation in parenterally alimented premature newborn infants. *J Pediatr 1982;100:260*

135. Schmidt-Sommerfeld E, Penn D, Wolf H: The influence of maternal fat metabolism on fetal carnitine levels. *Early Hum Develop 1981;5:233*

136. Schmidt-Sommerfeld E, Novak M, Penn D, et al: Carnitine and development of newborn adipose tissue. *Pediatr Res 1978;12:660*

137. Penn D, Schmidt-Sommerfeld E, Pascu F: Decreased tissue carnitine concentrations in newborn infants receiving total parenteral nutrition. *J Pediatr 1981;96:976*

138. Penn D, Schmidt-Sommerfeld E, Wolf H: Carnitine deficiency in premature infants receiving total parenteral nutrition. *Early Hum Develop 1980;4:23*

139. Borum P: Carnitine in neonatal nutrition. *J Child Neurol 1995;10:2S25*

BETA- HYDROXYBUTYRATE IN NEONATAL HYPOGLYCEMIA

Giuliana Trifiro. Endocrinology Unit. Sacco Hospital-   University . Milan,Italy

INTRODUCTION

The definition of hypoglycemia, the most common metabolic occurence in nurseries and neonatal intensive care units, is at present still controversial. A cut-off level has not yet been established and, therefore, its real incidence is difficult to ascertain. Signs and symptoms are not specific and may also be absent.Common methods of monitoring blood glucose concentrations at the bedside are imprecise and not consistently reliable, underestimating the true glycemic status whose importance is related to the cerebral metabolism (1). The neonatal brain has a very high glucose turn-over rate which is directly related to brain size. Glucose consumption in newborns is two-three times that of adults (2) and severe hypoglycemia causes brain damage up to both neuronal and glial death, resulting in severe handicap (3). Some studies have also demonstrated the potential danger of mild hypoglycemia. During the first hours of life, a counter-regulation (glycogenolysis, gluconeogenesis, proteolysis, lipolysis, ketogenesis) occurs as an adaptive response to extra-uterine life and hypoglycemia develops when these five metabolic adaptations fail. Among the main energy substrates of the neonatal brain, ketones have an unique role (2/3 of the brain's energy is supplied by ketones) (6). The aim of

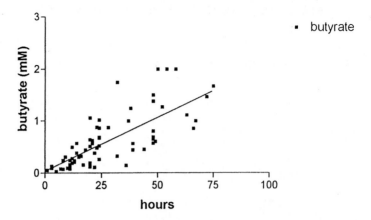

Figure 1 Linear increase of beta-hydroxybutyrate during the first hours of life.

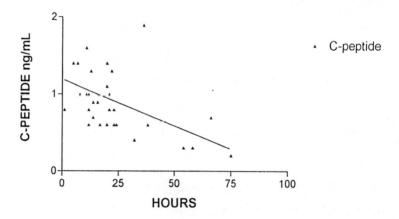

Figure 2 Decrease of C-peptide levels during the first hours of life.

this study is to evaluate the efficacy of the metabolic counter-regulation in newborns by detecting the beta-hydroxy-butyrate and C-peptide levels and to test the utility of a new reflectance photometer system (Ketosyte®) using special card planned for diabetes (7), which allows bedside determination of beta-hydroxybutyrate levels. We measured C-peptide because it has been found a more accurate index of pancreatic beta cell secretion than insulin concentrations (8).

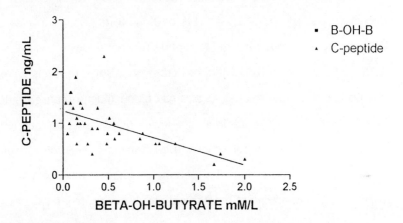

Figure 3 Inverse correlation between beta-hydroxybutyrate and C-peptide.

MATERIALS AND METHODS

We have studied 70 healthy newborns (35 males;35 females; gestational age 39 ± 0.16 weeks; mean birth weight 3515 ± 61 gms), born from vaginal delivery, exclusively breast-fed and undergone to partial fasting. All mothers had a normal carbohydrate metabolism. We measured beta-hydroxy- butyrate, glucose and C-peptide concentrations during the first 75 hours of life. KetoSyte® is a new reflectance-photometer-system in which the test for hy-droxybutyrate is based on the action of beta-hydroxybutyrate dehidrogenase and diaphorase enzymes (GDS Diagnostics,Elkhart, Inc.). C-peptide levels were determined by radioimminoassay (Myria, Technogenetics). Whole capillary blood glucose was measured by an oxidase method (Boehringer Mannheim Corp.).

RESULTS

Ten newborns (14 %) had blood glucose levels of less than 2.2 mmol/L (40 mg/dL) without clinical symptoms. Beta-hydroxybutyrate levels showed a significant linear correlation with age, increasing from birth to the third day of life (slope 0.024, r^2 0.55, p<0.0001) (fig.1). C-peptide levels significantly decreased (slope -0.0089, r^2 0.11, p=0.049) (fig.2). An inverse correlation between beta-OH-butyrate and C-peptide concentrations (slope -0.53, r^2 0.41, p<0.0001) was also found (fig.3). Beta-hydroxybutyrate levels were inversely, but not significantly, related to plasma blood glucose concentrations; when blood glucose levels were low, the levels of hydroxybutyrate were always detectable (i.e. >0.5 mmol) showing a satisfactory metabolic adaptation with an appropriate suppression of C-peptide. In the follow-up at 24 months all infants presented adequate mental and motor developmental scores.

CONCLUSIONS

Sexson et coll, using a cut-off value of 1.6 mmol/L (30 mg/dL), showed an incidence of hypoglycemia in 8% of full term neonates while by using a higher threshold (2.2 mmol/L; 40 mg/dL) the incidence of hypoglycemic newborns increased to 20 % (9). The differences among studies depend on heterogeneity of infants, assay methods, feeding policies. During the early adaptive response to extra-uterine life, glicogenolysis exhausts itself within 12 hours and the enzymatic activation for gluconeogenesis requires some hours, so, ketogenesis is a very important factor. In fact lipolysis releases free fatty acids which arrive to the liver and the hepatic beta-oxidation of these fatty acids produces ketones. The neonatal brain has an enhanced capacity to utilise ketones compared to infants (fourfold) and adults (40-fold) (10) and ketogenesis is already mature from the 35th week of gestational age (11). Within the brain, astrocytes, oligodendrocytes and neurons have an excellent capacity to utilise ketones (3). The presence of ketones (normal range 0.1-0.5 mmol/L) is a good indication that a metabolic adaptation is taking place (low insulin activity) while the absence of ketones during hypoglycemia is an abnormal finding and suggests the diagnosis of hyperinsulinism or inborn metabolic defects. The insulin control may be poor for a regulatory defect in beta cell function and this is the most likely explanation for functional hyperinsulinism. But during the neonatal period, basal insulin levels are phisiologically higher than in the following ages and the relationship between glucose and insulin concentration is not so close as later, in childhood. So, the diagnosis of hypoglycemia due to hyperinsulinism is not allowed by eva-luating the insulin concentration alone. In fact at the time of hypoglycemia, the infant may not have high insulin levels. Therefore undetectable levels of ketones are the best marker of hyperinsulinism. The full-term newborn is able to produce counter-regulatory ketogenesis as blood glucose levels fall and the capacity of healthy neonates to switch off insulin secretion and to initiate ketogenesis indicates good metabolic adaptation. The "safe" threshold value below which hypoglycemia becomes detrimental has not been recognized. According to Ainsley-Green, "physiologic hypoglycemia can be defined as the lowest concentration of bood glucose which, in combination with other metabolic fuels allows a normal brain function" (12). The evaluation of serum glucose levels should be supported by the determination of other metabolic fuels such as the beta-hydroxybutyrate. Infants who are able to mount an effective ketogenic counter-regulatory response are not at risk of brain da-mage during hypoglycemia. On the contrary, infants who fail to trigger the dual response are at risk of neural impairement. Therefore, the demonstration of low blood glucose levels alone does not justify an aggressive treatment in full-term neonates. Otherwise, invasive management with intravenous glucose, which separates mother and baby, is justified in presence of hypoketotic hypoglycemia (hypoglycemia associated with undetectable ketone levels). Ketosite® (blood ketone test) seems to be a simple and useful tool to distinguish the physiological hypoglycemia from the dangerous hypoketotic hypoglycemia.

REFERENCES

1. Aynsley-Green A. Glucose, the brain and the pediatric endocrinologist. *Horm Res* 1996, 46:8-25

2. Ogata ES. Carboydrate metabolism in the fetus and neonate and altered neonatal glucoregulation. *Pediatric Clinics North America* 1986, 33: 25-45

3. Land JM. Hypoglycaemia in the neonate: how and when is it important. *Dev Neurosci* 1994; 16: 307-12

4. Lucas A. Adverse neurodevelopment outcome of moderate neonatal hypoglycaemia. *Br Med J* 1988, 297:1304-8

5. Koh THHG. Neural dysfunction during hypoglycaemia. *Arch Dis Child* 1988,63:1353-8

6. Edmond J. Ketone body metabolism in the neonate: development and the effect of the diet. *Federation Proc* 1985; 44: 2359- 64

7. Gibson RG. .Accuracy of a rapid quantitative bedside beta-hydroxybutyrate test system.*Clin Lab Sci* 1996 , 9:282-7

8. Heding LG. Radioimmunological determination of human C-peptide in serum. *Diabetologia* 1975; 11:541-8

9. Sexson WR. Incidence of neonatal hypoglycaemia: a matter of definition. *J Pediatr* 1984; 105: 149- 50

10. Mehta a. Prevention and management of neonatal hypoglycaemia. *Arch Dis Child* 1994; 70: F54- F65

11. Hawdon JM. Patterns of metabolic adaptation for preterm and term infants in the first neonatal week. *Arch Dis Child* 1992; 67: 357- 65

12. Ainsley-Green A. Hupoglycaemia in the neonate: current controversies. *Acta Paed Japan* 1997; 39: S12- S16

FREE RADICALS IN NEONATAL BRAIN DISORDERS.
POSSIBLE BENEFITS OF ANTIOXIDANTS

R. Bracci

Istituto di Pediatria Preventiva e Neonatologia, Università di Siena, Italy

In the last decade free radicals have been demonstrated to play a role in the development of brain disorders. Reactive oxygen species (ROS) have been found to be harmful to the cells of the nervous system which, because of its high and constant oxygen requirements, produces superoxide radicals (O_2^-) as a product of normal aerobic metabolism. It has been calculated that approximately 2% of the oxygen used is converted to oxygen radicals[1]. ROS are released in the brain by various pathways. Damage to mitochondria may induce a vicious circle in which damaged mitochondrial DNA causes defective respiratory chain proteins which form ROS which further damage mitochondrial DNA. The vicious circle can be summarized as: ATP depletion, GSH deficiency, H_2O_2 accumulation, mitochondrial dysfunction[2,3], O_2^- release, hydoxyl radical (OH) formation by the Fenton/Haber Weiss reaction (which occurs in the presence of H_2O_2, O_2^- and free iron) and metabolisation of dopamine which induces formation of further H_2O_2. Other source of ROS are prostaglandin and catecholamine metabolism, the hypoxanthine-xanthine oxidase reaction and phagocyte activation[2,3]. Free radicals have been suggested to play a role in brain diseases, such as Parkinson's and Alzheimer's disease, stroke, progeria, Werner syndrome and lipofuscin deposits[2].

In the newborn infant, the role of free radicals in the development of hypoxic brain damage has been extensively investigated[4-9]. Possible sources of ROS in the newborn brain are those mentioned and particularly the hypoxia related mechanisms, such as ischemia reperfusion involving the hypoxanthine-xanthine oxidase reaction, mitochondrial dysfunction and prostaglandin metabolism[3]. Even the release of ROS by activated phagocytes cannot be ruled out[10]. ROS production in the fetal and neonatal brain during hypoxia has been demonstrated in vivo and in vitro[11,7]. Most experiments demonstrated membrane lipid peroxidation which is considered a marker of free radical production probably due to OH production[12-14]. The susceptibility of brain membrane lipids to peroxidation suggests that both premature and term infant are prone to oxidative cell damage. Indeed all neonates have lower antioxidant defences than adults, in terms of scavenger enzyme activities and antioxidant molecules, these defense systems are particularly deficient in premature infants[4]. However, the full term brain has a higher unsaturated lipid membrane content and therefore more peroxidizable substrate. This high peroxidizable membrane lipid content of the full term infant brain may be responsible for the higher rate of peroxidation after hypoxia in full term than in premature newborns[9].

Lipid membrane peroxidation seems to be the main event related to free radical release during fetal and neonatal asphyxia since high lipid peroxidation has been demonstrated in the hypoxic brain as well as in metabolic acidosis[9,15]. An increase in lipid peroxidation during hypoxia has been demonstrated in the fetus and in newborns[9,16]. Ischemia plays a key role in the release of ROS which are more crucial than oxygen tension during reperfusion[17]. Lipid peroxidation has been detected in the synaptosome membrane[18]. Synaptosome damage caused by hypoxia is complex. Recent research on tyrosine phosphorylation maps in synaptosomes of hypoxic guinea pigs suggests that hypoxia extensively remodels the signaling pathway, switching on Y-phosphorylation in some proteins and switching it off in others[19]. Decreased glutamate uptake by astrocytes and NMDA disorders also follow free radical release in the brain[20-22]. The decrease in inhibition by addition to the system of scavenger of ROS proves that ROS are responsible for reduced glutamate uptake by astrocytes[20]. Brain damage which follows lipid peroxidation therefore seems to be due to neurotransmitter disorders which lead to an increase in excitatory factors, a decrease in GABA, inhibitory molecules, ATPase, depolarization and the convulsion threshold[23].

Interesting studies have been made in an attempt to detect the reactions responsible for free radical release. Hydroxyl radical formation by the free iron-dependent Fenton reaction has been observed as a result of increased iron following hemolysis in intracranial hemorrhage or following cell damage due to severe hypoxia[24,25]. This reaction and the associated release of hydroxyl radicals is important in view of high free iron availability due to high saturation of transferrin in cerebrospinal fluid $(CSF)^{26}$. Experimental studies have also shown that hypo xanthine-xanthine oxidase source is an important of free radicals in hypoxic ischemic brain damage. Besides demonstration of high hypoxanthine content in CSF of anoxic animals and evidence that xanthine oxidase inhibitors such as allopurinol have a protective effectc[27,28], recent studies report that specific cerebral endothelial cell damage in ischemia reperfusion is reduced by xanthine oxidase inhibitors[29]. Furthermore, significantly higher extracellular concentrations of hypoxanthine were found in the cerebral cortex during an initial period of reoxygenation with 100% oxygen instead of 21% oxygen[30]. Although the role of the xanthine oxidase pathway in the release of ROS is still uncertain, there is now little doubt that postischemic reoxygenation is followed by release of ROS. Even normoxic reoxygenation after hypoxia has been found to be followed by permanent modification of the glutamate recognition site which may enhance NMDA receptor-mediated neuronal injury[31]. It is possible that post-ischemic release of ROS may depend on prostaglandin cascade[32]. Whatever the source, antioxidant enzyme activities appear to play a key role, reduction of SOD exacerbates neuronal cell injury and edema after transient focal cerebral ischemia[33]. The role of nitric oxide (NO·) the release of which seems to increase significantly in the brain during hypoxia, has also been investigated[34]. NO· is derived from conversion of arginine to citrulline by neuronal, endothelial or macrophage nitric oxide synthase (NOS). In the presence of ·O2·, NO· forms peroxynitrite, ONOO⁻, which is a strongly reacting molecule and can release ˙OH [34]. Several observations suggest that endothelial NO˙ production may be a protective factor against hypoxic ischemic brain damage because of its vasodilatatory effect[35-37] On the contrary, production of NO˙ by neuronal or macrophage NOS aggravates the brain injury[38]. The difference between the two NOS has been demonstrated by experiments with specific endothelial and neuronal NOS inhibitors[39]. Several observations in animals suggest that there is reduced NO˙ release in the brain of the fetus and newborn infant[40]. It is uncertain whether this deficiency could predispose the newborn to brain damage.

Another source of ROS to consider is phagocyte activation. It is well known that neutrophils and monocytes are activated by the endothelium and that the endothelium can be activated by phagocytes to release humoral factors and vasoactive substances[41]. Activation of microglial cells and accumulation of neutrophils in the brain capillaries has been demonstrated as well as relationships between hypoxia ischemia and inflammatory episodes[42]. Lipid peroxidation has been found in the endothelial cell during hypoxia ischemia[43]. Accumulation of neutrophils in capillary and post-capillaries venules after hypoxia - ischemia is associated with a pro-inflammatory cytokine increase in the spinal fluid of asphyxiated animals[44]. An increase in IL-6, IL-8 and TNF was recently reported in the spinal fluid of infants with asphyxia and poor outcome[45-47]. Phagocyte activation leads to a release of various molecules with potentially damaging CNS, of which ROS are among the most powerful.

The important role of ROS released during inflammation on the development of hypoxic-ischemic brain damage is suggested by the observation of relations between experimentally induced intrauterine infection and brain white matter lesions[48]. The finding of high cytokine secretion in hypoxia ischemia agrees with previous reports of high cytokine release and increased blood neurtrophil activation in vaginal and emergency deliveries in comparison with elective caesarean section[49,50].

Because of the complex mechanisms of ROS production, it is difficult to protect the brain against oxidative stress. This complexitiy is also demonstrated by the fact that although the markers of oxidative stress are correlated with the degree of hypoxia[51,52], the antioxidant status of the newborn does not appear to be correlated with outcome[53]. Nevertheless the importance of the possibility of limiting the effects of oxidative stress with antioxidant therapy justifies a number of studies in this field. Antioxidant therapy should be carried out before and during hypoxia and during reoxygenation. Any antioxidant treatment should have two fundamental aims: to increase free radical scavenging and to reduce free radical release by stopping the mechanism causing it. Many experimental studies have indicated that various molecules may have a protective effect on brain damage, limiting oxidative stress by acting on different steps of the pathway involved in the release of ROS. Unfortunately most of the drugs which demonstrated a fair protective effect against brain damage due to oxidative stress did not show a corresponding effect in clinical trials. The traditional antioxidant vitamin E, has been extensively studied in experimental animals and human newborns. This vitamin undoubtedly has some effect in protecting brain cell membranes from lipid peroxidation and brain cell membrane function [54]. However, in the human neonate, vitamin E administration seems to reduce the incidence of intraventricular hemorrhage, but no clear evidence for a corresponding reduction in intracerebral hemorrhage [55]. The limited results obtained with this powerful antioxidant may be due not only to the fact that oxidative damage may occur without lipid peroxidation but also to the mode of action of alphatocopherol which reacts with chain propagating peroxylradicals faster than ROS reacts with other targets. The relatively unreactive radical which is formed is removed by a mechanism involving ascorbate and ubiquinol, which is unclear in the adult and even more obscure in the neonate[56]. Recent experiments carried out with lazaroids, which have an antioxidant power 100 times greater than vitamin E, suggest that they protect mesencephalic neurons[57]. In particular, the molecule 21-aminosteroid has been demonstrated to be against hypoxia-ishemia in adult and immature animal models[58]. Another compound which limits lipid peroxidation is alpha-phenyl-tert-butylnitrone[59].

Other antioxidant molecules have been experimentally demonstrated to protect the nervous system against oxidative injury. These molecules include antioxidant enzymes, glutathione, cystine, alpha-lipoic acid and other compounds such as N,N-propylenedinicotinamide[60]. The antioxidant activity of ascorbic acid and the vitamin K cycle is complex and it is still unclear whether it prevents brain oxidative stress. SOD has been used with limited success although the experimental data has suggested some advantages[61]. Attempts have been made to modify the SOD molecule in order to obtain a longer half-life[62]. The administration of SOD conjugated to polyethylene glycol has been shown to reduce hypoxic-ischemic brain injury and to maintain the stability of the blood-brain barrier[63]. The prolonged half-life and large molecule of conjugated SOD has the disadvantage of precluding rapid penetration of the brain parenchyma[26]. Therapeutic effects have been obtained with SOD in experimental retinopathy[64].

Interesting results have also been obtained with molecules which reduce ROS release. Allopurinol, an inhibitor of xanthine-oxidase seems to reduce ROS release during ischemia-reperfusion[65]. Recent experiments suggest that allopurinol may also act as an antioxidant with a mechanism similar to that of deferroxamine. Experiments with animals have demonstrated protection of the brain from oxidative injury[66], but clinical trials have been negative[67]. Indomethacin, a cyclooxygenase inhibitor, also inhibited ROS release in experiments with animals[13]. Chelating agents inhibit ROS release by limiting formation of ·OH by the Fenton reaction[68]. Deferoxamine has been widely investigated and there is no doubt about its protective effect in experimental models[68,69]. Inhibition of the Fenton reaction even seems to be obtained with inositol[70]. Inhibition of adenosine reuptake by propentophylline may also reduce ROS release during hypoxia[71]. Finally, administration of magnesium seems to have promising effects in reducing brain injury during asphyxia[72-74]. This could be due to the reduction in formation of ROS demonstrated in experimental studies[73]. However the risks of Mg administration should be taken into account[74].

In conclusion, the key role of free radicals in the development of fetal and neonatal brain damage has been amply demonstrated. The free radicals are implicated in the complex mechanism of cell death together with excitatory amino acids, intracellular calcium regulation, gene activation, apoptosis and inflammatory reactions. The attempt to increase antioxidant factors in order to limit the effects of oxidative stress have provided interesting results in experimental studies, but clinical trials have not yet definitely confirmed the advantages of any type of antioxidant therapy.

REFERENCES

1. Boveris A, Chance B. The mitochondrial generation of hydrogen peroxide. General properties and effect of hyperbaric oxygen. *Biochem J* 1973;134:707-16.

2. Packer L. Prevention of free radical damage in the brain: protection by α-lipoic acid. In:Packer L, Hiramatsu M, Yoshikawa T (eds) *Free Radicals in Brain Physiology and Disorders* San Diego Academic Press 1996; 19-21.

3. Bracci R. Oxygen toxicity. In Kurjak A (ed) *Textbook of perinatal medicine*, LondonThe Parthenon Publishing Group 1998;78-89

4. Oka A, Belliveau MJ, Rosenberg PA, Volpe JJ. Vulnerability of oligodendroglia to glutamate: pharmacology, mechanisms, and prevention.*J Neurosci* 1993;13:1441-53

5. Yonezawa M, Back SA,Gan X, *et al*. Cystine deprivation induces oligodendroglial death: rescue by free radical scavengers and by a diffusible glial factor. *J Neurochem* 1996;67:566-73

6. Evans PJ, Evans P, Kovaar IZ, *et al*. Bleomycin-detectable iron in the plasma of premature and full-term neonates. *FEBS Lett* 1992;303:210-12

7. Goplerud JM, Mishra OP, Delivoria-Papadopoulos M. Brain cell membrane dysfunction following acute asphyxia in newborn piglets. *Biol Neonate* 1992;61:33-41

8. Delivoria-Papadopoulos M, Mishra OP. Mechanisms of cerebral injury in perinatal asphyxia and strategies for prevention. *J Pediatr* 1998;132:S30-4

9. Mishra OP, Delivoria-Papadopoulos. Lipid peroxidation in developing fetal guinea pig brain during normoxia and hypoxia. *Dev Brain Res* 1989;45:129-35

10. Hagberg H, Bona E, Gilland E. Mechanisms of perinatal brain injury. In: Kurjak A (ed) *Textbook of Perinatal Medicine* London: Parthenon Publishing Group Ltd 1998;90-106

11. Anderson CB, Ohnishi T, Groenedaal F, Mishra OP, Delivoria-Papadopoulos M. The in-vivo identification of free radicals in newborn piglet cerebral cortex during hypoxia. *Pediatr Res* 1995;37:41A

12. Rauhala P, Sziraki I, Chiueh CC. Peroxidation of brain lipids in vitro: nitric oxide versus hydroxyl radicals. *Free Rad Biol Med* 1996;21:391-4

13. McGowan JE, McGowan III JC, Misjhra OP, Delivoria-Papadopoulos M. Effect of cyclooxigenase inhibition on brain cell membrane lipid peroxidation during hypoxia in newborn piglets. *Biol Neonate* 1994;66:367-75

14. DiGiacomo JE, Pane CR, Gwiazdowski S, Mishra OP, Delivoria-Papadopoulos M. Effect of graded hypoxia on brain cell membrane injury in newborn piglets. *Biol Neonate* 1992;61:25-32

15. Waterfall AH, Singh G, Fry JR, Marsden CA. Acute acidosis elevates malonaldehyde in rat brain in vivo. *Brain Research* 1996;712:102-6

16. Maulik D, Numagami Y, Tsuyoshi Ohnishi, Mishra OP, Delivoria-Papadopoulos M. Direct detection of oxygen free radical generation during in utero hypoxia in the fetal guinea pig brain. *Pediatr Res* 1998;39:63A

17. Bagenholm R, Nilsson UA, Gotborg CW, Kjellmer I. Free radicals are formed in the brain of fetal sheep during reperfusion after cerebral ischemia. *Pediatr Res* 1998;43:271-5

18. Razdan B, Marro PJ, Tammela O, Goel R, Mishra OP, Delivoria-Papadopoulos M. Selective sensitivity of synaptosomal membrane function to cerebral cortical hypoxia in newborn piglets. *Brain Res* 1993;600:308-14

19. Buonocore G, Liberatori S, Bini L, Pallini V, Mishra OP, Delivoria-Papadopoulos M, Bracci R. Synaptosome protein tyrosine phosphorylation maps in hypoxic Guinea pig. *Pediatr Res* 1998;43:317A

20. Sorg O, Horn TFW, Yu NC, Gruol DL, Bloom FE. Inhibition of astrocyte glutamate uptake by reactive oxygen species: role of antioxidant enzymes. *Molecular Med* 1997;3:431-40

21. Aizenman E, Hartnett KA, Reynolds IJ. Oxygen free radicals regulate NMDA receptor function via redox modulatory site. *Neuron* 1990;5:841-46

22. Goel R, Mishra, Delivoria-Papadopoulos M. Effect of dithiothreitol on lipid peroxidation induced modification on NMDA receptor in fetal guinea pig brain. *Neuroscience Letters* 1994;169:109-13

23. Vannucci RC, Perlman JM. Interventions for Perinatal Hypoxic-ischemic encephalopathy. *Pediatrics* 1997,100:1004-14

24. Rosehnthal RE, Chanderbhan R, Marshall G, Fiskum G. Prevention of post-ischemic brain lipid conjugated diene production and neurological injury by hydroxyethyl starch-conjugated deferoxamine. *Free Rad Biol Med* 1992;12:29-33

25. Oubidar M, Boquillon M, Maric C, Bouvier C, Delcy A, Dralet J. Effect of intracellular iron loading on lipid peroxidation of brain slices. *Free Radical Biol Med* 1996;21:763-9

26. Gutteridge JMC. Iron and oxygen radicals in brain. *Ann Neurol* 1992;32:S16-S21

27. Poulsen JP, Oyasaeter S, Sanderud J, *et al.* Hypoxanthine, xanthine, and uric acid concentrations in the cerebrospinal fluid, plasma, and urine of hypoxemic pigs. *Pediatr Res* 1990;28:477-81

28. Palmer C, Vannucci RC, Towfighi J. Reduction of perinatal hypoxic-ischemic brain damage with allopurinol. *Pediatr Res.* 1990;27:332-6

29. Beetsch JW, Park TS, Dugan LL, Shah AR, Gidday JM. Xanthine oxidase-derived superoxide causes reoxygenation injury of ischemic cerebral endothelial cells. *Brain Res* 1998;786:89-95

30. Fee BA, Yu XQ, Rootwelt T, Oyasaeter S, Saugstad OD. Effects of hypoxemia and reoxygenation with 21% or 100% oxygen in newborn piglets: extracellular hypoxanthine in cerebral cortex and femoral muscle. *Crit Care Med* 1997;25:1384-91

31. Rosenkrantz TS, Hoffman DJ, Kubin J, Fritz KJ, Mishra OP, Delivoria-Papadopoulos M. Effect of reoxygenation on the glutamate binding site of the NMDA receptor following cerebral hypoxia in newborn piglets. *Pediatr Res* 1995;37:53A

32. Gucuyener K, Gur T, Oz E, Turkyilmaz C, Ozturk G, Erbas D, Atalay Y, Hasanoglu A. Biochemical alterations in neonatal hypoxic ischaemic brain damage. *Prostaglandins Leukot Essent Fatty Acids* 1997;57:567-70

33. Kondo T, Reaume AG, Huang TT, Carlson E, Murakami K, Chen SF, Hoffman EK, Scott RW, Epstein CJ, Chan PH. Reduction of CuZn-superoxide dismutase activity exacerbates neuronal cell injury and edema formation after transient focal cerebral ischemia. *J Neuroscience* 1997;17:4180-9

34. Groenendaal F, Mishra OP, McGowan JE, Hoffman DJ, Delivoria-Papadopoulos M. Cytosolic and membrane-bound cerebral nitric oxide synthase activity during hypoxia in cortical tissue of newborn piglets. *Neurosci Lett* 1996;206:121-4

35. Lipton SA, Kim W-K, Stamler JS. Neuroprotective and neuropathologic effects of nitric oxide: role of N-methyl-D-aspartate receptors. In:Packer L, Hiramatsu nM, Yoshikawa T (eds) *Free Radicals in Brain Physiology and Disorders* San Diego Academic Press 1996; 71-82.

36. Groenendaal F, Mishra OP, McGowan JE, Hoffman DJ, Delivoria-Papadopoulos M. Function of cell membranes in cerebral cortical tissue of newborn piglets after hypoxia and inhibition of nitric oxide synthase. *Pediatr Res* 1997;42:174-9

37. Utepbergenov DI, Mertsch K, Sporbert A, Tenz K, Paul M, Haseloff RF, Blasig IE. Nitric oxide protects blood-brain barrier in vitro from hypoxia/reoxygenation-mediated injury. *FEBS Lett* 1998;424:197-201

38. Huang Z, Huang PL, Panahian N, Dalkara T, Fishman MC, Moskowitz MA. Effects of cerebral ischemia in mice deficient in neuronal nitric oxide synthase. *Science* 1994;265:1883-5

39. Yoshida T, Limmroth V, Irikura K, Moskowitz MA. The NOS inhibitor, 7-nitroindazole, decreases focal infarct volume but not the response to topical acetylcholine in pial vessels. *J. Cereb Blood Flow Metab* 1994;14:924-9

40. Keelan J, Brand MP, Bates TE, Land JM, Clark JB, Heales SJR. Nitric oxide and antioxidant status in glucose and oxygen deprived neonatal and adult rat brain synaptosomes. *Neurochemical Research* 1996;21:923-7

41. Akopov S, Sercombe R, Seylaz J. Cerebrovascular reactivity: role of endothelium/platelet/leukocyte interactions. *Cerebrovasc Brain Metab Rev 1996;8:11-94*

42. Mcae A, Gilland E, Bona E, Hagberg H. Microglia activation after neonatal hypoxia-ischemia. *Dev Brain Res* 1995;84:245-52

43. Kunstmann S, Mertsch K, Blasig IE, Grune T. High metabolic rates of 4-hydroxynonenal in brain capillary endothelial cells during hypoxia/reoxygenation. *Brain Res* 1996;740:353-55

44. Hagberg H, Gilland E, Bona E, *et al.* Enhanced expression of interleukin (IL)-1 and IL-6 mRNA and bioactive protein after hypoxia-ischemia in neonatal rats. *Pediatr Res* 1996;40;603-9

45. Yoon BH, Romero R, Yang SH, Jun JK, Kim I-O, Choi J-H, Syn HC. Interleukin-6 concentrations in umbilical cord plasma are elevated in neonates with matter lesions associated with periventricular leukomalacia. *Am J Obstet Gynecol* 1996;174:1433-40

46. Yoon BH, Romero R, Kim CJ, Koo JN, Choe G, Syn HC, Chi JG. High expression of tumor necrosis factor-α and interleukin-6 in periventricular leukomalacia. *Am J Obstet Gynecol* 1997;177:406-11

47. Savman K, Blennow M, Gustafson K, Tarkowski E, Hagberg H. Cytokine response in cerebrospinal fluid after birth asphyxia. *Pediatr Res* 1998;43:746-51

48. Yoon BH, Kim CJ, Romero R, Jun JK, Park KH, Choi ST, Chi JG. Experimentally induced intrauterine infection causes fetal brain white matter lesions in rabbits. *Am J Obstet Gynecol* 1997;177:797-802

49. Buonocore G, Gioia D, De Filippo M, Picciolini E, Bracci R. Superoxide anion release by polymorphonuclear leukocytes in whole blood of newborns and mothers during the peripartal period. *Pediatr Res* 1994;36:619-22

50. Buonocore G, De Filippo M, Gioia D, Picciolini E, Luzzi E, Bocci V, Bracci R. Maternal and neonatal plasma cytokine levels in relation to mode of delivery. *Biol Neonate* 1995;68:104-10

51. Schmidt H, Grune T, Muller R, Siems WG, Wauer RR. Increased levels of lipid peroxidation products malondialdehyde and 4-hydroxynonenal after perinatal hypoxia. *Pediatr Res* 1996;40:15-20.

52. Buonocore G, Zani S, Sargentini I, Gioia D, Signorini C, Bracci R. Hypoxia-induced free iron release in the red cells of newborn infants. *Acta Paediatr* 1998;87:77-81

53. Drury JA, Nycyk JA, Baines M, Cooke RWI. Does total antioxidant status relate to outcome in very preterm infants? *Clinical Science* 1998;94:197-201

54. Shin SM, Razdan B, Mishra OP, Johnson L, Delivoria-Papadopoulos M. Protective effect of α-tocopherol on brain cell membrane function during cerebral cortical hypoxia in newborn piglets. *Brain Res* 1994;653:45-50

55. Law MR, Wijewardene K, Wald NJ. Is routine vitamin E administration justified in very-low birthweight infants? *Dev Med Child Neurol* 1990;32:442-50

56. Halliwell B, Gutteridge JMC, Cross CE. Free radicals, antioxidants, and human disease: where are we now?. *J Lab Clin Med* 1992;119:598-620

57. Hall ED, Braughler JM, Yonkers PA, *et al.* U-78517F: a potent inhibitor of lipid peroxidation with activity in experimental brain injury and ischemia. *J Pharm Exp Ther* 1991;258:688-94

58. Bagenholm R, Andine P, Hagberg AH. Effects of the 21-amino steroid tirilazad mesylate (U-74006F) on brain damage and edema after perinatal hypoxia-ischemia in the rat. *Pediatr Res* 1996;40;399-403.

59. Phillis JW. α-phenyl-tert-butylnitrone : inhibition of free radical formation and release from injured brain. In:Packer L, Hiramatsu M, Yoshikawa T (eds) *Free Radicals in Brain Physiology and Disorders* San Diego Academic Press 1996; 215-232.

60. Packer L, Hiramatsu M, Yoshikawa T (eds) Free Radicals in Brain Physiology and Disorders. San Diego Academic Press 1996.

61. Rice-Evans CA, Diplock AT. Current status of antioxidant therapy. *Free Radical Biol Med* 1993;20:675-705

62. Inoue M, Watanbe N, Toshihiko U, Sasaki J. Targetting SOD by gene and protein engineering and inhibition of free radical injury. *Free Radical Res. Comm.* 1991;12-13:391-9

63. Armstead WM, Mirro R, Thelin OP, *et al.* Polyethylene glycol superoxide dismutase and catalase attenuate increased blood-brain barrier permeability after ischemia in piglets. *Stroke* 1992;23:755-62

64. Niesman MR, Johnson KA, Penn JS. Therapeutic effect of liposomal superoxide dismutase in an animal model of retinopathy of prematurity. *Neurochem Res* 1997;22:597-605

65. Palmer C, Vannucci RC, Towfighi J. Reduction of perinatal hypoxic-ischemic brain damage with allopurinol. *Pediatr Res.* 1990;27:332-6

66. Shadid M, Buonocore G, Groenendaal F, Moison R, Ferali M, Berger HM, van Bel F. Effect of deferoxamine and allopurinol on non-protein bound iron concentrations in plasma and cortical brain tissue of newborn lambs following hypoxia-ischemia. *Neuroscience Lett.* In press

67. Russel GAB, Cooke RWI. Randomized controlled trial of allopurinol prophylaxis in very preterm infants. *Arch Dis Child* 1995;73:F27-31

68. Rosenthal RE, Chanderbhan R, Marshall G, Fiskum G. Prevention of post-ischemic brain lipid conjugated diene production and neurological injury by hydroxyethyl starch-conjugated deferoxamine. *Free Radical Biol Med* 1992;12:29-33

69. Palmer C, Rebecca L, Roberts BA, Bero C. Deferoxamine posttreatment reduces ischemic brain injury in neonatal rats. *Stroke* 1994;25:1039-45

70. Phyllippy BQ, Graf E. Antioxidant functions of inositol 1,2,3-trisphosphate and inositol 1,2,3,6-tetrakisphosphate. *Free Radical Biol Med* 1997;22:939-46

71. Numagami Y, Marro PJ, Kubin JA, Mishra OP, Delivoria-Papadopoulos M. Effect of propentoffyline (PPF) on free radical generation during hypoxia in newborn piglets. *Pediatr Res* 1996;39:378A

72. Hauth JC, Goldenberg RL, Nelson KG, *et al*. Reduction of cerebral palsy with maternal $MgSO_4$ treatment in newborns weighing 500-1000 g. *Am J Obstet Gynecol* 1995;172:419

73. Schendel DE, Berg CJ, Yeargin-Allsop M, *et al*. Prenatal magnesium sulfate exposure and the risk of cerebral palsy or mental retardation among very-low-birth-weight children aged 3 to 5 years. *J Am Med Assoc* 1996;276:1805-10

74. Maulik D, Naumagami Y, Xanelli S, *et al*. Effect of magnesium administration on oxygen free radical generation during *in utero* hypoxia in the fetal guinea pig brain. *Pediatr Res* 1997;41:57A

Evolution of new tests for the assessment of fetal lung maturity.

Piazze J.J., Brancato V., Marchiani E., Maranghi L., Anceschi M.M. and Cosmi E.V.

2nd. Dept. of Obst. and Gyn., Policlinico Umberto I, "La Sapienza University" Rome-Italy

Introduction

Many obstetrics situations including premature rupture of membranes, premature labor, management of pre-eclampsia, fetal distress and elective delivery at term require a rapid and ameliorate test available for the assessment of FLM (1-2). Occurrence of RDS is still the leading cause of death in preterm babies, amounting for 28% to 70% of neonatal death in the seven industrialised countries. It affects 10-15% of all preterm babies weighing less than 2.500 g at birth (3). Infants weighing less than 1.500 g and those below 30 weeks gestation are more at risk to develop RDS and to die from it (4-5). The tests currently available for FLM evaluation are based on the biochemical or biophysical analysis of pulmonary surfactant found in amniotic fluid (6). Among the biochemical techniques for testing FLM, the determination of Lecithin to Sphingomyelin Ratio (L/S) by thin-layer chromatography (TLC) (7) and the determination of Phosphatidylglicerol (PG) (8-9) are the more representative; among biophysical methods are the shake test (10) and the lamellar bodies (LB) concentration (11-12. Lamellar bodies (LB) count was tested as an alternative to other biophysical method, the shake test; the mini TLC as a modification of the classical TLC for the assessment of L/S ratio; and in those cases judged intermediate-borderline to FLM, the Biophysical x Biochemical marker (BxB) was performed.

Materials and Methods

Lamellar bodies (LB) count: On a total of 164 samples of AF delivered within 48 hour from amniocentesis and at <38 weeks' gestational age, for the very low incidence (<1%) of RDS in neonates born at $38 \geq$ weeks (n=109), LB density (13) was calculated by analysing the supernatant of AF samples after centrifugation at 300g x 10 min at 5°. Time for total procedure was about 10 min. In the same samples shake test, planimetric and stechiometric L/S ratio and the visualisation of phosphatidylglicerol (PG) by TLC were performed to compare diagnostic accuracy with LB count.

The mini thin layer chromatography (miniTLC): On a total of 102 AF samples we performed the classical L/S ratio for FLM diagnosis and its modification, the miniTLC for investigation purposes. In order to obtain a faster method respect to classical L/S ratio, a reduction of AF volume from 4ml used for the latter to only 1ml used to run the miniTLC was obtained using for lipid extraction a chloroform/methanol 2:1 mixture (3 ml vs 12 ml). Lipid extract was run in a 5x5 cm area instead of the original 10x10 cm area on silica gel plates using a total phases volume of 27.3ml instead of 54.7ml. After visualisation with iodine vapours an area-to area planimetry was performed for evaluation of L/S ratio. For a better discrimination of the spots generated by classical and miniTLC, we digitalized the plates, then images were interpreted by means of a computer software able to generate numeric values from chromatographic spots.

The Biophysical x Biochemical (BXB) marker: The BxB marker represents the combination of LB count and L/S planimetric ratio in a single formula. All cases with one or both intermediate (2.1:1 to 2.4:1 for L/S ratio and/or 15.000-19.000/µl for LB) or borderline (2.5:1 for L/S ratio and/or 20.000/µl for LB) FLM indices and PG absence, delivered within 72 hrs from amniocentesis were selected for the study. Any intermediate or borderline tests were combined one to each other in a total of n=105 cases. By multiplying each sample's L/S ratio for the corresponding LB count, then dividing by 10^3 we obtained the BxB marker.

Results

Lamellar bodies count: A positive correlation between LB count and gestational age (GA) was found (r^2=0.38, p<0.001), while it was not observed a variation of mean platelets volume with GA (P = 0.26, range 4.3-7.2 fl). A maturity cut-off of 20.000/µl was considered after performance of the best percentual agreement analysis for positive and negative results with respect to other tests (Shake test, planimetric L/S ratio, stechiometric L/S ratio and PG presence). Diagnostic accuracy for LB count was: sensitivity 92%, specificity 89%, positive predictive value (PPV) 56% and negative predictive value (NPV) 98%. All FLM tests showed specificity >82%, highest value was observed for planimetric L/S ratio (91%). The PPV was highest for stechiometric L/S ratio (61%), lower for the shake test (41%). The NPV was higher for LB counts (98%).

The mini thin layer chromatography (miniTLC): The reduction in AF volume samples allows using a silica plate area of 5x5 cm instead of the classical area plate of 10x10 cm. So we can diminished lipid solvents volume of 75% (from 12ml to 3ml) and running phases volume by a half (from 54.7ml to 27.3ml). Total time required for performing total procedure was only 55 minutes whereas 110 minutes for classical L/S ratio and the cost requires 10$ while 25$. The diagnostic accuracy of the tests shows a strong correlation between classical method and the modification: miniTLC sensitivity 89% vs classical L/S ratio 85%, miniTLC specificity 91% vs classical L/S ratio 91%.

The Biophysical x Biochemical (BXB) marker: After performing the ROC curve for BxB, a FLM cut-off at 50 was chosen. When we grouped BxB for diagnosis of RDS, BxB values were significantly lower in the RDS than in the not-RDS cases (30 [23-41] vs 52 [50-70], P<0.001) (median [25°-75° centile]). As shown in Figure 1, BxB

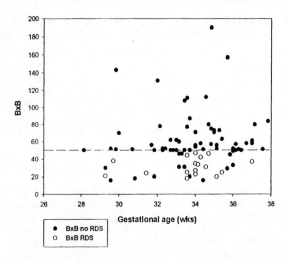

Fig.1: BxB values plotted against gestational age at the time of amniocentesis (wks) (P < 0.05, r=0.35). Dotted line represents BxB cut-off set at 50. Infants who developed RDS are depicted as open circles. Only cases delivered within 72 hours from amniocentesis were included.

cases had value <50. Regarding diagnostic accuracy were found: sensitivity 100% vs 73% for planimetric (plan) L/S ratio and 94% for LB; specificity 83% vs 68% for plan L/S ratio and 72% for LB; PPV 61% vs 35% for plan L/S ratio and 47% for LB; NPV 100% vs 90% for plan L/S ratio and 98% for LB. Sensitivity and positive predictive values were higher for BxB than L/S.

Conclusions

Clinical diagnostic tests are critical for the determination of FLM to provide timely prevention of premature. Many laboratory methods for the assessment of FLM are described worldwide, some are fully documented and commercially available while others are under research stages or clinical trial (14-15). The most broadly accepted test, which has become the "gold standard", is the L/S ratio in AF. However this chromatographic technique is labor intensive, requiring at least 5 hrs to completion. Several other procedures, including foam stability (10), the tap test (16), absorbance at 650 nm (17,18), and lamellar body number density measurement (19) have been proposed and used. The simultaneous performance on the same AF specimen of LB count in combination with a modified TLC (miniTLC) demonstrated high diagnostic accuracy (20). We have shown that both of them are able to successfully predict RDS in 89% of cases. Additional benefits of the use of combined LBs count and miniTLC include time and cost reduction, diminished volume of AF specimen, further to keep a good diagnostic accuracy. We suggest the combined use of LBs count and miniTLC is an option when accurate diagnosis of FLM is required and a choice provided that the hospital setting has a clinical laboratory and a Coulter counter equipment available. The combination of L/S and LB in a simple formula showed an excellent diagnostic accuracy as a predictor of neonatal RDS. The BxB marker successfully recognised all "immature" AF samples and represents the proportional increase of L/S and LB count along with gestational age and the dependence of one to each other as AF content of surfactant material increases. Surprisingly we observed a lower sensitivity and specificity of L/S and LB in group intermediate-borderline cases respect to the entire population observed in our laboratory. BxB is characterised by a 100% sensitivity but a relatively low specificity.

References

1) Herbert W.N.P., Chapman J.F. Clinical and economic considerations associated with testing for fetal lung maturity. *Am J Obstet Gynecol* 1986; 155: 820-3.
2) Maberry M.L. Methods to diagnose fetal lung maturity. *Semin Perinatol* 1993;7:241-6.
3) Avery M.E. Corticosteroids: the case for their use. In Preterm Labour (Elder M.G. & Hendricks CH eds), Butterworths, London 1981, 176-86.
4) Roberton N.R.C. Advances in respiratory distress syndrome. *Br Med J* 1982; 284: 917-18.
5) Saigal S., O' Brodovich H. Long term outcome of preterm infants with respiratory disease. *Clin Perinatol* 1987; 14: 635-50.
6) Dubin S.B. The laboratory assessment of fetal lung maturity. *Am J Clin Pathol* 1992; 97:836-49.
7) Gluck L., Kulovich M.V., Borer R.C. Jr. Diagnosis of the respiratory distress syndrome by amniocentesis. *Am J Obstet Gynecol* 1971; 109: 440-5.
8) Kogon D.P., Oulton M., Gray J.H., Liston R.M., Luther E.R., Peddle L.J., Yoh D. Amniotic fluid phosphatidylglycerol and phosphatidylcholine phosphorus as predictors of fetal lung maturity. *Am J Obstet Gynecol* 1986; 154: 226-30
9) Tsao F.H., Zachman R.D. Use of quantitative amniotic fluid phosphatidylglycerol as a criterion for fetal lung maturation. *Am J Perinatol* 1992; 9: 34-8
10) Clements J.A., Platzker A.C., Therney D.F., Hobel C.J., Creasy R.K., Margolls A.J., Thebeaulf W., Tooley W.H., Oh W. Assessment of the risk of respiratory distress syndrome by a rapid test for surfactant in amniotic fluid. *N Engl J Med* 1972; 286: 1077-81.
11) Ashwood E.R., Palmer S. E., Taylor J.S., Pingree S.S. Lamellar Body Counts for Rapid Fetal Lung Maturity Testing. *Obstet Gynecol* 1993; 81: 619-24.
12) Dalence C.R., Bowie L. J., Dohnal J. C., Farrell E. E., Neerhof M. G. Amniotic Fluid Lamellar Body Count: A Rapid and Reliable Fetal Lung Maturity Test. *Obstet Gynecol* 1995; 86: 235-9.
13) Dubin S.B. Determination of lamellar body size, number density and concentration by differential light scattering from amniotic fluid. Phisical significance of A650. *Clin Chem* 1988; 34: 938-43.
14) Spillman T., Cotton D.B. Current perspectives in assessment of fetal pulmonary surfactant status with amniotic fluid. *Crit Rev Lab Sci* 1989; 27:341-89.
15) Dubin S.B. Assessment of fetal lung maturity by laboratory methods. *Clin Lab Med* 1992; 12: 603-20.
16) Sepulveda W.H., Araneda H., Villanueva J., Vera E., Ciuffardi I., Donetch G. The tap test in the rapid evaluation of fetal lung maturity. *Rev Chil Obstet Gynecol* 1992; 57: 30-3.
17) Oulton M., Fraser M., Robinson S. Correlation of absorbance at 650 nm with presence of phosphatidylglycerol in amniotic fluid. *J Reprod Med* 1990; 35: 402-6.
18) Sbarra A.J., Chaudhury A., Cetrulo C.L., Mittendorf R., Shakr C., Kennison R. et al. A rapid visual test for prediction fetal lung maturity. *Am J Obstet Gynecol* 1991; 165: 1351-3.
19) Fakhoury G., Daikoku N.H., Benser J., Dubin N.H. Lamellar body concentration and the prediction of fetal pulmonary maturity. *Am J Obstet Gynecol* 1994; 170: 72-6.
20) Piazze J., Anceschi M.M., Brancato V., Cosmi E.V. Testing for fetal lung maturity. *Int J Gynecol Obstet* 1997; 59(3):255-6.

In utero surfactant for the prophylaxis of NRDS

Ermelando V. Cosmi, Renato La Torre, Maurizio M. Anceschi, Erich Cosmi Jr.and Juan Piazze

2nd Institute of Obstetrics and Gynecology, University 'La Sapienza' Rome, Italy

Introduction

It is well established that post-natal supplementary surfactant is effective for the treatment of neonatal respiratory distress syndrome (NRDS), although it is not devoid of complications, e.g., bronchopulmonary dysplasia (BPD); furthermore, the need of repeated doses make it an expensive and potentially hazardous method (vide infra).

This is why early or prophylactic treatment of NRDS is continuously sought. Antenatal steroids have been used quite frequently, depending on the country and the obstetric policy, with a success rate of about 90%. However, their efficacy before 28 wks' gestation on both the incidence and severity of NRDS still remains to be defined albeit a beneficial impact on neonatal mortality and on the reduction of IVH have been suggested [1]. This indicates that antenatal corticosteroids are not a panacea and that other pathophysiologic features are involved, such as the immaturity of the thoracic cage, and therefore the low compliance, and possibly of respiratory centers; in addition, there may be problems related to the lack of effectiveness due to insufficient placental transfer of betamethasone resulting from its inactivation by placenta 11-beta-ol-hydrysteroid dehydrogenase [2,3]; finally, corticosteroids are not devoid of possible maternal and fetal complications, e.g., acceleration of cell

145

differentiation at the expenses of their multiplication (see Table III in "Effect of

Corticosteroids on the Fetal Lung" by Cosmi *et al* in this book).

Administration of supplementary surfactant (SS) to neonates affected by RDS has become a

common method of treatment. However, endotracheal intubation and repeated doses of SS are

often required in order to facilitate its uniform distribution within the lung. It seems, therefore,

logical that the most rational approach would be the prevention rather than treatment of NRDS

and that the most natural way would be to instil SS into the fetal pulmonary liquid (FPL)

compartment, *i.e.*, either 1) at birth before the first breath after endotracheal intubation of the

extracted head from the vagina or from the incised uterine muscle during cesarean section (CS);

or 2) as we have found, in utero by direct injection of SS into amniotic fluid (IAF) close to the

fetal mouth and nostrils so that it will undergo uniform distribution within the FPL.

The scientific basis for this "prophylactic" IAF administration of SS spans three decades of

research on fluid dynamics and related biochemistry of FPL and amniotic fluid (AF)

compartments. Three lines of research have paved the way: a) Adams et al [4,5] provided the first

detailed and systematic studies of FPL. They defined organic and inorganic composition, surface

activity, fluid movement and comparison with other liquid compartments of the maternal-fetal

complex; b) Gluck et al [6,7], presented meticulous studies of the chemical development of FPL

and fetal pulmonary tissue; and c) Scarpelli [8,9] proved the metabolic origin of FPL surfactant

from pulmonary tissue and defined the lipid and protein gradients between FPL and AF. From

these data, Scarpelli suggested that AF phospholipids may be used to diagnose fetal lung maturity

(FLM); Gluck et al [10] later proved this to be correct. These studies had established the

biochemical interrelationship between FPL and AF. Two additional findings have reinforced our

appreciation of the importance of FPL surfactants to successful transition to air-breathing at birth:

1) FPL surfactants are the main substrate for formation of intra-alveolar bubbles from FPL at the

onset of air-breathing at birth [11]; surfactants form the ultra-thin films of bubbles that carry air to

the alveoli ("saccules") and establish normal gas exchange and alveolar stability; and 2) even after therapeutic intratracheal instillation of surfactant to the postnatal infant - first reported in the pioneering study of Fujiwara et al [12], significant clinical intervention is required. For example, multiple doses of SS may be needed and the positions of the neonate must be changed regularly to facilitate an even distribution of SS within the lungs. In addition, the untoward effects of endotracheal intubation and postnatal instillation of SS must be considered, including the associated hypoxia, bradycardia and barotrauma. It must be recalled that during the first breaths preterm babies may generate intrathoracic pressures up to -70 cm H_2O, thereby causing barotrauma.

IAF delivery of SS is subjected both to immediate dilution at the instillation site and to fetal swallowing, so that it may not enter the FPL compartment in sufficient concentrations [13,14]. Our observations on fetal sheep show that there is no net flow of FPL in and out of the lungs in the absence of FBMs [15, 16]. However, we have also found in pregnant sheeps and rabbits that aminophylline (A) given to the mother induces and/or increases FBMs [2,17]. The role of FBMs for inhalation of SS has been recently documented by Galan et al. in a study in pregnant rabbits where fetuses were paralysed with pancuronium and they did not inhale IAF labelled SS as opposed to non paralysed fetuses that inhaled IAF surfactant labelled with iron dextran [18]. Our observations in pregnant rabbits and ships have prompted us to combine the antenatal administration of A to the mother with IAF administration of natural SS. We anticipated that during FBMs, SS would enter the FPL and, hence, be distributed to the peripheral airways of the fetus [15,16]. Most of the data presented below have been reported in previous publications [19-22].

Material and Method

We have studied ten pregnancies complicated by impending fetal demise and/or imminent preterm delivery in which surfactant administration before birth was the only choice. Table I summarises maternal and fetal conditions of the study group. Four fetuses were affected by severe intra-

Table I: Summary of cases treated with intramniotic supplementary natural surfactant

Case#	Gest age (wks.)	Diagnosis	CTG	Doppler flow analysis	Pre - Surfactant Shake test	L/S	PG
1	28	I.U.G.R.	non-reactive	RED	Neg.	1.8	abs
2	32	I.U.G.R.	Reactive	AED	Neg.	2.0	abs
3	32	HELLP	Reactive	RI of uterine arteries	Neg.	1.9	abs
4	28	I.U.G.R.	Non-reactive	RED	Neg.	N.A.	
5	28	HELLP	Reactive	>PI Umb.art	Neg.	2.0	abs
6	24	Preterm labour-uncontrollable vaginal bleeding	Reactive	normal	Neg	10	abs
*7	33	Sjögren syndrome-IUGR <5 centile	Non reactive	ARED	ND	ND	
8	27	Placenta previa-uncontrollable bleeding	Reactive	normal	ND	2.0	abs
9	28	PIH	Non reactive	AED	Neg	1.0	abs
10	32	PIH, polyhydramnios	Non reactive	normal	Neg.	2.4	abs

* in spite of A to the mother at high dosage, it was impossible to elicit FBMs.

uterine growth retardation (IUGR); two mothers had presented also with HELLP syndrome (hemolysis, elevated liver enzymes, and low platelets). The indication for C.S. in 9 cases was the rapid deterioration of the fetal conditions. The 6th case was affected by vaginal bleeding which contraindicated further treatment with the utero inhibitor, ritodrine. Because labor proceeded rapidly without signs of fetal distress and the presentation was cephalic, it was decided to deliver the fetus vaginally.

After obtaining informed consent from all patients, amniocentesis was performed under ultrasound (US) guidance to collect AF for testing FLM; the needle was directed near the fetal nares and mouth and was kept in place. FLM was assessed by a rapid test, the shake test, and later on by L/S determination and phosphatydylglicerol (PG) measurements using the method of Gluck et al. [10], and lamellar bodies count [23]. If the shake test indicated fetal lung immaturity, a bolus of 240 mg of A was administered over 10 minutes to the mother followed by I.V. infusion at the rate of 0.02-0.1 mg/kg/min. The fetus was continuously monitored with Doppler velocimetry and intermittently with external cardiotocography (CTG). Five to fifteen minutes after the bolus dose of A, FBMs first appeared as vortexes of nasal fluid waveforms through the fetal nostrils, then began at a rate of 10 to 12/min as documented both by chest wall movements and inspiratory and expiratory flows of liquid through the nares. This activity was recorded continuously with colour Doppler equipment (Aloka SD 2000). Natural Surfactant (80-120 mg in 1 ml normal saline solution)* was then instilled through the amniocentesis needle directed toward the fetal mouth and nares. In 9 cases C.S. was performed under epidural anesthesia 60 to 150 min after the administration of SS. Before the incision of amniotic membranes a sample of AF was collected for further analyse FLM.

*Curosurf purchased from Chiesi Pharmaceutics, Parma , Italy.

Results

After IAF injection of SS, entry of the surfactant was seen by US as a sonolucent material that moved down the trachea and upper airways during FBMs, which from 10 to 12/min. had increased in depth and frequency up to 88/min. during A infusion. Some of SS was swallowed by the fetus. Following A infusion to mother, fetal heart rate (FHR) increased 10-15 beats/min. Treatment with SS resulted in a significant increase of the L/S. PG was also identified in the AF samples taken at C.S., T.S.R., Apgar score at 1 and 5 min, sex and weight are shown in Table II. The neonates were transferred to the neonatal ward. Six newborn infants (case 1-4 and 7-8) followed an uneventful clinical course to the time of discharge from the hospital. Case No. 5 showed radiological signs of mild RDS and at 3 hrs after birth received a dose of 120 mg of Curosurf. He was extubated 72 hrs later. Case No. 6 (birth weight = 630 g) was born at 24 wks' gestation in good conditions and was administered a prophylactic dose of 120 mg Curosurf, in accordance with the protocol in use in our Neonatology Department for all babies weighing less than 900 g. Because of the above protocol, she was artificially ventilated for 13 days and then extubated. At 35 days of life she died because of a disseminated CMV infection acquired following a blood transfusion for the treatment of anemia of prematurity. Because fetus No. 9, whose mother was suffering from pregnancy induced hypertension (PIH), was gasping in utero, we wrongly decided not to give A to the mother. At birth he showed some signs of respiratory distress and required 2 doses of SS in the neonatal period. Fetus No.10 was born to a mother affected by hypertension and polyhydramnios; even after a second dose of IAS before delivery, the neonate died 12 hrs after birth at 32+4 wks' gestation because of severe pulmonary hypoplasia.

Table III summarises laboratory and clinical data of two neonates whose mothers refused IAS therapy. The first one was born by emergency C.S. from a mother who underwent in vitro

Table II: Outcome of cases treated with intraamniotic supplementary natural surfactant

Case#	Mode of delivery	Post shake test	Surfactant L/S	PG	Weight (g)	Sex	T.S.R. (sec.)	Apgar at 1 and 5 min	Clinical outcome
1	CS	Pos.	5.0	pres.	1,035	M	30	8/10	Uneventful
2	CS	Pos.	3.5	pres.	1,650	M	25	8/9	Uneventful
3	CS	Pos.	2.5	pres.	1,700	M	45	8/10	Uneventful
4	CS	Pos.	NA		1,095	M	30	7/10	Uneventful
5	CS	Pos.	2.4	pres.	970	M	20	5/8	Mild RDS*
6	VD	ND		ND	630	F	35	6/9	Uneventful§
7	CS	ND		ND	675	F	45	6/9	Uneventful
8	CS	ND		ND	950	F	35	6/9	Uneventful
9	CS	Pos	2.0	pres.	1,228	M	40	6/9	RDS**
10	CS	Pos.	3.0	pres.	1,950	M	50	7/7	Pulmonary hypoplasia°

Umbilical artery ; RI, resistance index; RED, reversed end-diastolic flow; AED, absent end-diastolic flow; Pre-surf , fetal lung maturity tests (shake test, lecithin/sphyngomyelin (L/S) and phosphatidylglycerol levels (PG) before intraamniotic surfactant injection; Post-surf, fetal lung maturity tests (shake test, lecithin/sphyngomyelin and phosphatidylglycerol levels) in AF taken at CS after surfactant injection; N.A. not analyzed; I.U.G.R., intra-uterine growth retardation; HELLP, hemolysis, elevated liver enzymes, low platelets;neg, negative; pos, positive, pres, present; abs, absent; P.I.H., pregnancy induced hypertension;T.S.R., time to sustained respiration (normal values≤60 sec); C.S., cesarean section; V.D., vaginal delivery.

* treated at birth with one dose of supplementary natural surfactant and extubated after 72 hrs.

§ the same as case #5, extubated after 13 days. Died at 35 days of life following a blood-born CMV infection.

** The mother did not receive A because of fetal gasping. At birth he was treated with 2 additional doses of SS, a complete recovery followed.

°The neonate died 12 hrs after birth of severe pulmonary hypoplasia, after a second dose of IAS before delivery.

Table III: Characteristics of patients who refused treatment with intraamniotic surfactant

Case	Gest age (wks.)	Diagnosis	CTG	Doppler flow analysis	L/S	PG	Mode of delivery	Weight (g)	Sex	T.S.R (sec.)	Apgar 1/5	Clinical outcome
1	26	HELLP	React.	AED	1.0	abs	C.S.	630	F	120	1/6	4 doses of SS to neonate, interstitial emphysema, died following 36 hrs. after birth
2	26	PROM/ bleeding	React.	AED	ND	ND	V.D.	960	M	50	6/8	2 doses of SS to neonate, 48 hrs. under HFV, CPAP for 4 wks. Severe BPD, died at 8 months of age.

fertilisation and was affected by HELLP; the newborn, developed signs of RDS; for this reason after birth she was given four doses of SS. The infant developed interstitial emphysema and died 36 hrs following delivery. The other neonate was delivered vaginally because of bleeding that contraindicated further tocolytic therapy. He was treated for RDS with 2 doses of SS, with HFV for 48 hrs and CPAP for 4 wks. He died at 8 months of age from severe BPD.

Discussion

The present study follows our previous reports [19-22] and shows a successful outcome following prenatal administration of natural surfactant to the human fetus. Whereas definitive demonstration of distribution of surfactant into distal airways was not expected, several lines of evidence suggest that effective intrapulmonary distribution was achieved: 1) The surfactant was injected at the level of mouth and nares of the fetus and seen to be distributed into the upper airways; 2) FBMs induced by the IV administration of A to the mother were sustained and deep and increased in frequency up to 88 per min. 3) At the beginning nasal fluid waveforms were synchronous with chest wall breathing movements as documented by US and colour Doppler. Entry of surfactant into and distribution by diffusion throughout all potential airspaces are promoted by the agitation produced by FBMs [13,14]; this is analogous to the mixing of added substrates in lamb fetal lungs [13]. 4) It is also possible that smooth muscle relaxation induced by A may lower the resistance to the movement of SS through the airways; 5) Some of the SS was seen to be swallowed by the fetus which was expected particularly since gastric fluid at birth often reflects surfactant content of the lung. 6) Continued FBMs favour rapid dispersion and uniform distribution of the surfactant into the smallest airways and saccules as suggested by our studies in the sheep fetus and also by Adams et al [4,5]; 7) Consequently, the previously surfactant- poor FPL (see first AF L/S and PG analyses) had been enriched by the prophylactic surfactant at sites required for successful adaptation to air-breathing at birth.

8) The uneventful clinical course of most newborn infants in our study, is consistent with the

known role of FPL as the first substrate for normal surfactant function at birth [11]. Studies in baboons [13,14] indicated that antenatal IAF instillation of surfactant can be an effective prophylactic therapy. 9) IAF administration of Curosurf with a suspension of microparticles of charcoal in pregnant rabbits is followed by inhalation of the surfactant into the peripheral airways of the fetuses as documented at birth [24]. 10) Petrikovsky et al [25], have also shown the feasibility of intrauterine administration of surfactant. However, in their study SS was injected into the mouth of human fetus under direct vision through a fiberoptic endoscope, which had been passed through the cervical canal during active preterm labor after spontaneous rupture of the membranes. The authors found no fetal, maternal or neonatal complications in the three cases reported. Solana C. from Buenos Aires- Argentina, labelled SS with Tc99 and methylene-blue and injected this material into rabbits AF and found labelled SS uniformly distributed in peripheral airways of the fetus [26]. Galan *et al.* had similar findings in rabbit fetuses using SS labelled with iron dextran [18]

If we rephrase the NIH Consensus Development Conference Statement [27], intraamniotic surfactant is particularly useful in pregnancies where delivery is expected to be imminent and there is no time for corticosteroids to elicit their effect, reminding also that betamethasone crosses the placenta to the extent that fetal concentrations are about 33% of those in maternal circulation [2,3]. In any event, direct prenatal administration of SS appears to be a potentially powerful and unambiguous clinical approach. In one of our cases (No.9), the mother was affected by severe PIH with absent end diastolic flow (AED) and non-reactive CTG. Because the fetus was gasping, we did not administer A to the mother. We anticipated that the SS instilled into AF might be inhaled into the airways as a result of the fetal respiratory movements, *i.e.*, gasps. This fetus was delivered by C.S., weighed 1,228 g, had T.S.R. of 40 seconds and an Apgar score of 6 at 1 min and 9 at 5 min, but showed signs of respiratory distress. Thus, after birth he received 2 additional doses of SS, which were followed by full recovery after 14 days of intubation and CPAP. It should be noted that, whereas fetal gasping may favour the influx of SS into the potential airspaces of the fetus, some of it may be extruded following a subsequent grunt. Therefore, we speculate that administration of A or of another analeptic drug may be essential to induce the vortexes and regular FBMs, and thereby favour the influx of SS into the lungs (see Table I in "Effect of Corticosteroids on the Fetal Lung" by Cosmi *et al* in this book).

According to the suggestion of Szabo et al. (28) we also have started the administration of betamethasone directly I.M. or I.V. to the human fetus in cases of mild distress and potential preterm delivery (See article by Szabo *et al.* in this volume). We found that after the administration of betamethasone to 5 patients there was an increase of uterine artery blood flow and of FBMs, and a decrease of FHR, with no changes in middle cerebral artery blood flow. The patients delivered uneventfully.

Acknowledgements

This work was supported in part by the Italian CNR and MURST, Italy.

References

1. Crowley P, Chalmers I and Keirse MJN. The effects of corticosteroid administration before preterm delivery: an overview of the evidence from controlled trials. Br J Obstet Gynaecol 1990; 97:11-25.

2. Cosmi EV and Caldeyro-Barcia R. Fetal Homeostasis. In: Cosmi EV (Ed) Obstetric Anesthesia and Perinatology. Appleton-Century-Crofts. New York 1980; Chap. 7, Part I.

3. Marinoni E, Korebrits C, Di Iorio R, Anceschi MM, Cosmi EV, Challis JRG. Effect of betamethasone in vivo on placental corticotropin releasing hormone (CRH) in human pregnancy. J Soc Gynecol Invest 1997; 4(Suppl 1)Abstr 124,110A.

4. Adams FH, Fujiwara T: Surfactant in the fetal lambs tracheal fluid. J Pediat 1963; 63:537-542.

5. Adams FH, Fujiwara T, Rowshan G: The nature and origin of the fluid in the fetal lamb lung. J Pediat 1963; 63:881-888.

6. Gluck L, Motoyama EK , Smits HL , Kulovich MV :The biochemical development of surface activity in mammalian lung. I. Pediat Res 1967; 1:237-246.

7. Gluck L, Scribney M, Kulovich MV. The biochemical development of surface activity in the mammalian. II. Pediat Res 1967; 1:247-265.

8. Scarpelli EM (Ed). The lung tracheal fluid, and lipid metabolism of the fetus. Pediatrics 1967; 40:951-961.

9. Scarpelli EM. The Surfactant System of the Lung. Lea & Febiger Publ. Philadelphia, 1968.

10. Gluck L, Kulovich MV, Borer RC Jr, Brenner PH , Anderson GG, Spellacy WN. Diagnosis of respiratory distress syndrome by amniocentesis Am J Obstet Gynecol 1971; 109:440-445.

11. Scarpelli EM: Intrapulmonary foam at birth: an adaptional phenomenon. Pediat Res 1978; 12:1070-1080.

12. Fujiwara T, Chida S ,Watabe Y, Maeta H, Morita T, Abe T. Artificial surfactant therapy in hyaline membrane disease. Lancet 1980; 1:155-159.

13. Galan HL, Cipriani C, Coulson JJ, Bean JD, Collier G, Kuehl TJ. Surfactant replacement therapy in utero for the prevention of hyaline membrane disease in the preterm baboon. Am J Obstet Gynecol 1993; 169:817-824.

14. Galan HL, Cipriani C, Coalson JJ, Bean-Lijewski JD, Collier G, Kuhel TJ: Hyaline membrane disease surfactant prophylaxis in the preterm baboon: a comparison of postpartum versus *in utero* therapy. Prenat Neonat Med 1996, 1:122-130.

15. Scarpelli EM, Condorelli S, Cosmi EV. Fetal pulmonary fluid. I. Validation and significance of a method for determination of volume and volume change. Pediatr Res 1975: 9:190-195.

16. Scarpelli EM, Condorelli S, Cosmi EV. Lamb Fetal Pulmonary Fluid. II Fate of phosphatidylcholine. Pediatr Res 1975: 9:195-201.

17. Cosmi EV, Felli F, Grossmann G, Lachmann B, Robertson B. Improved survival in the in the premature rabbit neonate following antenatal treatment with aminophylline. IRCS Med Sci 1979; 7:115-122.

18. Galan H.L., Tennant L.B., Marsh D.R., Creasy R.K. Paralysis of the preterm rabbit fetus inhibits the pulmonary uptake of intraamniotic iron dextran. Am J Obstet Gynecol 1997; 177:42-49.

19. Cosmi EV, La Torre R, Di Iorio R, Anceschi MM. A novel treatment of fetal lung immaturity. Society for Perinatal Obstetricians, 16th Annual Meeting. Am J Obstet Gynecol 1996; 174:1(2): 487 Abstract No.653.

20. Cosmi EV, La Torre R, Di Iorio R, Anceschi MM. Surfactant administration to the human fetus in utero: a new approach to prevention of neonatal respiratory distress syndrome (IRDS). J Perinat Med 1996;24:191-193.

21. Cosmi EV, La Torre R, Di Iorio R. Intraamniotic instillation of surfactant for prevention of neonatal respiratory distress syndrome (IRDS): a preliminary report. Appl Cardiopulm Pathophysiol 1996; 6:3-5.

22. Cosmi EV Prenatal administration of surfactant. Editorial Prenat Neonat Med 1996; 1:109-11.

23. Anceschi MM, Piazze JJ, Rizzo G, Di Pirro G, Maranghi L, Cosmi EV. Amniotic fluid lamellar bodies density: a comparison with classical methods for the assessment of fetal lung maturity. Prenat Neonat Med 1996; 1:343-348.

24. Tannuri U, Maksoud F, Diniz EMA, Santos MM, Tannuri ACA, Rodrigues CJ, Rodrigues Jr. Intraamniotically infused surfactant is aspirated by the fetus and improves functional and morphometric parameters in an animal model of congenital diaphragmatic hernia (CDH). 12th International Worshop on Surfactant Replacement. Stockholm May 29-June 1, 1997. Book of Abstracts.

25. Petrikovsky BM, Lysikiewicz A, Markin LB, Slomko Z. In utero administration to preterm human fetuses by endoscopy. Fetal Diag Therap 1995; 10:127-130.

26. Solana C. Buenos Aires, Argentina. Personal communication 1997.

27. National Institutes of Health Consensus Development Conference Statement. Effect of corticosteroids for fetal maturation on perinatal outcomes. Am J Obstet Gynecol 1995; 173:246-252.

28. Szabo I, Vizer M., Ertl T., Arany A., Gàacs E. New therapeutic approaches for the antenatal prevention of respiratory distress syndrome. Proceedings of the 2nd World Congress on Labor and Delivery. Cosmi E.V. (Ed). Parthenon Publ. 1997 pp. 522-525.

Effects of Corticosteroids on the Fetal Lung

Cosmi EV, Anceschi MM, Cosmi E Jr., Piazze JJ.

2nd Institute of Obstetrics and Gynecology – University of Rome "La Sapienza"

Introduction

The state of maturation of the fetal lung is one of the most important factors for the survival of premature infants. If fetal lungs are immature; the infant will develop respiratory distress syndrome (IRDS), which is the leading cause of death in preterm neonates, accounting for 28 to 70% of neonatal deaths. Untreated (around 25%) babies with IRDS born before 28 weeks of gestation will die within 28 days of birth and another 25% will develop bronchopulmonary dysplasia (BPD).

In the pathophysiology of IRDS a deficit of pulmonary surfactant, as a result of immaturity of type II pneumocytes in fetal lung, plays an important role; nevertheless, other factors, such as the immaturity of lung structure, may be involved.

Therefore, fetal lung maturity (FLM) is mainly the result of the enhancement (either quantitative and qualitative) in the synthesis and secretion of pulmonary surfactant and structural changes of the lung parenchyma. The development of fetal lung begins at about 3 weeks after conception and continues for about 8 years after birth, throughout three phases: glandular period (3-16 weeks' gestation); canalicular period (16-24 weeks' gestation), characterized by the development of early bronchioles and the vascularization and differentiation of the epithelium; alveolar period (24 weeks' gestation-childhood), in which bronchiolar division leads to the development of thin spherical saccules (alveoli) that are lined by type II pneumocytes. The concomitant proliferation of capillaries around these alveoli makes effective gas exchange possible after delivery.

The type II pneumocytes produce intracellular stores, or "packages" of phospholipids called lamellar bodies, which are released into the alveolar spaces. Surfactant is the name given to this group of "surface-active" phospholipid becouse following delivery they can reduce the surface tension close to zero within the alveolar spaces during expiration of the newborn. Low surface tension within the alveoli allows these sacs to remain expanded during respiratory activity permitting continuous and effective gas exchange.

The most abundant of these surfactants is lecithin (phosphatidylcholine). Phosphatidylglycerol (PG) appears later and the documentation of its presence is the basis of several of the commonly used test for FLM. Other phospholipids (phosphatidylinositol, phosphatidylethanolamine), lung specific proteins (SP-A, SP-B, SP-C, SP-D) contribute to this group of surface-active substances within the lung.

Surfactant synthesis and/or secretion is affected by a number of hormones and pharmacological agents, including ACTH, GC, TRH, T3; agents influencing the intracellular content of cAMP, such as β-adrenergic agonists, aminophylline, substances increasing intracellular calcium or acting on protein kinase C and other compounds (e. g., heroin) (Table I).

The findings by Liggins et al. in 1969 that antenatal administration of GC or ACTH prevents the development of RDS in premature newborn lambs have stimulated a great deal of interest in the pharmacological enhancement of FLM (1); similar results have been obtained in 1972 in humans (2). For review see Cosmi and Roberston.(3).

Table I. Agents affecting fetal lung maturity

Stimulation	Inhibition
Glucocorticoids	*Maternal Diabetes*
ACTH	(Insulin,
	Hyperglycemia,
	Butyric acid)
Thyroid hormones	*Male sex*
	(Testosterone)
Thyrotropin releasing	*Transforming growth*
hormone	*factor-β*
(TRH)	*Barbiturates, prolactin*
Epidermal growth factor	
Heroine	
Aminophylline	
c-AMP	
γ-Interferon	
Estrogen?	
Fibroblast Pneumocyte	
Factor (FPF)	

Pharmacokynetics and pharmacodynamics

Glucocorticoids can be administered I.V., reaching a rapid increase in their plasma concentration, or i.m., in wich case they undergo slower absorption with a prolonged action (4,5). The i.m. administration is the most adequate for clinical use, because of the relatively rapid absorption of the drug depending on its hydrosolubility. The most common hydrosoluble esters are 21-phosphate (dexamethasone and betamethasone). The use of "Celestone Cronodose[®]" from Schering-Plough (21-phosphate/21-acetate betamethasone), allows to obtain a continuous relapse with a prolonged therapeutic effect and a rapid absorption. GC are metabolised by several tissues, particularly by maternal and fetal liver, although their relative contribution is unknown, and also by the placental 11 β-hydroxysterods dehydrogenase (11β-HSD) which converts active steroids into inactive 11-ketosteroids. This pathway is more active early in pregnancy (8-10 weeks' gestation) and its importance decreases progressively during gestation (6). For eliciting their action in the fetus GC must cross the placenta; therefore the question has been posed as to whether certain GC administered to the mother reach the fetus in sufficient quantities to elicit their biological effects.

Dexamethasone and betamethasone are the preferred corticosteroids used for antenatal therapy; they have identical biological activity and cross readily the placenta in their biological form. They are ligands for type 2 glucocorticoid receptors but both are relatively poor substrates for placental 11β HSD-2 enzyme, so escape inactivation. Betamethasone crosses the placenta to the extent that fetal concentration is about 33% of that in maternal circulation (7). Both hormones are devoid of mineralocorticoid activity, have a relatively weak immunosuppressive action and are more resistant to inactivation with a prolonged plasma half-life and a longer duration of biological activity than cortisol and prednisolone. In term of GC potency betamethasone and desamethasone are pharmacologically equivalent, whereas as inductor of pulmonary surfactant in the fetus, betamethasone is more potent (8). Biological action of GC depends upon tissues distribution, metabolism, delivery to target cells and receptors' affinity. Cytoplasmatic receptors for GC are present in all fetal tissues, particularly in liver, bowel, pancreas, stomach, skin, retina, brain, placenta, adrenal cortex and medulla, breast and lung, promoting cell differentiation (9). In some tissues, such as breast, bowel and stomach, receptor activity appears at birth, while in other tissues begins during fetal development.

In the fetal lung specific receptors for GC are present since 9 weeks and their concentration increases progressively during gestation, showing a greater affinity for exogenous GC. The pharmacologic effect of GC depends on receptor affinity, pharmacokynetic properties of the drugs and the gestational age. Strong evidence exists of neonatal benefits from antenatal GC therapy between 29 to 34 weeks (10).

In vitro and in vivo activity

The administration of exogenous GC modifies biochemical, morphological and physiological FLM parameters. In the animal model, antenatal administration of GC may affect different aspects of the maturation process of the fetal lung (11). They may influence the mechanical properties of the isolated lung in vitro, as measured by quasi-static pressure volume diagrams that show a lower opening pressure during insuflation (analogous to inspiration) and higher volumes of air retaines during desuflation (analogous to expiration), suggesting an improvement of lung stability. Treated lungs showed lower opening pressures and higher maximal volumes of air during desuflation than controls; however at the end of deflation limb they did not significantly retain more air (Fig.1). Furthermore, betamethasone administered to pregnant rabbits before delivery significantly increased the content of elastin in the fetal lung (Fig.2) and decreased serum protein leaking into the airspaces (12). These findings suggest that betamethasone acts particularly on the mechanical properties of the lung and less on pulmonary surfactant. It has also been demonstrated that GC act as transcriptional

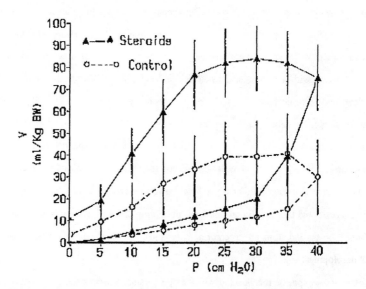

Figure 1. Quasi-static pressure volume curves in controls and beatamethasone treated rabbit fetuses at 22 days' gestation.

From Anceschi et al; Exp Lung Dis 1990; 16:593-605

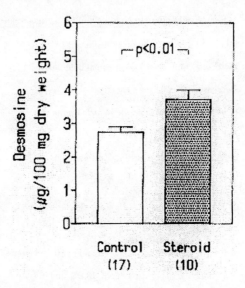

Figure 2. Effect of betamethasone administered to pregnant rabbits before delivery, increasing significantly the content of elastin in fetal lung and decreasing serum protein leaking into the airspaces. *From Anceschi et al; Exp Lung Dis 1990; 16:593-605*

activators for the synthesis of surfactant associated proteins (SP-A and SP-B). In addition, prenatal administration of GC primes the immature lungs, making them more responsive to exogenous surfactant (13) (Table II).

There is evidence that lung fibroblasts are the primary site of GC action and that fibroblasts, in response to the hormone, elaborate a factor (fibroblast pneumocyte factor) that subsequently acts on type II cells and stimulates surfactant synthesis (14).

Betamethasone has been shown to stimulate corticotropin releasing hormone (CRH) output by the human placenta (15,16).

Recently it has been shown that human fetal lung cells express GC receptors in term and preterm labor, demonstrating that these tissues are capable of responding to GC derived from maternal blood (17). Interestingly, it has been suggested that administration of GC for enhancing FLM to patients with multiple pregnancy may predispose to earlier delivery (18). These data could suggest that under certain conditions the administration of GC may lead to the stimulation of uterine contractility.

Table II. Summary of physiologic effects of GC in developing lung

1. Increased tissue and alveolar surfactant

2. Increased compliance and maximal lung volume

3. Decreased vascular permeability

4. Enhanced maturity of parenchymal structure

5. Enhanced clearance of lung water

6. Enhanced response to surfactant treatment

7. Improved respiratory function and survival

Clinical studies

Among hormones tested for the accelerating FLM, GC administered prenatally to the mother have proven to be effective in reducing the incidence of IRDS and of other complications, such as intraventricular hemorrhage (IVH), periventricular leukomalacia, retinopathy of prematurity (ROP), necrotising enterocolitis (NEC), patent ductus arteriosus (PDA) (19-21).

The clinical efficacy of prophylactic treatment with GC has been shown in several clinical trials. A meta-analysis (22) carried out on 12 controlled trials involving more than 3,000 women demonstrated that antenatal GC administration was associated with 50% reduction of IRDS and that its effectiveness was more evident when delivery occurred after 24 hours and within 5 days of drug administration. Data are not sufficient to establish the clinical benefit beyond 5 days after GC therapy and the potential benefit or risk of repeated administration. In vitro experiments (23) in human fetal lung explant demonstrated that inducible biochemical effects had dissipated by 7 days but structural changes persisted. A recent study has demonstrated in preterm lambs that the minimal interval from fetal exposure to GC to delivery for the improvement of postnatal lung function was between 8 to 15 hours (24). This approach is clearly beneficial in infants who are born between 30 to 34 weeks' gestation, but there has been some controversy on its effecacy for those born before 28 weeks; in these infants antenatal GC do not decrease the incidence of RDS, although they seem to reduce its severity. Nevertheless, Kari et al. (25) in a randomised multicenter study on dexamethasone versus placebo treatment in preterm pregnancies (< 32 wks' gestation) showed that treated neonates had higher mean blood pressure during the first 3 days after birth. In the treated group there was also a decreased incidence of IVH and periventricular leukomalacia. The cerebral protection confered by dexamethasone occurred in neonates born < 24 hours after administration, thereby rising the possibility that prenatal steroids are beneficial even when delivery is imminent. These findings are suggestive of the fact that the protective effect of dexamethasone against cerebral complications is independent from that of induction of fetal lung maturity, possibly because they enhance the maturation of the vessels of germinal matrix and the maturation of the cardiovascular system, thereby preventing neonatal hypotension that in turn predisposes to cerebral ischemia and hemorrhage. In a related study it was shown that incidence of germinal matrix hemorrhage is reduced in low birth weight newborns exposed antenatally to GC.

Recently the National Institute of Health Consensus Conference of U.S.A., (1995) (10) stated a general recommendation on the use of GC for the induction of FLM in fetuses at risk of preterm delivery. The optimal dose to administer was fixed in two doses of 12 mg of betamethasone given i.m. 24 hours apart,or four doses of 6 mg of dexamethasone given i.m. 12 hours apart. These therapeutic regimens result in about 75% of corticosteroid receptor occupacy, providing a near maximal induction of antenatal corticosteroid receptor-mediated response in fetal tissue (26).

For infants born at 29 to 34 weeks' gestation, treatment with antenatal GC clearly reduces the incidence of RDS and of overall mortality. While antenatal GC do not clearly decrease the incidence of RDS in infants born at 24 to 28 weeks' gestation, they reduce its severity; more important, antenatal GC clearly reduce mortality and the incidence of IVH in these group. All fetuses between 24 and 34 weeks' gestation should be considered candidates for this treatment, unless immediate delivery is imminent (<24 hrs) or GC may have an adverse effect on the mother. In infants born beyond 34 weeks' gestation the risk of neonatal mortality, of IRDS and of IVH is low. The use of GC in mothers expected to deliver at more than 34 weeks is, therefore, not recommended unless there is evidence of pulmonary immaturity as assessed by FLM tests or an intrauterin approach is feasible with the use of supplementary surfactant, according to our method (37-39).

The use of antenatal GC to reduce infant morbidity in the presence of premature rupture of membranes (PROM) remains controversial, particularly for the possible maternal and fetal adverse effects. Because of the efficacy of antenatal GC in reducing IRDS and IVH in fetuses of less than 30 to 32 weeks' gestation, the use of antenatal GC is appropriate in the absence of chorioamnionitis (10). Garite et al. have presented combined data from seven randomized trials concerning GC and PROM, and have found that the risk of maternal infection after treatment with GC was increased by 70% over those women with PROM, who did not receive steroids (27).

Nevertheless, a meta-analysis has shown that the rate of endometritis was significantly higher in women with PROM, who received GC compared to untreated controls (28).

According to the Crowley meta-analysis, it does not seem to be a significant increase in neonatal infection after GC treatment in pregnancies with PROM (29). In PROM at <32 weeks, repeated courses of steroids is not associated with an increase in the prevalence of clinical or histologic evidence in infectious outcome (30). In a recent meta-analysis, the combined use of GC and antibiotics for the treatment of preterm PROM, appears to diminish the beneficial effects of antibiotics (31).

Piazze et al. (32) observed decreased FLM indices in pregnancy induced hypertension (PIH), particularly between 24 to 33 weeks' gestation. Glucocorticoid administration increases significantly FLM in cases with the same gestational ages, showing the greatest effectiveness between 29 to 33 weeks, no significant effect was observed in the period between 34 to 38 weeks, apart from increased lamellar bodies count.

The benefits of antenatal GC therapy are still debated. In fact, Spinillo et al.(33), in a retrospective study, showed a significant reduction in the incidence of RDS in 21 pairs of twins treated with antenatal GC therapy. The reduction in IRDS could be the result of a significantly long gestational age and birth weight, noted in the treated group as compared to the non treated group. Ardila et al. (34) reviewed 134 pairs of twins between 24 to 34 weeks' gestation and found a significant reduction in IRDS only for a gestational age between 28-32 weeks; no significant difference was found for the other gestational age group. Conversely, Turrentine et al. (35) did not find any difference in the incidence of IRDS in 21 pairs of twins delivered between 24 to 34 weeks' gestation, compared to controls.

For eliciting their action on FLM, GC must be administered at least 48 hours before delivery; if this time interval between hormone administration and delivery of the infant is not available, GC are not clinically effective in reducing the incidence of IRDS. But it is not always possible to prolong the time of delivery, particularly in the presence of severe fetal hypoxia and/or asphyxia or imminent preterm labor. In the latter situation, in fact, the combined use of GC and betamimetics may induce maternal pulmonary edema.

Mechanisms of betamimetics and GC interaction include (36):

1. Increased electrolyte and water retention within the lung; 2. increase in mean pulmonary arterial pressure; 3. disturbance of membrane properties; and 4. decreased vascular resistance.

The incidence of pulmonary edema seems to be particularly relevant in twin pregnancies and in severely infected women, or in any other circumstance in which fluids are administered unjudiciously to the mother.

In cases where benefical effects of GC therapy may not be achieved, we suggest the direct injection of supplumentary surfactant in utero after the documentation of fetal lung immaturity and the induction of fetal breathing movements, as first suggested by us (37-39). In vitro studies in human fetal lungs have shown that GC, in combination with prolactin and/or insulin, increase the rate of lamellar body phosphatidylcoline synthesis and the molar ratio of surfactant phosphatidylglycerol/phosphatidylinositol to a value similar to that of surfactant secreted in vivo by human fetal lung at term (40, 41). According to the ACTOBAT Study Group on 1234 women between 24 to 31 weeks' gestation, the combined use of GC and TRH up to four doses of 200 μg was not effective in reducing the incidence of IRDS and the need for assisted ventilation. Instead, the incidence of maternal symptoms, such as nausea, vomiting and hypertension, were significantly higher. Moreover, TRH treatment was associated with an increased risk of motor and psychosocial delay and language disturbance in the baby (42).

Concerns have been expressed for the potential short- and long-term adverse side effects on the fetus and the neonate of GC therapy (Table III) (43). Although some animal studies have suggested that

Table III. Side effects of pharmacological therapy for the induction of fetal lung maturity

	GLUCOCORTICOIDS	AMINOPHYLLINE	BETASTIMULANTS
F **E** **T** **A** **L**	↓CELLULAR GROWTH ↑CELLULAR DIFFERENTIATION ↓SOMATIC DEVELOPMENT IMPAIRED MYELINIZATION ↓PLACENTAL TRANSFER OF GLUCOSE ↑UDP-GLUCORONIL TRANSFERASE AGED PLACENTA? LABOR INDUCTION	↑FHR VARIABILITY ↑GLICEMIA ↑GLUCAGON ↑INSULIN	↑GLICEMIA ↑GLUCAGON ↑INSULIN HYPOXIA METABOLIC ACIDOSIS ↑FHR
N **E** **O** **N** **A** **T** **A** **L**	↑THYMUS INVOLUTION ↓T LYMPHOCYTES ↓EOSINOPHYLES ↓IgG ↓IgM ↓ANTIBODY RESPONSE ↑CHOLESTEROL ↑TRYGLICERIDES ↑O2 TOXIXICTY ↓SOMATIC DEVELOPMENT IMPAIRED EEG NEUROLOGICAL- BEHAVIOURAL ALTERATIONS	↑FHR ↑GLICEMIA ↑GLUCAGON ↑INSULIN ATRIUM- VENTRICULAR ARRHYTMIAS ↑DIURESIS	↑FHR ↓POTASSIUM ↓CALCIUM ↓PTH METABOLIC ACIDOSIS ↑GLICEMIA ↑GLUCAGON ↑INSULIN ↑SIDEREMIA ↑HAEMATOPOYESIS

antenatal GC treatment might promote impairment in the response to hypoxia, data from human trials do not give evidence of such effect or of increased incidence of infection in treated infants, as well as no adrenal suppression (44). One or three doses of maternal GC begun at an early gestational age, caused symmetric growth retardation in lambs delivered prematurely; the decreased fetal size persisted until term (45). Follow-up of children up to 12 years shows that antenatal GC treatment does not adversely affect physical growth or psychomotor development, although long-term effects on the onset of puberty are not fully known (46).

It is well recognized that GC determine a significant alteration in the circadian rhythm of the fetal hormonal secretion. Several studies have demonstrated a suppression of fetal pituitary and adrenal axis for the secretion of ACTH and cortisol in the born baby when treating mothers with repeated doses of dexamethasone (47). There was a recovery within three days of life with no evidence of chronic suppression; cortisol rose appropriately in infants with IRDS or asphyxia (48).

It has been suggested that betamethasone produces a reduction of fetal breathing movements, body movements and/or fetal heart rate (FHR) variability; such effects were transient and returned to normality upon discontinuation of therapy; conversely, dexamethasone causes an increase in FHR variation (49).

On the contrary, we have found that the i.v. or i.m. administration of betamethasone or dexamethasone directly to the human fetus induces or enhances fetal breathing movements, increases umbilical artery blood-flow and decreases FHR (50).

This discrepancy needs a careful prospective investigation, since both GC are believed to act on the same pulmonary receptors, while apparently their actions on the central nervous system elicit different responses. The only absolute contraindications to the use of GC are: chorioamnionitis, peptic ulcer, and tuberColosis.

Polk et al. (51) evaluated the efficacy of a second administration of GC on FLM. Additional physiological effects were not found; nevertheless the SP-A, SP-B, SP-C and m-RNA levels were increased; a variation of these results was observed, that was related to gestational age. For this reason, the routine use of a second GC dose still needs a proper evaluation.

In conclusion, GC are effective in promoting lung maturity in fetuses >28 weeks troughout 34-35 weeks' gestation. Before 28 weeks GC reduce the incidence of IVH and neonatal mortality. Their use seems to be safe and devoid of contraindications.

References

1) Liggins GC. Premature delivery of foetal lambs infused with glucocorticoids. J. Endocrinol 1969;45:515-523.

2) Liggins GC, Howie RN. A controlled trial of antepartum glucocorticoid treatment for prevention of the respiratory distress syndrome in premature infants. Pediatrics 1972;50:515-525.

3) Cosmi EV and Robertson B. Morphologic and functional aspects of neonatal lung adaptation. In: Cosmi EV (Ed.): Obstetric Anesthesia and Perinatology 1981. Appleton-Century-Crofts. NewYork, 625-76.

4) Whitt GG, Buster JE, Killam AP, Seragg WH. A comparison of two glucocorticoid regimens for acceleration of fetal lung maturation in premature labor. Am. J. Obstet. Gynecol 1976; 124:479-482.

5) Anderson GG, Rotchefl Y, Kaiser DG. Placental transfer of methylprednisolone following maternal intravenous administration. Am. J. Obstet. Gynecol. 1981;140:699-701.

6) Cosmi E.V., Caldeyro Barcia R. Fetal Homeostasis . In Cosmi E.V. (Ed.): Obstetric Anesthesia and Perinatology 1981. Appleton-Century-Crofts. NewYork, Chapter 7, Part 1.

7) Gross I. Regulation of fetal lung maturation. Am J Physiol 1990;259:337-44.

8) Anderson GG, Lamden MP, Cidiowski JA, Ashicaga T. Comparative pulmonary surfactant-inducing effect of three corticosteroids in the near term rat. Am J Obstet Gynecol 1981;139:562-564.

9) Ballard PL. Glucocorticoids and differentiation. In: Baxter JD, Rousseau GG, (Eds.): Glucocorticoid hormone action. Heidelberg: SpringerVerlag; 1979, p.493-515.

10) NIH Consensus Conference: Corticosteroids For Fetal Maturation on Perinatal Outcome. JAMA. 1995; 275:413-417.

11) Anceschi MM, Luzi P, Broccucci L, Di Renzo GC, Cosmi EV. Effects of corticosteroids on fetal lung maturation. In: "The Surfactant System of the Lung" (EV Cosmi, GC Di Renzo, MM Anceschi, Eds), London: The Mac Milan Press;1991;p23-27.

12) Anceschi MM, Palmerini M, Codini M, Luzi P, Cosmi EV. Collagen and elastin in rabbit fetal lung: ontogeny and effects of steroids. J Dev Physiol 1992;18:233-236.

13) Robertson B. Corticosteroids and surfactant for the prevention of neonatal IRDS. Ann Med 1993;25:285-288.

14) Post M, Smit BT. Effect of fibroblast pneumocyte factor on the synthesis of surfactant phospholipids in type II cells from fetal rat lung. Biochem Biophys Acta 1984;793:297-299.

15) Jones SA, Challis JRG. Local stimulation of prostaglandin production by corticotropin-releasing hormone in human fetal membranes and placenta. Biochem Biophys Res Commun 1989;159:186-192.

16) Marinoni E, Korebrits C, Di Iorio R, Anceschi MM, Cosmi EV, Challis JRG. Effect of betamethasone in vivo on placental corticotropin releasing hormone (CRH) in human pregnancy. J Soc Gynecol Invest 1997; 4(Suppl 1)Abstr 124,110A.

17) Sun M, Ramirez M, Challis JRG, Gibb W. Immunohistochemical localization of the glucocorticoid receptor in human fetal membranes and decidua throughout gestation. J Endocrinol 1996;149:243-248.

18) Elliott GP, Radan TG. The effect of corticosteroid administration on uterine activity and preterm labor in high-order multiple gestations. Obstet Gynecol 1995;85:250-254.

19) Di Renzo GC, Anceschi MM, Cosmi EV. Lung surfactant enhancement in utero. Eur J Obstet Gynecol Reprod Biol 1989;32:1-12.

20) Cosmi EV. New frontiers in prenatal prevention of respiratory distress syndrome. J Perinat Med 1991;19(Suppl 1):170-175.

21) Anceschi MM, Di Iorio R, Soulakis G, Piazze JJ, Cosmi EV. New advances in prenatal prevention of IRDS: time for combinations. J Perinat Med 1994;22(Suppl 1):88-92.

22) Crowley P, Chahners I, Keirse MJNC. The effect of corticosteroids administration before preterm delivery: an overview of the evidence from controlled trials. Br J Obstet Gynaecol 1990; 97:11-25.

23) Gross I, Wilson CM. Fetal lung in organ culture. IV. Supra-additive hormone interactions. J Appl Physiol 1982;32:1420-1425.

24) Ikegami M, Polk D, Jobe A. Minimum interval from fetal betamethasone treatment to postnatal lung responses in preterm lambs. Am J Obstet Gynecol 1996;174:1408-1413.

25) Kari MA, Hallman M, Eronen Teramo K, Virtanen M, Koivisto M, Ikonen RS. Prenatal dexamethasone treatment in conjunction with rescue therapy of human surfactant: a randomised placebo controlled study. Pediatrics 1994; 93:730-736.

26) Gross I, Ballard PL, Ballard RA, Jones CT, Wilson CM. Corticosteroids stimulation of phosphatidylcholine synthesis in cultured fetal rabbit lung: evidence for de novo protein synthesis mediated by glucocorticoid receptors. Endocrinology 1983;112:829-837.

27) NIH Consensus Development Panel on the Effect of Corticosteroids for Fetal Maturation on

Perinatal Outcomes: Efficient of corticosteroids for fetal maturation on perinatal outcome. JAMA 1995; 273: 413-418.

28) Ohlsson A. Treatments of preterm premature rupture of the membranes: a meta-analysis. Am J Obstet Gynecol 1989;160:890-906.

29) Crowley P. Antenatal corticosteroid therapy: a meta-analysis of the randomized trials, 1972 to 1994. Am J Obstet Gynecol 1995;173:322-335.

30) Ghidini A, Salafia CM, Minior VK. Repeated courses of steroids in preterm membrane rupture do not increase the risk of histologic chorioamnionitis. Am J Perinat 1997;14:309-313.

31) Leitich H, Egarter C, Reisenberger K, Kaider A and Berghammer P. Concomitant use of glucocorticoids: a comparison of two meta-analyses on antibiotic treatment in preterm premature rupture of membranes. Am J Obstet Gynecol, 1998;178:899-908.

32) Piazze JJ, Maranghi L, Nigro G, Rizzo G, Cosmi EV, Anceschi MM. The Effect of glucocorticoid therapy on fetal lung maturity indices in hypertensive pregnancies. Obstet Gynecol 1998; 92:220-225.

33) Spinillo A, Capuzzo E, Ometto A, Stronati M, Baltaro F, Iasci A. Value of antenatal corticosteroid therapy in preterm birth. Early Human Dev 1995;42:37-47.

34) Ardila J, Le Guennec JC, Papageorgiou A. Influence of antenatal betamethasone and gender cohabitation in outcome of twin pregnancies 24 to 34 weeks of gestation. Semin Perinatol 1994;18:15-18.

35) Turrentine MA, Dupras-Wilson P, Wilkins IA. A retrospective analysis of the effect of antenatal steroid administration on the incidence of respiratory distress syndrome in preterm twin pregnancies. Am J Perinat 1996;13:351-354.

36) Cosmi EV. Role of beta-symphatomimetics and aminophylline on fetal lung maturation. In: Vignali M, Cosmi EV, Luerti M (Eds). Diagnosis and Treatment of Fetal Lung Immaturity. Italy: Masson;Publ.1985.p.127-133.

37) Cosmi EV, La Torre R, Di Iorio R, Anceschi MM. A novel treatment of fetal lung immaturity. Society for Perinatal Obstetricians, 16th Annual Meeting. Am J Obstet Gynecol 1996; 174:87 Abstract No.653.

38) Cosmi EV, La Torre R, Di Iorio R, Anceschi MM. Surfactant administration to the human fetus in utero: a new approach to prevention of neonatal respiratory distress syndrome (IRDS). J Perinat Med 1996;24:191-193.

39) Cosmi EV, La Torre R, Di Iorio R. Intraamniotic instillation of surfactant for prevention of

neonatal respiratory distress syndrome (IRDS): a preliminary report. Appl Cardiopulm Pathophysiol 1996; 6:3-5.

40) Mendelson CR, Johnston JM, MacDonald PC, Snyder JM.. Multihormonal regulation of surfactant synthesis by human fetal lung in vitro. J Clin Endocinol metab 1981;53: 307-317.

41) Snyder JM, Longmuir KJ, Johnston JM, Mendelson CR. Hormonal regulation of the synthesis of lamellar body, phosphatidylglycerol and phosphatidilinositol in fetal lung tissue. Endocrinology 1983;112:1012-1018.

42) ACTOBAT Study Group. Australian Collaborative trials of antenatal thyrotropin-releasing hormone (ACTOBAT) for prevention of neonatal respiratory disease. Lancet 1995;345:877-882.

43) Cosmi E.V., Anceschi M.M., Piazze Garnica J., Marinoni E. Prevention of Fetal and Neonatal Lung Immaturity. In: Kurjak A. (Eds) Textbook of Perinatal Medicine Parthenon Publ.1998 Vol.2,Chap.130, 382-1392.

44) Cotterell M, Balazs R, Johnson AC. Effects of corticosteroids on the biochemical maturation of rat brain: postnatal cell formation. J Neurochem 1972;19:2151-2167.

45) Jobe AH, Wada N, Berry LM, Ikegami M, Ervin MG. Single and repetitive maternal glucocorticoid exposures reduces fetal growth in sheep. Am J Obstet Gynecol 1998;178:880-885.

46) Shmand B, Neuvel J, Smolders-De Haas, Hoeks J, Tretters PE, Koppe JA. Psychological development of children who were treated antenatally with corticosteroid to prevent respiratory distress syndrome. Pediatrics 1990;86:58-64.

47) Terrone DA, Smith LG, Wolf EJ, Uzbay LA, Sun S, Miller RC. Neonatal effects and serum cortisol levels after multiple courses of maternal corticosteroids. Obstet Gynecol 1997;90:819-823.

48) Ballard PL, Gluckman PD, Liggins GC, Kaplan SL, Grumach MM. Steroid and growth hormone levels in premature infants after prenatal betamethasone therapy to prevent respiratory distress syndrome. Pediatr Res 1980;14:122-127.

49) Dawes GS, Serra V, Moulden M, Redman CWG. Dexamethasone and fetal heart rate variation. Brit J Obstet Gynaecol 1994;101:675-679.

50) Cosmi E.V., La Torre R., Fusaro P., Patella A. and Anceschi M.M. The influence of development of certain hormones and drugs on fetal respiration. In: Kurjak A. and Di Renzo G.C. Eds Modern methods of the assessment of fetal and neonatal brain. CIC Edizioni Internazionali,1997,pp.51-68.

51) Polk DH, Ikegami M, Jobe AH, Sly, P, Kohan R, Newnman J. Preterm lung function after retreatment with antenatal betamethasone in preterm lambs. Am J Obstet Gynecol 1997;176:308-315.

Effects of vasoactive agents on utero-placental and fetal blood flow and on fetal breathing movements

E.V. Cosmi, E. Cosmi Jr., L. Maranghi, R. La Torre

2nd Institute of Gynecology and Obstetrics, University "La Sapienza", Rome

Fetal behavior and fetal breathing movements (FBMs) are closely interwoven, responding to different physiologic, (e.g., sleep states, supply of suitable substrates) and pathologic conditions, e.g., circulatory changes including diving reflex induced by hypoxia, and to drugs, which may affect the fetus indirectly through alteration of maternal circulation and/or directly by altering FBMs and fetal circulation following their placental transfer. Because FBMs are closely interrelated with sleep states, or more specifically with the behavioral states of the fetus, they may, in conjunction with body movements, condition not only fetal lung growth and development but possibly fetal brain growth and development (1). We have studied the response of FBMs to various pharmacologic agents.

BACKGROUND

Rhythmic periodic FBMs were described and recorded for the first time in humans between 1888 and 1911 by Ahlfeld, Weber, Ferroni and Reiflerscheid, and in animals from 1871 until 1941 (for review see Cosmi [2]). Subsequent studies have in general denied that FBMs are normally present in utero, provided the fetus is not disturbed by physical stimuli or asphyxia.

Recent studies both on the animal and human have demonstrated that FBMs are a phenomenon of intrauterine development; in fact, normally the fetus does make episodic, irregular respiratory movements in utero (3-7). In the animal fetus, FBMs have been studied extensively by recording

173

intratracheal, intraesophageal and/or intrapleural pressure changes, phrenic nerve impulses, diaphragmatic electromyograms and the activity from respiratory center neurons (2-7). These studies have demonstrated that normally there are two patterns of FBMs: [1] A predominant pattern of rapid, irregular (in rate and amplitude) episodic movements, with interspersed episodes of apnea, is present more than 50 percent of time and accounts for more than 90 percent of the breathing activity. Interestingly, periodic sighs are often seen during these FBMs; [2] There is also a less frequent pattern of sporadic, slow (1 to 4 movements/min), deep inspiratory movements, like sighs or gasps, or expiratory efforts which resemble grunting, coughing, or panting. The first pattern, which represents normal fetal respiratory activity, only occurs during rapid eye movement (REM) sleep, and it is unrelated to changes in blood gases and pH values and to afferent impulses from aortic and carotid bodies (3-6); FBMs may produce intrathoracic pressure swings of 35 Torr or more and are independent of Hering-Breuer reflexes (6). This pattern is usually accompanied by increased FHR beat-to-beat variability and increased systolic and diastolic pressure and blood flow (3,4). Therefore they may influence the velocimetric appearance in the humans, e.g., RED and ARED of umbilical artery, which do not necessarily indicate impending fetal demise. There is also a circadian rhythm in maternal plasma estriol concentrations, which is inversely related to the circadian rhythm of cortisol levels at 30-35 weeks gestation (11). The second pattern is unrelated to the fetal behavioral state and blood gas tensions. The incidence of FBMs (expressed as minutes of breathing each hour) varies among species, ranging from 40 to 80 percent (3,4), it is two or more times greater in the evening hours than in the morning and increases with gestation. Interestingly, in the lamb fetus, FHR and beat-to-beat variability show a similar diurnal variation and therefore FBMs may provide an index of fetal well-being (2-4,9,10). Increased FBMs are observed overnight when the mothers are asleep (9,10). The causes of this circadian rhythm are unknown. This is consistent with the hypothesis that maternal cortisol or its placental metabolites may reach the fetus and affect the fetal hypothalamic-pituitary and adrenal function. In fact, the overnight increase in maternal cortisol levels coincides with the overnight increase in FBMs (10). In women receiving exogenous corticosteroids and with suppressed or absent circadian rhythms in cortisol concentration (12), the overnight increase in FBMs was not seen (13), thereby suggesting that during the last 10 wks of pregnancy the increase in FBMs is modulated by the circadian rhythm of maternal corticosteroids (10). Nevertheless, we have recently found that the i.m. or i.v. administration of betamethasone to pregnant women induces FBMs and an increase in umbilical blood flow (see below).

Some investigators have surmised that FBMs *in utero* are essential for the normal development of respiratory muscles and lungs (3,5,14,15). Pulmonary hypoplasia has been induced in lamb fetuses after either experimentally produced diaphragmatic hernia or bilateral phrenic nerve division (16,17). Sectioning of the cervical spinal cord, but not of the vagus nerve in the lamb fetus, inhibits lung growth (18). It has also been suggested that FBMs may play an important role in the synthesis and secretion of pulmonary surfactants (6); the negative pressure associated with FBMs may influence the production of FPL (17) which is a repository of pulmonary surfactant. We suggest they influence the appearance and disappearance of RED and/or ARED and that the latter are not invariably reliable parameters of impending fetal demise (19,20).

We have found that regular, rhythmic, and spontaneous FBMs can be induced in the lamb fetus by electric stimulation of peripheral somatic nerves and/or by cutaneous stimulation of the fetus. Following the stimulation, the fetus may continue to breathe in utero for several hours (8). Unlike the intermittent and irregular breathing movements described above, this activity simulates the pattern of the normal onset of breathing at birth; thus somatic sensory stimuli from the skin may be important determinants of the onset of breathing in the fetus and newborn (6). Experimental results in the lamb fetus are summarized in Table I. The first trials of electrical stimulation of the intact sciatic nerve generated spontaneous regular breathing movements in each fetus which lasted up to 25 min (1-25 min). The fetuses were refractory to this kind of stimulation for the first 30-60 min after the induction of anesthesia with 4 mg/kg thiopental given I.V. to the ewe. Unlike our previous observations in the ewe in which the sciatic nerve of the fetus had been severed before stimulation of the central end, stimulation of the intact nerve produced sustained contraction of the muscle of the limb which relaxed when stimulation was withdrawn.

Electric stimulation of the skin of the limb of the lamb fetus invariably generated spontaneous, regular breathing movements which were sustained for up to 30 min (2-30 min) (8). The rhythm,

175

Table I. Mechanisms inducing spontaneous regular breathing in apneic mature lambs fetuses

		Electric stimulation		Mechanical stimulation		
Ewe	Fetus	Sciatic nerve	Skin	Scratch	Rub	Vibration
1	1	2(+)	3(+)	3(+)	3(+)	3(0)
	1	2(+)	2(0)	2(0)	2(0)	2(0)
2	2	2(+)	3(+)	3(+)	3(+)	3(0)
	2	2(+)	3(0)	2(0)	2(0)	2(0)
3	3	3(+)	3(+)	2(+)	2(+)	2(0)
	3	3(+)	3(+)	2(+)	2(+)	3(0)
4	5	3(+)	3(+)	2(+)	2(+)	2(0)
	6	3(+)	3(+)	2(+)	2(+)	2(0)
Total		16(+)	18(+)	14(+)	14(+)	15(0)

From Scarpelli EM et al (8)

frequency, and intratracheal pressure (ITP) swings of these breathing efforts were indistinguishable from those elicited by direct stimulation of the sciatic nerve. Scratching and rubbing the skin of the lower leg of the fetus invariably induced sustained spontaneous regular breathing, which lasted a few sec to 5 min, whereas vibration of the skin (with the barrel of electric shear), under the restricted conditions of the study, had no effect (Table I) (8).

FBMs are reduced or suppressed by surgical stress, temperature changes, manipulation of the fetus (4,21). This probably explains the failure of some investigators to observe FBMs in the laboratory. FBMs are reduced or abolished in the presence of uterine hyperactivity, fetal hypoxemia of a moderate degree, fetal acidemia, infection, maternal and/or fetal hypoglycemia, maternal hyperventilation, hemorrhage, and cigarette smoking, and the administration of ethanol and certain sedatives, including diazepam, hypnotics and anesthetics to the mother, e.g., tiobarbitutates (19,20,22). Conversely, hypercapnia, the administration to the mother or the fetus of glucose (2), methylxanthines (2,23), doxapram or catecholamines induce FBMs or enhance their rate and amplitude (for review see Cosmi [22,23]). Sustained intrauterine asphyxia initially stimulates rhythmic FBMs which continue at fairly constant rate until they become weaker and slower; then an apneic pattern followed by deep inspiratory efforts ensues (24,25). The most common mechanisms capable of stimulating the respiration in the fetus and newborn are shown in Table II (26).

Table II. Mechanisms of respiratory stimulation in the fetus and newborn

	IN FETUS	*AT BIRTH*
NONSPECIFIC		
SOMATOSENSORY		
Cold	*	+
Proprioceptive	*	+
Tactile pain	**	+
SPECIAL SENSORY		
Visual	**	+
Auditory	**	+
SPECIFIC		
PULMONARY STRETCH	**	+
CHEMORECEPTOR		
Central	***	+
Peripheral	***	+

+ significant stimulus* not elicited in utero** of unknown or doubtful significance in utero***threshold to CO_2 is high in fetus: hypoxia usually depresses fetal breathing
From Scarpelli and Moss (26)

ANIMAL AND CLINICAL STUDIES

In two pregnant sheep in labor we have found that uterine activity exerts variable effects on FBMs. In fact, during regular uterine contractions (normal frequency, duration and intensity), FBMs decrease in amplitude and frequency, but tend to reappear in the interval between uterine contractions. On the contrary, in the presence of intensive and frequent uterine contractions of labor and delivery, or uterine hyperactivity FBMs disappears (19,20,25); thus indicating that fetal hypoxia and/or asphyxia inhibits FBMs.

Since 1970 a variety of ultrasonographic (US) methods (A-scan, real time B-scan, Doppler flow analysis) have been used to monitor FBMs in the human. Boddy et al in 1971 using an ultrasonic technique (27) recorded FBMs of the chest wall at the frequency of 40-70/min from 26 to 42 weeks' gestation. Like the FBMs of the sheep fetus, they were episodic, normally present 70% of the time, irregular and rapid. In 1985 Chiba et al (28) elaborated a method for US analysis of FBMs. In 1991 Isaacson and Birnholtz (29) recommended 2-D US combined colour flow and spectral Doppler analysis; they studied the anatomy and dynamics of respiratory function in the oro-pharynx, larynx and trachea of 10 normal fetuses. FBMs were recorded by observation of the longitudinal fetal axis (30). Fetal nasal fluid flow velocity was determined also by Badalian et al (31), and by our group (32) using a modification of the method of Isaacson and Birnholtz, which consists in scanning the nose in several serial sagittal and transverse planes, during FBMs the Doppler colour flow was activated. After detecting color signals, the sample volume was placed over the coloured area to obtain fluid flow velocities waveforms (spectral Doppler); the angle of insonation was maintained below of 50 degrees relative to the direction of nasal colour flow. The flow moving toward the transducer was coded red and the frequency of the waveform was displayed above the baseline (expiratory phase of nasal flow). The blue color indicated flow in the opposite direction (i.e., away from the transducer), and the frequency waveform was displayed below the baseline (inspiratory phase of nasal flow). We have used a similar method to study FBMs initially in 10 pregnant women starting before 22 wks' gestation up to term (19,32) and then in more than 50 pregnant women. The study performed in uncomplicated pregnancies, in pregnancies complicated by IUGR and preterm labor and bronchial asthma. After 25 wks' gestation the records were evaluated by obtaining more than 20 consecutive fetal breathing-related nasal flow cycles. With hard copies of each measurement in each case the averages of all cycles from that case were analysed for each of the following parameters: mean nasal peak inspiratory flow velocity, acceleration of the inspiratory velocity, expiratory fetal breathing-related nasal fluid flow velocity, acceleration and peak expiratory velocity and duration of the inspiratory phase, (i.e., time between the beginning of inspiration and the beginning of expiration) and the duration of the inspiratory peak phase, (i.e., the time between the beginning of the inspiration and the peak of inspiration), according to the method described by Badalian et al (31). A continuous video-tape of the spectral Doppler imaging of fluid flow velocity at the nose, of chest breathing movements and of FHR, and intermittent flow velocimetry of uterine, umbilical and middle cerebral artery was taken during each study. All studies were performed in the morning at least 2 hrs. after a light breakfast.

Rhythmic fetal breathing movements were detected in normal pregnancies from 10 wks' gestation onward (32). Characteristically, in our study the breathing episodes were brief and breathing frequency was relatively short in the younger fetuses; in addition they were not synchronous with thoracic movements. With fetal development, particularly >25 wks' gestation, breathing activity increased significantly both in terms of the duration of each episode and of frequency and amplitude of individual breaths; furthermore, they were synchronous with thoracic movements. In all cases, movements of the fetal thorax, which denoted a fetal breathing pattern, were associated with increased velocity of flow of fluid in the nostrils. The oscillatory flow velocity peaked during each half of the breathing cycle (viz., inspiration and expiration); the amplitude of the velocity tracings increased with advancing gestational age.

Effects of hormones

Conjugated estrogens (Premarin) administered to the mother as a 10 mg bolus enhanced FBMs, as documented by thoracic cage movements; this response was associated an increase of umbilical blood flow (19).

Betamethasone (4 mg bolus to the mother at 38 wks' gestation) was shown to induce FBMs while umbilical artery blood flow increased. In a tween pregnancy with preterm delivery, betamethasone was injected i.m. to one fetus in a dose of 0.5 mg/kg and i.v. to the other fetus in a dose of 0.5 mg/kg (Fig. 1-2).

Dexamethasone (4.85 mg bolus to mother at 29 weeks) had a similar effect but of smaller magnitude (19).

Effects of uteroinhibitory drugs

The I.V. infusion of 0.60 mg/min of hexoprenaline to a pregnant women at 41 wks' gestation induced fetal chest wall movements and inspiratory nasal fluid flow followed by expiratory fluid flow

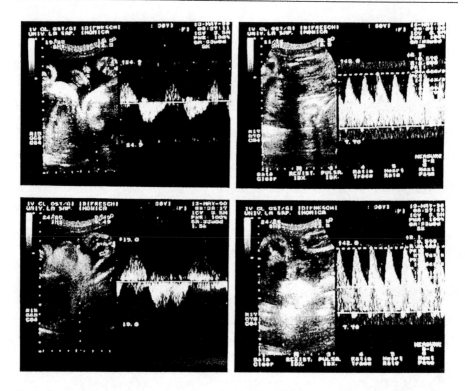

Fig. 1. Tween pregnancy in a women at 33 weeks gestation with preterm delivery. From left to right, fetal breathing movements (FBMs) before betamethasone was given to the fetuses and umbilical artery blood flow.

of small magnitude and short duration (19,20). On the contrary, the I.V. infusion of 0.8-1.4 mg/kg/hr of aminophylline to the mother induced prompt and sustained fetal chest wall movements which were accompanied and followed by sustained nasal fluid flow whose inspiratory and expiratory phases increased in frequency (up to 88/min) and amplitude; after a bolus of aminophylline to mother nasal fluid flow was in the form of vortexes. We have also found that the depression created by a vorticous fluid may promote the inhalation of surfactant, when administrated prophylactically in proximity of fetal mouth/nose (19,32).

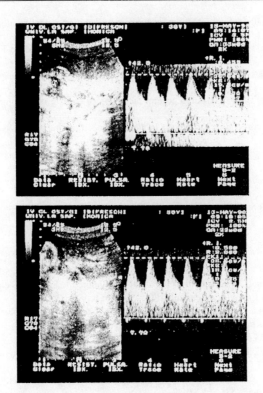

Fig. 2. Same cases as Fig. 1. The i.v. injection of betamethasone to one fetus induces FBMs and an increase on umbilical artery velocimetry. The i.m. injection of 0.5 mg/kg of betamethasone to the other fetus produced 30 min after the injection similar effects on FBMs and umbilical artery velocimetry.

Conclusions

Several animal and human studies indicate that in the fetus there is a progressive maturation of respiratory regulation. The role of FBMs in lung growth and development, and possibly brain growth, and in the transition at birth from placental exchange to air-breathing is unknown. FBMs are related to fetal sleep states and may be inhibited or induced by many factors, hormones and pharmacologic agents. During profound hypoxemia gasping occurs independent of the control of peripheral chemoreceptors; it is ominous, because it precedes fetal demise (6). Mechanisms controlling gasping are poorly understood. Somatosensory stimulation, sciatic nerve and cutaneous stimulation, elicit somatic respiratory reflex in the mature lamb fetus that results in FBMs. During

REM sleep FBMs are activated by somatosensory stimulation; in REM sleep FBMs are either in

phase with the stimulus or are not responsive to it (2,6,24,25). NREM sleep appears to be a

significant inhibitor of FBMs (33). An important factor which cause a reduction and then inhibition

of FBMs are uterine contractions, particularly in the presence of uterine hyperactivity.

There are many endogenous modulators of FBMs, including glucose, catecholamines, opiates,

prostaglandins and serotonin, and exogenous modulators of FBMs, including estrogens,

corticosteroids, beta-stimulants and aminophylline.

REFERENCES

1. Prechtl HRF. Prenatal development of postnatal behaviour. In: Rauh H, Steinhausen E (Eds): Psychobiology and Early Development. Elsevier Science Pbl, 1987
2. Cosmi EV, Caldegno-Bercia R. Fetal homeostasis. In: Cosmi EV (Ed): Obstetric Anesthesia and Perinatology, Appleton Century Crofts, New York, Chap 7, 1981
3. Boddy GS and Dawes DS. Fetal breathing. Brit Med Bull 31:3, 1975
4. Dawes GS, Fox HE, Leduc BM et al. Respiratory movements and rapid eye movements sleep in the foetal lamb. J Physiol (London) 220: 119, 1972
5. Dawes GS. Revolutions and cyclical rhythms in prenatal life: Fetal respiratory movements rediscovered. Pediatrics 51: 965, 1973
6. Cosmi EV and Condorelli S. Onset of breathing. In: Mushin WW, Severinghaus JW, Tiengo M, Gorini S (Eds): Physiologic Basis of Anaesthesiology. Theory and Practice. Piccin Medical Books, Padua, Italy 1973, p 239
7. Duhenhoelter JH, Pritchard JA. Fetal respiration: A review. Am J Obstet Gynecol 129: 326, 1977
8. Scarpelli EM, Condorelli S and Cosmi EV. Cutaneous stimulation and generation of breathing movements. Pediatr Res 11: 24, 1977
9. Dalton KJ, Dawes GS, Patrick JE. Diurnal, respiratory, and other rhythms of fetal heart rate in lambs. Am J Obstet Gynecol 127: 414, 1977
10. Richardson BS and Gagnon R. Fetal breathing and body movements. In: Maternal-Fetal Medicine. Principles and Practice. Creasy RK (Ed) W.B. Saunders, 1994, Chap 17
11. Patrick J, Challis J, Campbell K, et al. Circadian rhythms in maternal plasma cortisol and estriol concentrations at 30 to 31, 34 to 35, and 38 to 39 weeks gestational age. Am J Obstet Gynecol 136: 325, 1980
12. Challis J, Patrick J, Richardson B et al. Loss of diurnal rhythm in plasma estrone, estradiol and estriol in women treated with synthetic corticosteroids at 33 to 35 weeks gestation. Am J Obstet Gynecol 139: 338, 1981
13. Patrick J, Challis J, Campbell K, et al. Effects of synthetic glucocorticoid administration on human fetal breathing movements at 34 to 35 weeks' gestational age. Am J Obstet Gynecol 139: 324, 1981
14. Snyder FF, Rosenfeld M. Intrauterine respiratory movements of the human fetus. JAMA 108: 1946, 1937
15. Potter EL, Bohlender GP. Intrauterine respiration in relation to development of fetal lung. Am J Obstet Gynecol 42: 14, 1941

16. Alcorn D, Adamson TM, Maloney JE et al. Morphological effects of phrenicectomy in the fetal lamb lung. J Anat 124: 526, 1977

17. Fewell JE, Lee CC, Kitterman JA. Effects of phrenic nerve section on the respiratory system fetal lambs. J Appl Physiol 51: 293-6, 1981

18. Wigglesworth JS. Experimental growth retardation in the foetal rat. J Pathol Bacteriol 88: 1 , 1964

19. Cosmi EV, La Torre R, Fusaro P, Patella A and Anceschi MM: The influence of development, of certain hormones and drugs on fetal respiration. In: A. Kurjak and G.C. Di Renzo Eds. "Modern methods of the assessment of fetal and neonatal brain" CIC Edizioni Internazionali, 1997, pp.51-68.

20.

21. Martin CB Jr, Murata Y, Petrie RH, Parer JT. Respiratory movements in the fetal Rhesus monkey. Am J Obstet Gynecol 119: 939, 1974

22. Cosmi EV. Effects of anesthesia on the uteroplacental blood flow and the fetus. In: Cosmi EV (Ed), Obstetric Anesthesia and Perinatology, Appleton-Century-Crofts. New York, 1981 Chap 10

23. Cosmi EV. Effects of anesthesia on labor and delivery. In: Cosmi EV (Ed), Obstetric Anesthesia and Perinatology, Appleton-Century-Crofts. New York, 1981 Chap 11

24. Cosmi EV. Fetal homeostasis. In: Scarpelli EM (Ed) Pulmonary Physiology of the Fetus, the Newborn and Child, Lea & Febiger, Philadelphia, 1975, p 61

25. Condorelli S, Scarpelli EM. Fetal breathing: Induction in utero and effects of vagotomy and barbiturates. J Pediatr 88: 94, 1976

26. Scarpelli EM, Moss IR. Control of fetal and neonatal breathing and its disturbances. Clin Chest Med 1: 145, 1980

27. Boddy K, Robinson JS. External method for detection of fetal breathing in utero. Lancet 2: 1231, 1971

28. Chida Y, Utsu M, Kanzaki T, Hasegawa T. Changes in venous flow and intra-tracheal flow in fetal breathing movements. Ultrasound Med Biol 11: 43, 1985

29. Isaacson G, Birnholz JC. Human fetal upper respiratory tract function as revealed by ultrasonography. Ann Otol Rhinol Laryngol 100: 743, 1991

30. Fox HE, Inglis J, Steinbrecker M. Fetal breathing movements in uncomplicated pregnancies: relationship to gestational age. Am J Obstet Gynecol 134: 544, 1979

31. Badalian SS, Chao CR, Fox HE, Timor-Tritsch IE. Fetal breathing-related nasal fluid flow velocity in uncomplicated pregnancies. Am J Obstet Gynecol 169: 563, 1993

32. Cosmi EV, La Torre R, Di Iorio R, Anceschi MM. Surfactant administration to the human fetus in utero: a new approach to prevention of neonatal respiratory distress syndrome. J Perinat Med 24: 191, 1996

33. Yee WFH. Developmental physiology of respiratory control. In: Scarpelli EM (Ed). Pulmonary Physiology. Lea & Feboger, Philadelphia, 1990 Chap 16

The effect of direct fetal steroid treatment on fetal heart rate variation

I. Szabó, M. Vizer, T. Ertl, A. Arany and E. Gács

University Medical School of Pécs, Department of Obstetrics and Gynecology,
Édesanyák útja 17, H-7624 Pécs, Hungary

Maternal antenatal corticosteroid treatment is widely accepted for the prevention of respiratory distress syndrome in expectation of preterm birth. Glucocorticoid therapy is effective if delivery occurs at least 24-48 hours after the first dose was given. Recent data suggest, that antenatal corticosteroid administration causes considerable but transient changes in fetal heart rate (FHR) variation. Short term variation (STV) increases after maternal dexamethasone treatment for up to a day (1). In contrast, FHR variation is reduced for 3 days after maternal betamethasone therapy (2).

Animal studies have shown that single direct fetal intramuscular injection of betamethasone improved functional lung maturity (3). Beneficial effects of direct fetal corticosteroid was observed in human pregnancies as well (4).

In our department when impending or indicated preterm delivery was expected to occur within 24-48 hours after admission, we administered intramuscular betamethasone to the fetus (0.5 mg/kg-estimated fetal weight) under continuous ultrasound-guidance in 21 pregnancies (gestational age: 26-34 weeks) complicated with preterm premature rupture of membranes, oligohydramnios or preeclampsia and intrauterine growth retardation. Fourteen of these women had 134 cardiotocograph records that were complete (daily or more for one day before and three days after drug administration). Clinical data of patients are listed in the table.

	steroid
Cases (n)	14
Gestational age at intervention (weeks)	28.4 (26-34)
PPROM / intact membranes	5/9
Geastational age at delivery (weeks)	29.7 (26-35)
Birth weight (g)	1280 (600-2210)
Apgar score (5-min)	8.9 (7-10)
Severe RDS (n)	3
28-day survival (n)	12

PPROM, preterm premature rupture of membranes; RDS, respiratory distress syndrome. Data are expressed as absolute values or mean (range).

One day before fetal treatment the mean STV was 6.13 ± 0.48 msec. Subsequently we observed a downward trend in the mean STV value measured immediately, one day and 2 days after fetal betamethasone injection (5.02 ± 0.67, 5.43 ± 0.37, and 4.95 ± 0.23 msec, respectively). The mean STV value 48 hours after fetal betamethasone was significantly decreased compared with the initial value ($p < 0.02$). In more than one third of these cases (35.7%) STV fell transiently below the normal range for gestational age. All values returned to baseline on day 3.

Inspite of this transient reduction in STV, fetal betamethasone treatment did not induce any FHR deceleration or abnormal doppler flow-velocimetry result suggesting that these alterations are not mediated through fetal hypoxaemia.

Glucocorticoid receptor occupancy affects the neural activity of the presumptive sleep centre in the fetal pons (5). Reduction in body movements after betamethasone administration may be the result of prolonged periods of fetal quiescence and to a lesser extent due to shorter activity periods (2). The transiently decreased FHR variation may be related to the reduction in body movements.

It seems that after direct fetal betamethasone administration the changes in FHR variation are more rapid probably because the action does not depend on placental

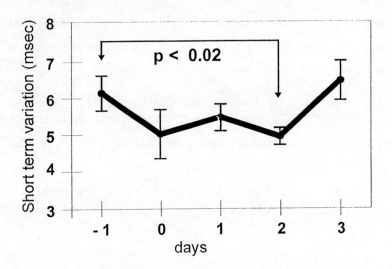

transfer and metabolism, single dose is used and the dosage is more exact.

Knowledge of this phenomenon both after maternal and fetal betamethasone treatment is important in assessment of fetal well-being. Clinicians should be aware that the reduction in fetal activity and heart rate variation following betamethasone treatment may have nothing to do with fetal distress and should not necessarily prompt immediate delivery.

Sponsored by the EEC Biomed 2 program - EURAIL (Europe Against Immature Lung)

References

1. Dawes GS, Serra-Serra W, Moulden M, Redman CWG. Dexamethasone and fetal heart rate variation. *Br J Obstet Gynaecol* 1994; 101: 675-9

2. Derks JB, Mulder EJH, Visser GHA. The effects of maternal betamethasone administration on the fetus. *Br J Obstet Gynaecol* 1995; 102: 40-6

3. Polk DH, Ikegami M, Jobe AH, Newnham J, Sly P, Kohen R, Kelly R. Postnatal lung function in preterm lambs: Effects of a single exposure to betamethasone and thyroid hormones. *Am J Obstet Gynecol* 1995; 172: 872-81

4. Szabó I, Ertl T, Vizer M, Arany A, Gács E. In utero fetal steroid or surfactant treatment and perinatal outcome. *Acta Obstet Gynecol Scand* 1997; 76, 167: 12

5. de Kloet ER, Reul JMHM, Sutanto W. Corticosteroids and the brain. *J Steroid Biochem Mol Biol* 1990; 37: 387-94

COLOR DOPPLER AND 3-D ULTRASOUND IN THE STUDY

OF UTERINE ANOMALIES

Sanja Kupesic and Asim Kurjak

Department of Obstetrics and Gynecology, Medical School, University of Zagreb,

Sveti Duh Hospital, Sveti Duh 64, Zagreb, Croatia

INTRODUCTION

Congenital uterine malformations are variable in frequency and are usually estimated to represent 3-4%, although less than half have clinical symptoms[1-3]. Uterine anomalies can be organized into the following categories: unicornuate uterus, uterus didelphus, the bicornuate uterus and the septate uterus. Unicornuate uterus is due to a failure of development in one Muellerian duct. A rudimentary horn may be present and implantation in this horn is followed by a very high rate of pregnancy wastage or tubal pregnancies. This anomaly can be precisely diagnosed using three-dimensional ultrasound. Uterus didelphus is characterized with lack of fusion of the two Muellerian ducts. This results in duplication of the corpus and cervix. These patients usually have no difficulties with menstruation and coitus. Pregnancy in this anomaly is associated with increased risk of malpresentations and premature labor. Partial lack of fusion of the two Muellerian ducts produces a single cervix with a varying degree of separation in the two uterine horns. This anomaly is called "bicornuate uterus" and has a high rate of early abortion, preterm labor and breech presentations. Partial lack of resorption of the midline septum between the two Muellerian ducts results in defects that range from a partial midline septum to a significant midline division of the endometrial cavity. A total failure in resorption results in a longitudinal vaginal septum, so called "double vagina".

UTERINE ANOMALIES: COMPLICATIONS AND DIAGNOSIS

The respective frequency of symptomatic malformations is dominated by septate uterus (close to 50%) compared with other malformations[3,4].

During the first trimester of pregnancy, the risk of spontaneous abortion in this group is between 28% and 45%, while during the second trimester the frequency of late spontaneous abortions is approximately 5%[3]. Premature deliveries, abnormal fetal presentations, irregular uterine activity and dystocia at delivery are likely to prevail in cases of septate uterus[5]. Poor vascularization of the septum was proposed as a potential cause of miscarriages[4]. Electron microscopy study of Fedele et al[6] indicated a decrease in the sensitivity of the endometrium covering the septa of malformed uteri to preovulatory changes. This could play a role in the pathogenesis of primary infertility in patients with septate uterus.

It is clear that unfavorable obstetric prognosis can be transformed by surgical correction of the intrauterine septum. Formerly, removal of the septum was performed by transabdominal metroplasty[7]. Hysteroscopic treatment was currently proposed as the procedure of choice for the management of these disorders. This simple and effective treatment has an obvious advantage that uterus is not weakened by a myometrial scar. Cararach et al[8] and Goldenberg et al[9] reported 75% and 88,7% pregnancy rates after operative hysteroscopy.

Clearly, simplicity and effectiveness of the hysteroscopy have faced the clinician with need of an early and correct diagnosis of the uterine anomalies. When used as a screening test for detection of congenital uterine anomalies transvaginal ultrasound had a sensitivity of almost 100%[10,11]. However, clear distinction between different types of abnormalities was impossible and operator dependent[12,13].

X-ray hysterosalpingography (X-ray HSG) is an invasive test which requires the use of contrast medium and exposure to radiation. Although HSG provides a good outline of the uterine cavity, the visualization of minor anomalies and clear distinction between different types of lateral fusion disorders is sometimes impossible. More recently hysterosonography has been introduced[14]. In these patients transvaginal ultrasound is carried out after distension of the uterine cavity by instillation of a saline solution. This simple and minimally invasive approach allows anatomical images of endometrium and myometrium, accurate depiction of the septate uterus and even the measurement of the thickness and height of the septum[15].

Although some reports have indicated a high diagnostic accuracy of magnetic resonance imaging[16,17] and three dimensional ultrasound[18] in the diagnosis of congenital uterine anomalies, these techniques are rarely routinely used for this indication. In patients scheduled for corrective surgery the evaluation is usually completed by another invasive procedure - CO_2 diagnostic hysteroscopy[19].

ULTRASOUND IMAGING IN DIAGNOSIS AND TREATMENT OF SEPTATE UTERUS - OWN RESULTS

Our study attempted to evaluate the combined use of transvaginal ultrasound, transvaginal color and pulsed Doppler sonography, hysterosonography and three-dimensional ultrasound in the preoperative diagnosis of septate uterus[20].

Second part of the study analyzed obstetrical and perinatal complications of septate uterus, and assessed the reproductive outcome after the hysteroscopic treatment.

A total of 420 infertile patients undergoing operative hysteroscopy were included in

Table 1

Intraoperative findings in 420 infertile patients undergoing hysteroscopy

HYSTEROSCOPIC FINDING	NUMBER
submucous leiomyoma	46
endometrial polyp	35*
intrauterine synechiae	19*
septate uterus	278
arcuate uterus	28
bicornuate uterus	16+
TOTAL	422

* One patient with endometrial polyp and one with intrauterine synechiae had intrauterine septum

+ Diagnosis made by combined use of laparoscopy and hysteroscopy

this study. Table 1 summarizes intraoperative findings in 420 infertile patients undergoing hysteroscopy. The final diagnosis of the uterine disorder was confirmed by hysteroscopy, and 278 patients had intrauterine septum corrected surgically. Forty three of the patients with septate uteri had a history of repeated spontaneous abortion, 71 had one spontaneous abortion (56 in first trimester, while 15 reported spontaneous abortion during the second trimester), 82 had primary sterility and 20 had premature delivery, including 6 with breech and 2 with transverse presentation. A positive history of ectopic pregnancy was noticed in 76 patients.

Each patient underwent transvaginal ultrasound and transvaginal color Doppler examination during the luteal phase of their cycle. A systematic examination of the uterine position, size and morphological characteristics was performed. With the use of B mode transvaginal sonography, the morphology of uterus was carefully explored with emphasis to endometrial lining in both sagittal and transverse sections. The septum was visualized as an echogenic portion separating the uterine cavity into two parts. Once B mode examination was completed by experienced sonographer, transvaginal color Doppler examination was performed by another skilled operator who was unaware of the previous finding.

Color and pulsed Doppler was superimposed to visualize intraseptal and myometrial vascularity. Flow velocity waveforms were obtained from all the interrogated vessels. For each recording, at least five waveform signals of good quality were obtained. During each procedure the resistance index (RI) was automatically calculated. The RI was calculated from the maximum frequency envelope and was: peak systolic velocity minus end-diastolic velocity divided by peak systolic velocity.

Instillation of isotonic saline (hysterosonography) was carried out on a gynecological examination table. In 76 patients the uterine cervix was exposed with a speculum disinfected with iodine solution. A catheter with external diameter of 1,6 mm and internal diameter of 1,1 mm was slowly introduced into the cervix. The balloon was insufflated with 1,5 to 2 ml of sterile saline to avoid outflow of the fluid. A syringe containing 20 ml isotonic saline solution was attached to the catheter and fluid was slowly injected. For distension of the uterine cavity about 10 to 20 ml of the contrast was required. The speculum was then withdrawn and the endovaginal probe introduced. Transverse and sagittal sections were carefully explored, and septum was visualized as an echogenic portion separating the uterine cavity into two parts.

Eighty six women undergoing hysteroscopy were examined by three dimensional ultrasound. They all had transvaginal scan, and color and pulsed Doppler evaluation performed prior to 3-D examination. Twelve of these patients underwent additional

Table 2

Sensitivity, specificity, positive (PPV) and negative predictive (NPV) values of transvaginal ultrasound, transvaginal color Doppler, hysterosonography and three dimensional ultrasound for the diagnosis of septate uteri in 420 patients with history of infertility and recurrent abortions

Imaging modality	Sensitivity (%)	Specificity (%)	PPV (%)	NPV (%)
Transvaginal sonography	94,96	92,86	95,65	91,77
Transvaginal color Doppler	99,28	99,30	99,64	98,60
Hysterosonography	100,00	95,65	98,18	100,00
Three dimensional ultrasound	93,55	96,55	98,31	87,50

examination: instillation of the isotonic saline into the uterine cavity. The results of the previous diagnostic tests were not available to the ultrasonographer. Three perpendicular planes of the uterus were simultaneously displayed on the screen, allowing a detailed analysis of the uterine morphology. Frontal reformatted sections were particularly useful for detection of the uterine abnormalities.

Table 2 summarizes the sensitivity, specificity, positive and negative predictive values of transvaginal sonography, transvaginal color and pulsed Doppler ultrasound, hysterosalpingography and three-dimensional ultrasound for the diagnosis of the septate uterus.

In 264 cases septate uterus was suspected by transvaginal ultrasound, while normal finding was reported in 14 patients. The sensitivity of transvaginal sonography in the diagnosis of septate uteri was 94.96%.

Transvaginal color and pulsed Doppler enabled the diagnosis of septate uterus in 276 cases, reaching the sensitivity of 99,28%. In one patient with endometrial polyp and one with intrauterine synechiae, septate uteri were not correctly diagnosed. Therefore, the reliability of color and pulsed Doppler examination was reduced if other intracavitary structures (such as endometrial polyp or submucous leiomyoma) were present.

Color and pulsed Doppler studies of the septal area revealed vascularity in 198 (71,22%) patients. The RI values obtained from the septum ranged from 0,68 to 1,0 (mean RI=0,84±0,16). Eighteen patients demonstrated absence of diastolic blood flow, while in the rest a continuous diastolic flow was present.

In 76 patients intrauterine injection of an isotonic saline solution was advised before entering the hysteroscopic procedure. In 54 (71,05%) patients septate uteri were clearly identified. Sensitivity and NPV of hysterosonography following transvaginal color Doppler examination reached 100%. However, in one patient with extensive intrauterine synechia hysterosonography did not detect intrauterine septum.

Good quality 3D images were obtained in 86 patients. Three dimensional ultrasound agreed with hysteroscopy in 58 patients with septate uteri. However, in 4 patients with septate uteri 3D ultrasound indicated the arcuate one. Distortion of the uterine cavity by a fundal fibroid was shown in these four patients. One false positive diagnosis of septate uterus with 3D ultrasound was obtained in a patient with intrauterine synechiae.

One hundred eighty eight patients underwent X ray HSG within 12 months prior to our examination. X-ray HSG made a diagnosis of septate uteri in 49 patients according to the Reuter's criteria[15]. A septate uterus was suspected if the angle between the two cavities was <75°, while a bicornuate uterus was suspected for

195

angles >105°. In 15 cases (7,98%) hysterosalpingography indicated deformed uterine cavity, but congenital anomaly of the uterus was not suspected. The sensitivity of X ray HSG in the diagnosis of septate uteri was only 26.06%.

The second part of our study attempted to evaluate the obstetrical complications in a population of 278 patients with septate uterus and to compare it with general population which considered a control group during the 5 years' period (1992 to 1996). Early abortions appeared at a rate of 114/278 (41,01%) as compared to a rate of 15% for controls. Late abortions and premature deliveries appeared at a rate of 35/278 (12,59%) as compared to a rate of 7% for normal pregnancies. Intrauterine growth retardation appeared in 2 (8,7%) pregnancies with septate uterus as compared to 6% among the general population. Intrauterine fetal death occurred in one (4,35%) patient as compared to 0,5% in our control population. Abruptio placentae was found in one (4,35%) patient with septate uterus, as well as placenta praevia (4,35%). Breech presentation was found in 6 (26,09%) pregnancies complicated by intrauterine septum, while transverse presentation occurred in 2 (8,70%) patients. Since abnormal fetal presentation was significantly more frequent in patients with septate uterus, a remarkably higher rate of Caesarean section (34,78%) occurred. Cervical incompetence during pregnancy appeared in nine (25.71%) women with intrauterine septum.

Extrauterine pregnancy appeared in 76 patients at a rate of 27,34% which was 2 times higher incidence than in our control group (13.3%). Bilateral ectopic pregnancy was noticed in seven patients with septate uterus.

We assessed the reproductive outcome in 116 patients (32 with primary sterility, 16 with one spontaneous abortion, 12 with premature deliveries and 26 with recurrent abortions) following the operative hysteroscopy for an intrauterine septum. A prospective follow-up period was 24 months for each patient. The pregnancy rate in the studied group was 50.86%: 44 patients (74.58%) had term deliveries, 11 (18.64%) had first trimester abortion and 4 (6.78%) reported preterm delivery. Other patients (n=162) are followed in the same manner, but follow-up period is less than 24 months and therefore is not reported in this study.

NEW IDEAS ON OLD PROBLEM

Until now at least two procedures have been used for detection of the congenital uterine anomalies. The gynecologists should be aware that long diagnostic evaluation delays the treatment, increases the cost, patient's discomfort and risk associated with each of the diagnostic procedures[15]. Therefore, quick and reliable diagnosis is important in patients with septate uterus since surgical correction should be recommended. Fedele et al[6] recently indicated that intrauterine septum may be a cause of primary infertility. They demonstrated significant ultrastructural alterations in septal endometrium compared with endometrium from the lateral uterine wall in samples obtained during the preovulatory phase. The ultrastructural alterations included a reduced number of glandular ostia distributed irregularly, ciliated cells with incomplete ciliogenesis, and reduced ciliated : non-ciliated ratio. The ultrastructural morphological alterations were indicative of irregular differentiation and estrogenic maturation of septal endometrial mucosa. Since the hormonal levels of the patients enrolled in this study were normal for the cycle phase, the most convincing hypothesis was that endometrial mucosa covering the septum was poorly responsive to estrogens probably due to scanty vascularization of septal connective tissue.

March[21] stated that the septum is built from a fibroelastic tissue, while Fayez[22] believed that in the septum there are fewer muscle fibers and more connective tissue. However, our study did not confirm this statement. Color and pulsed Doppler revealed septal vascularity in 71,22% of the patients giving the fact that most of the septa comprised myometrial vessels.

Dabirashrafi et al[23] performed histologic study of the uterine septa from 16 patients undergoing abdominal metroplasty. Four biopsy specimens were taken from the uterus in each case: from the septum near the serosal layer, at the midpoint of the septum, at the level of the tip of the septum and from the left posterior aspect of the uterus away from the septum. Their findings of less connective tissue in the septum were confirmed by the Bonferroni criterion for multiple comparisons and the mean ridit results for the amount of muscle tissue, amount of muscle interlacing and vessels with a muscle wall and were contradictory to the classic view about the histologic features of the uterine septum.

Less connective tissue in the septum can be the reason for poor decidualization and placentation in the area of implantation[22,23]. Increased amounts of muscle tissue and muscle interlacing in the septum can cause an abortion by the higher and uncoordinated contractility of these muscles.

Recent study from our Department[24] found no correlation between septal height and occurrence of obstetrical complications ($p>0.05$). Abortions and late pregnancy complications occured with the same rate in patients with small septa that were dividing less than one third of the uterine cavity, and those with division of more than two thirds of the uterine cavity. The same was related to septal thickness: obstetrical complications were found in the same proportion of the patients with tiny and those with thick septa ($p>0.05$). Indeed, pregnancy loss correlated significantly with septal vascularity. Patients with vascularized septa had significantly higher incidence of early pregnancy failure and late pregnancy complications than those with avascularized septa ($p<0.05$).

By using transvaginal ultrasound it is possible to perform a precise assessment of the uterine morphology, including the endometrial lining and outer shape of the uterine muscle. Color Doppler technique allows simultaneous visualization of morphology and vascular network giving full information on the type of anomaly and the extent of the defect. The visualization of the myometrial portion is further enhanced by detection of the myometrial vessels by color Doppler technique. Furthermore, Doppler imaging can detect deficient intraseptal vascularity and/or inadequate endometrial development in patients with septate uteri[24,25].

Three dimensional ultrasound enables planar reformatted sections through the uterus which allow precise evaluation of the fundal indentation and the length of the septum. Based on our experience, this technique may give a wrong impression of an arcuate uterus in patients with fundal location of the leiomyoma. In these cases uterine cavity has a concave shape, while fundal indentation is more shallow. Furthermore, shadowing caused by the uterine fibroids, irregular endometrial lining and decreased volume of the uterine cavity (in cases of intrauterine adhesions) are obvious limitations of 3-D ultrasound.

Our study[20] clearly proved that obstetric complications were more frequent among patients with septate uterus than among other women. Furthermore, it demonstrated that ectopic pregnancy occurred at double rate (27.34%) in these patients, when compared to controls (13.3%). A possible etiology for this finding is the menstrual reflux, commonly present in patients with uterine anomalies, which sequelae may interfere with passage of the fertilized egg into the uterine cavity. Our study clearly demonstrated the benefit of removing the intrauterine septum in patients suffering from infertility and recurrent pregnancy wastage. Furthermore, it is expected that cumulative pregnancy rate will be even higher, since some of the primary infertile patients who are involved in IVF program due to male factor await for the procedure.

Conventionally it has been agreed not to intervene until the first obstetrical accidents have occurred, because a great proportion of septate uteruses have no obstetrical pathology[3]. However, hypofecondity in this group of patients and good results achieved by endoscopic surgical treatment obligate us to propose hysteroscopy as soon as we diagnose septate uterus even prior to any pregnancy[20,24,26]. It seems that septal incision eliminates an unsuitable site of implantation, through revascularization of the connective uterine fundal tissue or elimination of the unfavourable uterine contractions[6]. Since both of these events can be detected by color and pulsed Doppler ultrasound, this technique can be efficiently used for detection of the congenital uterine malformations and follow-up of the patients undergoing hysteroscopy.

REFERENCES:

1. Ashton, D., Amin, H. K., Richart, R. M. and Neuwirth, R. S. (1988). The incidence of asmyptomatic uterine anomalies in women undergoing transcervical tubal sterilization. Obstet. Gynecol., 72, 28-30

2. Sorensen S. (1988). Estimated prevalence of mulerian anomalies. Acta Obstet. Gynecol. Scand., 67, 441-5

3. Gaucherand, P., Awada, A., Rudigoz, R. C. and Dargent, D. (1994). Obstetrical prognosis of septate uterus: a plea for treatment of the septum. Eur. J. Obstet. Gynecol. Reprod. Biol., 54, 109-12

4. Fedele, L., Arcaini, L., Parazzini, F., Vercellini, P. and Nola, G. D. (1993). Metroplastic hysteroscopy and fertility. Fertil. Steril., 59, 768-70

5. Heinonen, P. K., Saarikoski, S. and Pystynen, P. (1982). Reproductive performance of women with uterine anomalies. An evaluation of 182 cases. Acta Obstet. Gynecol. Scand., 61, 157-62

6. Fedele, L., Bianchi, S., Marchini, M., Franchi, D., Tozzi, L. and Dorta, M. (1996). Ultrastructural aspects of endometrium in infertile women with septate uterus. Fertil. Steril., 65, 750-2

7. McShane, P. M., Reilly, R. J. and Schiff, L. (1983). Pregnancy outcome following Tompkins metroplasty. Fertil. Steril., 40, 190-4

8. Cararach, M., Penella, J., Ubeda, J. and Iabastida, R. (1994). Hysteroscopic incision of the septate uterus: scissors versus resectoscope. Hum. Reprod., 9, 87-9

9. Goldenberg, M., Sivan, E. and Sharabi, Z. (1995). Reproductive outcome following hysteroscopic management of intrauterine septum and adhesions. Hum. Reprod., 10, 2663-5

10. Valdes, C., Malini, S. and Malinak, L. R. (1984). Ultrasound evaluation of female genital tract anomalies: a review of 64 cases. Am. J. Obstet. Gynecol., 149, 285-90

11. Nicolini, U., Bellotti, B., Bonazzi, D., Zamberleti, G. and Battista, C. (1987). Can ultrasound be used to screen uterine malformation? Fertil. Steril., 47, 89-93

12. Reuter, K. L., Daly, D. C. and Cohen, S. M. (1989). Septate versus bicornuate uteri: errors in imaging diagnosis. Radiology, 172, 749-52

13. Randolph, J., Ying, Y., Maier, D., Schmidt, C. and Riddick, D. (1986). Comparison of real time ultrasonography, hysterosalpingography, and laparoscopy/hysteroscopy in the evaluation of uterine abnormalities and tubal patency. Fertil. Steril., 5, 828-32

14. Richman, T. S., Viscomi, G. N., Cherney, A. D. and Polan, A. (1984). Fallopian tubal patency assessment by ultrasound following fluid injection. Radiology, 152, 507-10

15. Salle, B., Sergeant, P., Galcherand, P., Guimont, I., De Saint Hilaire, P. and Rudigoz, RC. (1996). Transvaginal hysterosonographic evaluation of septate uteri: a preliminary report. Hum. Reprod., 11, 1004-7

16. Marshall, C., Mintz, D. I., Thickman, D., Gussman, H. and Kressel, Y. (1987). MR evaluation of uterine anomalies. Radiology, 148, 287-9

17. Carrington, B. M., Hricak, M. and Naruddin, R. N. (1990). Mullerian duct anomalies: MR evaluation. Radiology, 170, 715-20

18. Jurkovic, D., Giepel, A., Gurboeck, K., Jauniaux, E., Natucci, M. and Campbell, S. (1995). Three dimensional ultrasound for the assessment of uterine anatomy and detection of congenital anomalies: a comparison with hysterosalpingography and two-dimensional sonography. Ultrasound Obstet. Gynecol., 5, 233-7

19. Taylor, P. J. and Cumming, D. C. (1979). Hysteroscopy in 100 patients. Fertil. Steril., 31, 301-4

20. Kupesic, S. and Kurjak, A. (1998). Pregnancy after diagnosis and treatment of uterine anomalies. Croat. Med. J., submitted

21. March, C. M. (1983). Hysteroscopy as an aid to diagnosis in female infertility. Clin. Obstet. Gynecol., 26, 302-12

22. Fayez, J. A. (1986). Comparison between abdominal and hysteroscopic metroplasty. Obstet. Gynecol., 68, 399-403

23. Dabrashrafi, H., Bahadori, M., Mohammad, K., Alavi, M., Moghadami-Tabrizi, N. and Zandinejad, R. (1995). Septate uterus: New idea on the histologic features of the septum in this abnormal uterus. Am. J. Obstet. Gynecol., 172, 105-7

24. Kupesic, S. and Kurjak, A. (1998). Comparison of B-mode, color Doppler, three-dimensional ultrasound and hysterosonography in detection of septate uteri. Am. J. Obstet. Gynecol. (submitted)

25. Kupesic, S. and Kurjak, A. (1993). Uterine and ovarian perfusion during the periovulatory period assessed by transvaginal color Doppler. Fertil. Steril., 3, 439-43

26. Keltz, M. D., Olive, D. L., Kim, A. H. and Arici, A. (1997). Sonohysterography for screening in recurrent pregnancy loss. Fertil. Steril., 67, 670-4

Prevention and management of female genital cancer at the beginning of the third millennium after a century of clinical experience

A. Onnis

Montreal CND (Past head professor of Padua University)

SUMMARY

On the basis of his long experience as a gynecologist oncologist the author makes some considerations on the evolution of prevention and management of female genital cancer. Looking back and moving forward the author suggests some guidelines with respect to the cost-benefit balance in cancer treatment and to the patients' quality of life.

PREVENTION AND MANAGEMENT

What about prevention and management of female genital cancers at the beginning of the third millennium? What has happened in this century?

Undoubtedly, the prevention and management of female genital cancer have greatly improved in the last decades, particularly after the second world war.

In the first half of our century neither prevention nor early detection were applied. Female genital cancer management was based solely on extensive surgical operations – such as Wertheim, Shauta, Haltstead – on internal or external radiotherapy or on radio-surgical combined strategies.

> I am an old oncologist who has been practising our discipline since 1950, when genital cancers were nearly always diagnosed at advanced stages. In that time surgery started to improve, after the long period of serious limitations because of the lack of anesthesia, blood transfusions and because of the vast spread of cancer at diagnosis; *radiotherapy* also started to improve after its first steps, which began in the twenties, heavy, without enough knowledge of the biological effects of ionisating radiation on healthy and cancerous tissues; *antimitotic chemotherapy* on the contrary, was completely unknown.

After 1950 adequate staging (TNM and FIGO), progress in early detection and clinical application of antimitotic drugs have allowed more and more adequate treatments.

In western countries, today, at the beginning of the third millennium, the gynaecological oncological situation is, in my opinion, satisfactory, particularly for uterine (cervical and endometrial) and breast cancers because of the adequate screening and early detection and also because of women's new health education.

What about the clinical experiences of gynecologic oncology in the century we are now leaving behind? The development of gynecologic oncology in every western country resulted in important progress in the management of female genital cancers. We now can face the new millennium with the best optimistic perspective.

Screening is now unrenounciable to preserve the progress already achieved in our discipline, even if mass screening programs now face organizational and financial problems in welfare countries. In my opinion gynecologists and not only oncologic gynecologists continue to have the leadership of prevention and early detection of female genital cancer.

They only can perform simultaneous adequate screening for uterine, ovarian, vulvar and breast tumors during every outpatient consultation.

Simultaneous combined ultrasound and gynecological examinations for a more in-depth clinical diagnosis are precious. In fact, cervical, ovarian, endometrial, vulvar and breast controls can be performed at the same time by the same gynecologist who will perform specific examinations (on the basis of age, sexual activity, familiar and personal risks for every neoplasia).

Separate screenings in different centres by different physicians – who are often not expert enough in genital female pathology and endocrinology – are more expensive, less reliable and very heavy for women.

Following this strategy, in many countries the incidence of advanced stages in cervical, endometrial, vulvar and breast cancers is reducing year by year. Consequently, also the therapeutical strategies have changed and now in the majority of cases radical non-mutilating surgical operations are possible. In cervical cancer conization is now more frequent than Wertheim's operations, in breast cancer quadrantectomy is more frequent than Haltstead's operation, in vulvar cancer skin vulvectomy or radical enlarged non-mutilating vulvectomy are more frequent than Way's operation; in endometrial cancer simple hysterectomy, often without lymphadenectomy is preferred.

Not only survival rate but also quality of life have improved profoundly for these cancer patients.

On the contrary, for ovarian cancer we have not yet either a correct strategy for early detection or an adequate knowledge of tumor aggressivity. In fact now we have the same incidence of advanced stages as thirty years ago: 75%.

All over the world this dangerous situation was and is stressed; screening programs were and are done; epidemiologists, sociologists, politicians were and are involved with us: still, the situation remains unchanged.

It is not only because of the lack of early diagnostic programs but also because of the high aggressiveness, speed of diffusion and invasion of ovarian cancer. In the peritoneal cavity, which is its home, the ovarian tumor can gallop like a horse in the open and large prairie where no rock, no mountains, no fences stop its course.

Malignant epithelial ovarian tumors that appear at a young age, in the largest number of cases in early stages and borderline forms support the hypothesis of a preclinical phase of ovarian carcinoma with low malignancy.

WHAT CAN WE DO?

Neither special expensive medical organization, like OVARIAN SCREENING CENTERS, not the heavy involvement of women is necessary.

I believe that when the gynecologist begins to systematically apply simultaneous combined ultrasound and gynaecological examination, earlier detection of ovarian cancer will be more and more easy and frequent.

Anyway, the progress of our discipline has been great even in advanced stages, because combined treatments often allow good results for survival rates and quality of life, with a good cost-benefit balance.

We now know very well what is really useful and what is useless for the patients. We have learned to avoid many large mutilating operations which more and more can qualify the surgeons' image but less and less the patient's life.

We have worked for many decades all over the world, experimenting even with heroic treatments: we have reached conclusions on what we believe is the best management today, with respect to the cost-benefit balance.

The new generation of gynaecologists, oncologists and surgeons who follow us will undoubtedly go ahead, sometimes verifying and also repeating our experiences but carefully avoiding to repeat our mistakes.

Only in this way, in my opinion , will it be possible to improve the management of every genital cancer, even advanced stages, with integrated therapies.

Unfortunately the anticancer agents we have today are always the same and we know how to reach the best results, how to combine the best associations and how to avoid harmful complications.

WHAT IS THE BEST MANAGEMENT OF FEMALE GENITAL CANCER TODAY?

In my opinion surgery continues to be the cornerstone for every gynaecological cancer but only in personalised operations, avoiding, when possible, every unnecessary mutilation and extensive demolition.

Radiotherapy and chemotherapy, in adequate sequences, today sufficiently tested in every advanced tumor, must respect the cost-benefit balance and the quality of life of patients.

As is well-known, a 5-year survival rate is correlated not only with surgical stage and with tumoral aggressiveness factors (histotype, grading, proliferating cell nuclear antigen positivity – Ki67 – and mutant p53 protein pattern levels in tumoral cells) but it is also correlated with the quality of surgery – and the quality of integrated therapies.

We are now able to avoid over or undertreatments both harmful for quality of life and with the same survival rate.

Consequently we are facing the new millennium with the most optimistic visions to improve and improve again the results of prevention and management of female genital cancers.

TREATMENT OF OVARIAN TUMORS

PAVEŠIC D, HALLER H, MATEJCIC N; RUPCIC S.

Department of Obstetrics & Gynecology,University Hospital of Rijeka

Cambierieva 17/5

51000 Rijeka (CROATIA)

Tel : + 385-51-338-555

E-mail :herman.haller@ri.tel.hr

When in a gynecologic routine an ovarian neoplasm is encountered, the first question arises from the everpresent fear of malignancy. Nowadays, in spite of great progress in the field of medical equipment and techonology, the answer to this simple question in certain number of cases remains uncertain.

DIAGNOSTICS

Histologic specimen analysis represents unique and undoubtly definitive confirmation regarding the nature of ovarian neoplasms. Various reported preoperative diagnostic tools have different percentage of precision in precluding the histologic nature of the ovarian neoplasm, but none of the reported methods is free of inaccuracy.

Among these diagnostic methods, transvaginal ultrasound and color Doppler (in the future perhaps 3 D ultrasound) offer the best possibilities to differentiate preoperatively benign and malignant ovarian neoplasms.

In our Department since more than 7 years transvaginal and color Dopper techniques have been used as routine methods in everyday gynaecological practice. The results of one prospective clinical trial conducted in our institution where only ovarian mass less than 10 cm were included, showed

sensitivity 98 %, specificity 92 % and positive predictive value 80 %. The add of tumor markers as

CA 125 did not increase reported diagnostic accuracy.

BENIGN OVARIAN NEOPLASMS

In the cases of presumed benign ovarian pathology, when minor operative procedure is sufficient,

the decision of the way of action, **i.e.** laparoscopy or laparotomy is made after analysing eventual

risk factors and concomitant diseases , genital and extragenital.

The operative techniques during ablative laparoscopic procedures used in our Department in

resolving benign ovarian neoplasms include the use of instrument known as three-function

instrument - Trisector. The triple action includes grasping, electrocoagulation and cutting.

Ovariectomy as wells as adnexectomy is performed very easily and quickly. Mean time is 2 minutes

and practically whithout blood loss. In the cases when concomitant hysterectomy is planned,

following release of ovary or ovaries or adnexis, laparoscopy assisted vaginal hysterectomy (LAVH)

of type 1 or 2 can be performed.

Removal of ovarian neoplasms from abdominal cavity after dissection from the ligamentar and

vascular pedicles during laparoscopic procedure represents the final problem in significant number

of cases. The way of ovarian neoplasm removal could include trocar channel, umbilical or incision

in lower part of abdominal wall as posterior colpotomy. Every presented way for neoplasms

removal has advantages as well as disadvantages. However , the simpler as well as the faster and

less invasive technique should be attempted. Dermoid cysts management requires few additional

explanatory words. In our practice smaller dermoid cysts (less than 6 cm) could be removed through

the plastic bag. In the cases of dermoid cysts of greater diameter laparoscopical treatment is also

suitable. Evacuation can be safely performed through the posterior colpotomy with inevitable spillage of the content into the pelvis. After evacuation of the tumor mass, the abdomen is washed thoroughly pouring the line through upper trocar-port, while the liquid containing material from the cyst is washed away through the posterior colpotomy. In our experience (until now we removed 37 dermoid cysts with dimension greater than 10 cm) applying the abundant washing of abdominal cavity results in uncomplicated postoperative period.

MALIGNANT OVARIAN NEOPLASMS

Surgery represents the cornerstone in the ovarian cancer treatment. Surgery has a critical role in diagnosis and staging, removal of tumor, assessment of response to chemotherapy and palliation of symptoms. At the same time, both chemotherapy and radiotherapy depend heavily for their success on appriopiate surgery.

In the apparent early ovarian cancer, our standard treatment policy include total abdominal hysterectomy, bilateral salpingoophorectomy and infracolic omentectomy whit comprehensive staging procedures; where cytologic analysis of free fluid lavage is obtained, any suspicious lesion are histologicaly defined, multiple blind byopsis of peritoneum are obtained and finally sistematic pelvic and aortic lymphadenectomy is performed.

In the cases of advanced ovarian cancer, surgical dogma " to remove all or doing nothing " is not valid. The maximal reduction of residual tumor mass as we well know, represents the only factor we can influence. Many techniques are applied to obtain maximal cytoreduction, such as deperitonisation of the pelvis or diaphragm, resection of the rectum and, in minor number of cases, small intestine, elimination of peritoneal deposits with various techniques, but the final effectiveness currently is not completely known, and further studies are required to determine the precise role of such surgery.

Gravitational Vario flow system with deficit indicator - for safe fluid delivery in hysteroscopic operations

T Tomaževič, L Savnik, M Dintinjana

Department of Obstetrics and Gynecology, University Medical Centre, Ljubljana, Slovenia

INTRODUCTION The automated gravitational Vario Flow system was constructed in order to reduce the risk of fluid intravazation while using gravity for uterine distention during continuous flow hysteroscopic procedures1,2. It provides linear regulation, definition and measurement of intrauterine pressure by simply pressing the pedal and changing the height difference between the fluid level and the operative area. The zero point is set by height of the operating table. Three height ranges are marked in different colours on the elevating bar: the safe range of 100 - 140 cm H2O (73-100 mm Hg) is marked green, the intermediate range 140 - 150 cm H20 (100-110 mm Hg) is marked yellow and extreme range 150 -190 cm H2O (110-140 mm Hg) is marked red. Fluid outflow to the receptacle is also driven by height difference of 100 H20 (73 mm Hg). The weighing based electronic fluid deficit indicator was built into the second version of the Vario Flow system in order to provide the utmost control of fluid dynamics and to further improve safety for the patient. In August 1996 it was introduced into daily clinical work. The electronic weighing system indicates the weight of the whole system, including inflow bag and outflow receptacle and shows the overall fluid deficit in ml on the display. The scales on the display determine the weight of the whole system as zero reference weight at the beginning of the procedure and as real weight during the procedure. If the liquid that was discharged from the endoscope is not collected in the fluid receptacle, the weight of the system is reduced and the difference between the two values is shown on the display as liquid loss. If the loss exceeds a preset critical amount of liquid (1000 –1500 ml) a warning signal sounds. Long ago It was presumed that a fluid deficit indicator could provide major safety for the patient during continuous flow hysteroscopic procedures (3).

Figure 1. Schematic of the Vario flow with fluid deficit indicator

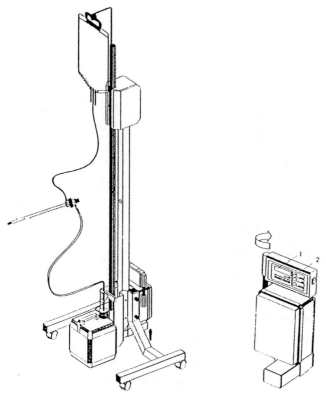

PATIENTS AND METHODS Between August 1996 and July 1997, the fluid deficit indicator with the alarm system was used in 203 hysteroscopic operations. Early experiences with the use of the fluid deficit indicator are reported. They are compared to experiences between January 1994 and August 1996 when the Vario Flow System without the fluid deficit indicator was used in 240 hysteroscopic operations. In this period of time the volumetric method was used to control the fluid deficit. In all there were 443 hysteroscopic operations: 301 metroplasties, 20 endometrial ablations, 10 cases of lysis of synechiae, 58 myomectomies and 54 polypectomies.

Most women received danazol 400 mg starting on day 1 of the menstrual cycle for endometrial preparation. Vaginal ultrasound and diagnostic continuous flow hysteroscopy were performed for preoperative diagnosis. Dextrose 5% was the distending medium. In normal circumstances the fluid-filled bag of the Vario Flow was raised between 1 and 1.4 m above the patient according to individual conditions permitting good visualization and considering the danger of fluid intravasation. Higher pressure ranges were used according to individual surgical needs. Volumetric and weighing method were used for final fluid deficit evaluation. T-test comparing two samples assuming equal variances was used for statistical evaluation.

RESULTS In our patients accurate visualization and good control of fluid dynamics were always obtained during operative hysteroscopies. The fluid deficit indicator proved to be highly efficient in providing information on the fluid deficit at any moment during the procedure as well as the actual information on the final fluid deficit. In the first series of our hysteroscopic procedures before the introduction of the fluid deficit indicator there were two uterine perforations. No general complications occurred. Retrospective data on the final fluid deficit before and after the introduction of the fluid deficit indicator are presented in Table 1.

Table 1. Data on final fluid deficit without (group 1) and with the fluid deficit indicator (group 2) - N.S.

Fluid deficit	Number of observations	Avarage value	Standard deviation
GROUP 1	240	440 ML	310
GROUP 2	203	375 ML	369

DISCUSSION

The fluid overload is the major complication related to the uterine distension (3,4,5,6,7,8,9). The control of intrauterine pressure was shown to reduce the risk of fluid intravasation (7,8). The ideal system for delivery of low viscosity media would also measure the inflow and outflow of the fluid and sound an alarm if an excess of fluid deficit is detected (4). It is this feature, and not the intrauterine pressure, that should guide the conduct of any case (5).

By combining the non expensive (2) automated gravitation to control the intrauterine pressure with the fluid deficit indicator and alarm system (1) we tried to reach this goal and to furthe reduce the risk of uncontrolled fluid intravasation during our hysteroscopic procedures. According to early experiences in our series of patients, the real weight based fluid deficit indicator proved to be highly efficient in providing information on the fluid deficit at any moment during the procedure as well as the information on the final fluid deficit. If fluid deficit exceeded critical amount of liquid - preset at 1000 to 1500 ml as an upper limit for a safe procedure - a warning signal would be activated. The reassuring or alarming information about fluid deficit at any moment during hysteroscopic procedures was specially important in operations where higher intrauterine pressure ranges were needed for uterine distention. Except in cases with abundant spillage, the fluid intravasation was easily controlled. In these cases any of commercially available drape systems works well, if properly applied to the patient perineum (9).

Thus in our hands the fluid deficit has become one of the leading parameters of the fluid dynamics at any moment during our hysteroscopic procedures. There were no significant differences between the data on the final fluid deficit in both series of patients. This is not surprising because the lowest possible pressure providing good vision was used in both groups of patients. Compared to volumetric assessment, monitoring the real weight on the display seems to be an easier way of following the fluid deficit in hysteroscopic suurgery . We conclude that the real weight based fluid deficit indication further improves safety for patients while using automated gravitational continuous flow system during hysteroscopic procedures

REFERENCES

1. Tomaževič T. Savnik L, Dintinjana M. An Automated Gravitational system for Deliverry of Low Viscosity Media During Continuous- Flow Hysteroscopy. J Am Assoc Gynecol Laparosc 3:617-621,1996

2. Tomaževič T, Savnik L, Dintinjana M et al. Attempt to reduce the costs of irrigation in endoscopic surgery. 12th Congress of European Association of Gynaecologists and Obstetricians, June 1997, Dublin.

3. Indman PD. Instruments and video cameras for operative hysteroscopy. Clin Obstet Gynecol 35:211-224, 1992

4. Loffer FD. The need to monitor intrauterine pressure - myth or necessity. J Am Assoc Gynecol Laparosc 2:1-2,

5. Loffer FD. Complications from uterine distention during hysteroscopy In Complications of Laparoscopy and Hysteroscopy. Edited by Corfman RS, Diamond MP, DeCherney A. Oxford, London, Edinburgh, Melbourne, Paris, Berlin, Vienna, Blackwell Scientific Publications, 1993, 177-186

6. Shirk GJ, Kaigh J. The use of low-viscosity fluids for hysteroscopy. J Am Assoc Gynecol Laparosc 2:11-21, 1994

7. Hamou J, Fryman R, MCLucas B et al. A uterine distention system to prevent fluid intravasation during hysteroscopic surgery. Gynaecol Endosc 5:, 131-136, 1996

8. Garry R, Mooney P, Hashman F et al. A uterine distention system to prevent fluid absorption during Nd Yag laser endometrial ablation. Gynaecol Endosc 1:23-27, 1992

9. Corson SL. Hysteroscopic Fluid Management J Am Assoc Gynecol Laparosc 4: 375-379, 1997

Complications during laparoscopically assisted vaginal hysterectomy (LAVH)

A. Scarfi* and E.V. Cosmi**

*Clinic of Obstetrics and Gynecology of Hospital Ruit, Department School of Medicine and School of Specialization, University of Tübingen, Esslingen, Germany and Visiting Professor, University 'La Sapienza' Rome; **II Institute of Obstetrics and Gynecology Clinic, University of Rome, Italy

SUMMARY

Hysterectomy is one of the most frequently performed surgical procedures among women of reproductive age in the USA. Between 1970 and 1978, more than 3.5 million women aged 15 to 44 underwent nonradical hysterectomy, 28% by a vaginal approach and 72% by an abdominal approach. We have examined the incidence of morbidity after hysterectomy. Laparoscopically assisted hysterectomy (LAVH) was compared with abdominal hysterectomy as a necessary step before its acceptance by the medical community. From 1990 onwards this procedure has modified significantly the approach to laparoscopic surgery. The operation was claimed to be a laparoscopic method superior to abdominal hysterectomy (AH), being associated with less postoperative pain, a better cosmetic result and perhaps reduced costs, and with less complications. The severe complications amount altogether to 3.24%; most of the complications concern the surgical lesion of the urinary tract (1.43%) and reintervention for hemorrhage (0.78%). The exact rate of the complications is not really known, and is derived from the papers already published. This surgical technique is relatively new and is not uniformly standardized. In fact, altogether the number of LAVH obtained until now from the international literature, is very small considering the total number of hysterectomies, carried out in the USA approximately 600 000 yearly and increasing. Compared with the USA results, we have a lower percenage rate of abdominal hysterectomy.

INTRODUCTION

In the USA, altogether 3 500 000 hysterectomies were carried out from 1970 to 1978; in 72% of the cases, the abdominal method was preferred, whereas the other 28% were done the vaginal way. With 750 000 cases in the year 1975, this year was the one with the greatest number of hysterectomies. In 1985, in a population of 97 000 000 women, about 18 500 000 patients underwent a hysterectomy. During the twenty years period from 1965 to 1984, about 12 500 000 women underwent a hysterectomy, the average

217

age of these patients being 40.9 years. In the USA, from 1981 to 1985, the hysterectomy represented the most frequent type of the principal operations of gynecological surgery and was only exceeded by the Cesarian sections. Every year, 600 000 hysterectomies were carried out; these numbers are identical in all the other nations with industrial development. The preceding information was obtained by the National Center for Health Statistics (NCHS), on the collective data from the National Hospital Discharge Survey (NHDS). In the USA, every year an average of seven hysterectomies on 1000 women were carried out, the youngest woman being 15 years old. The indications for a hysterectomy, which have constantly increased during the last 50 years, in the meantime caused some amount of criticism regarding the necessity, and brought into discussion the application of these operations. The hysterectomy is just incriminated by the importance of the rate of morbidity. The rate of mortality is reduced; this rate still amounts to 8.6 cases out of 10 000 abdominal hysterectomies, and to 2.7 cases out of 10 000 vaginal hysterectomies, where all of the patients were free of risks[1].

THE EVENT OF MINIMAL SURGERY ACCESS

The end of the eighties represents a historic period for the minimal invasive surgery. In France, in Lyon, cholecystectomy was applied and the results published by Mouret, although this method of minimal invasive surgery was applied for the first time in Germany by Muhe, who carried out six cases of cholecystectomy, using the pneumoperitoneum from September to December 1985.

The results of hysterectomy by the laparoscopic method, were published for the first time by Harry Reich *et al.* in 1989. This minimal invasive surgery technique, was not immediately regarded as an efficient method or as an alternative to the usual abdominal hysterectomy.

IS THE INDICATION FOR LAVH ALWAYS AN OPPORTUNE OR AN OPPORTUNISTIC CHOICE?

An 'opportunistic' surgical operation, has to be distinguished from an opportunity to operate. A very small mobile uterus, does not represent an indication for the laparoscopic method, but can better be extracted by the vaginal method, with less trauma, and in real surgical times. A randomized trial of Summit *et al.*[2] and of Richardson *et al.*[3], concludes, that a laparoscopic hysterectomy (LH) is not appropriate, if a vaginal hysterectomy is practicable. But it is true as well, that due to an excessively large uterus, or restricted pelvic space, some laparoscopic surgical maneuvres are difficult.

To propose the laparoscopically assisted vaginal hysterectomy as an alternative to the traditional abdominal hysterectomy, there were some authors who intended to reduce the frequency and the type of those complications which were especially caused by laparotomy.

It is statistically known that, if the abdominal wall and the parietal peritoneum are saved, the frequency of complications is reduced, while some typical abdominal hysterectomy complications disappear completely. The most frequent complications following an abdominal hysterectomy are:

(1)   Sub- and prefascial haematoma;
(2)   Hemorrhage;
(3)   Dehiscence;
(4)   Laparocele;
(5)   Hemias;
(6)   Lesion of the urinary tract;
(7)   Infection;
(8)   Ileus;
(9)   Postsurgical scar;
(10) Thrombose.

For this reason there is an increase, in hospitalization, in convalescence, and in the public expense. By applying the vaginal hysterectomy, there will not be the laparocele, the dehiscences, the hernias, and the sub- and prefascial hematomas.

In the USA, the hysterectomy through a transabdominal laparotomic access was applied to 75% of the women less than 65 years old.

HOSPITALIZATION IN RELATION TO SURGICAL TIMES

Until 1965, the hospitalization after hysterectomy amounted to 12 days; in 1984, the hospitalization was reduced to 7 days. According to the data previously reported, this substantial reduction of hospitalization led to fewer complications, that resulted from: an improvement of surgical technique; a preventive use of some antibiotics, especially for patients at great risk; and an early mobilization of the patients in the immediate postoperative stage.

Until today the surgical time of LAVH cannot be compared to the surgical time of abdominal hysterectomy; in fact doing the LAVH the necessary preparation time increases. For the LAVH we need an average of 140 min of operation time, whereas the surgical time is only half this.

STATE OF THE ART

LAVH may cover a whole range of procedures, and a classification system is needed. From now on we refer to Tables 1 and 2, which show different classification systems of laparoscopic hysterectomy[4–6].

From all the techniques and the variants of laparoscopic hysterectomy till now proposed, 76.1% of LAVH-procedures ligated the uterine vessels laparoscopically; but the total fraction of LH (laparoscopic hysterectomy) is only 1.5%. These results are derived from a collection of data gathered on 4502 cases, and put together from the English, German and French international literature until 1995, and published in the same year by J.A. Deprest and colleagues[7].

A large number of hysterectomies, involving the presentation of abdominal wall using laparotomy, can be terminated in the vaginal way, after having explored the abdominal cavity and after treatment in the laparoscopical manner. The laparoscopic

Table 1 Different classification systems of LH, based on anatomy of uterus, vascular pedicles and support apparatus

Johns and Diamond[4]	Munro and Parker[5]	Garry, Reich and Liu[6]
Stage 0: diagnostic laparoscopy and vaginal hysterectomy	not considered as laparoscopy hysterectomy	not considered as laparoscopy vaginal hysterectomy
Stage 1: laparoscopic adhesiolysis and/or excision of endometriosis	type 0: laparoscopically directed preparation for vaginal hysterectomy	vaginal hysterectomy assisted by laparoscopy
Stage 2: either or both adnexa freed laparoscopically	type I: dissection up to but not including uterine artery**	laparoscopically assisted vaginal hysterectomy
Stage 3: bladder dissected from the uterus*	type II: type I, and uterine artery and vein occlusion**	laparoscopic hysterectomy
Stage 4: uterine artery transected laparoscopically*	type III: type II and portion of cardinaluterosacral ligament complex**	total laparoscopic hysterectomy
Stage 5: anterior and/or posterior colpotomy or entire uterus freed*	type III: type II and total cardinaluterosacral ligament complex	

When the extent of the procedure varies on the right and left, the most advanced side defines the stage or the type of the procedure.
*stages has subscript O if no ovary is excised, subscript I if one ovary is excised, and subscript 2 when both ovaries are excised.
**types has subscript A when only the support or vascular structures are divided, subscript B when anterior structures are included, C when posterior structures are included and D when both anterior and posterior structures are included. E is only applicable to type IV hysterectomies and means that the entire uterus has been removed laparoscopically.

Table 2 Classification of laparoscopic hysterectomies

Type of hysterectomy	Abbreviation	Description
Total laparoscopic hysterectomy	TLH	Total hysterectomy, all steps performed endoscopically
Subtotal laparoscopic hysterectomy	SLH	Subtotal (supracervical) hysterectomy, all steps performed endoscopically
Vaginally assisted laparoscopic hysterectomy	VAHL	Total hysterectomy, four or more steps performed endoscopically, procedure completed vaginally
Laparoscopically assisted vaginal hysterectomy	LAVH	Total hysterectomy, less than four steps performed endoscopically, procedure completed vaginally

assisted vaginal hysterectomy (LAVH), as an alternative to the laparotomy for saving the abdominal wall, has the purpose of reducing the mortality and the morbidity.

During the surgical time of LAVH the first laparoscopic stage involves the resection of the uterus under direct visible control. In fact, the laparoscopic approach has diverse objectives, which must be treated first:

(1) The adhesions treatment;
(2) The ovarian cyst;
(3) To differentiate the pathology or exclude it;
(4) To facilitate the resection of the first uterine ligaments (round ligament of uterus, utero-ovarian and uterotubal ligaments, large ligaments, parametry).

The incidence of the complications is already low in the vaginal hysterectomy, if compared with abdominal hysterectomy; all these facts diminish the social costs. The rate of complications is variable according to the indications and contraindications. Every surgical step includes the potentiality of specific complications.

LAVH is carried out at two different times: the intrabdominal time, and the vaginal time. The first intrabdominal time, includes certain surgical steps:

(1) Laparoscopic access at the abdominal cavity;
(2) Inspection of cavity and of the organs;
(3) Surgical resection of round ligament of uterus;
(4) Surgical resection of the uterus from or with adnexa;
(5) Surgical resection of the vesicouterine peritoneum;
(6) Surgical resection of the uterine arteries.

But the second surgical time, the vaginal time, is completed with the extraction of the uterus, through the vaginal canal, but first the following steps have to be performed:

(1)   The opening of the posterior vaginal fomix (posterior couldotomy) and the access at the Douglas cul-de-sac;
(2)   The resection of the uterosacral and cardinal ligaments on both right and left side;
(3)   The resection of the uterine arteries, in case the uterus has not been previously removed.

LAVH ought to be understood as the first laparoscopic surgical stage, which is completed in the second vaginal stage. In the first laparoscopic stage the following can be carried out:

(1)   The omentum and/or intestinal adhesiotomy;
(2)   The examination and the enucleation from miomas, especially when intra-ligamentary;
(3)   The annessiectomy;
(4)   The treatment of endometriosis, especially in cul-de-sac of Douglas and vesicouterine pouch to vesicovaginal tract.

In chronological order, the complications can be subdivided into: intraoperative complications and postoperative complications. The postoperative complications, in turn, can be subdivided into immediate complications and complications later on.

WHICH FACTORS HAVE REPERCUSSIONS ON THE FREQUENCY OF COMPLICATIONS?

The frequency of intra- and postoperative complications depends on factors of common and specific risks; among the principal factors of risk, first the patient's age has to be considered. Because of senile involution and postmenopausal vaginal atrophy the hysterectomy can, in this case, lead to an abdominal method. The senility of the introitus vagina, is generally associated with the senility of all the genital tract; in this case the uterus itself is small and atrophic. As risk factors the following items have to be taken into account:

(1)   The general condition;
(2)   The presence of metabolic disease (diabetes, adiposity),
(3)   Cardiovascular disease;
(4)   Hypertension;
(5)   Endometriosis;
(6)   Mioma, and in particular the intralegamentary miomas
(7)   Previous laparotomies, and in particular the iterative cesarean section, because it is difficult to dissect the bladder from the uterus;
(8)   Hemias;
(9)   Adipocele;
(10) Cholecystectomies;
(11) The adhesions valuation;
(12) The intraoperative general sight.

The frequency of complications is depends on the intraoperative situation and on the indication, while the type of complication is determined by the surgical method and is specific to the organ.

The complications include unpredictable ones, but they are basically specific to the operative process (complications step by step).

During a hysterectomy, the techniques, the applied technologies and the surgical experiences are decisive to prevent the number and the gravity of the complication in the course of the operation.

The surgical techniques we apply are the following:

(1) Suture;
(2) Loops;
(3) Forceps;
(4) High frequency bipolar scissors[8,9].

In addition to these techniques, there exist:

(1) Experiences of laparotomy and abdominal hysterectomy;
(2) Experiences of vaginal surgery and colpohysterectomy;
(3) Experiences of diagnostic and operative gynecologic laparoscopy;
(4) Knowledge of instrumental technology and of energy with high frequency (HF).

Our specialized school of Obstetrics and Gynecology, includes the teaching of the gynecologic laparoscopy in its complete process, which lasts 5 years[10].

There are some more factors, which influence the rate of complications: the team's experiences and the meticulousness of the operating surgeon, the hysterectomy and the plastic reconstructive vaginal surgery benefits.

The intraoperative complications are not determining factors, when opportunely underlined; the severe complications are those which cannot be identified at once. As a consequence severe postoperative complications can follow, which sometimes are so serious, that they involve the general well-being of the patient and even her life expectancy and quality of life. Among the postoperative complications the following have to be mentioned too: the thrombosis, the pulmonary embolism, cardiovascular complications, disorders of coagulation, anemia and infections. The intra- and postoperative complications exclusively concern the morbidity, but even lethality is not a rare phenomenon. The major intra- and postoperative complications are:

(1) Severe hemorrhage, requiring transfusion;
(2) Infections;
(3) Lesion of adjacent organs (uro-genital tract).

In addition there are also late complications and dyspareunia. The conversion to laparotomy must not be considered as a complication. The laparotomy breach, because of its amplitude, was always considered as a better access, as it is much more simple in terms of application especially in the field of demolishing surgery. We now present in Table 3 the rate of the complications for the vaginal hysterectomy on the one hand and for abdominal hysterectomy on the other hand; the numbers are taken from a publication about women from 15 to 44 years, who underwent a hysterectomy between 1978 and

Table 3 Rate of the complications in comparison between vaginal and abdominal hysterectomy. Breakdown of categorical complication rates among women aged 15 to 44 years undergoing abdominal and vaginal hysterectomy by surgical approach. CREST 1978–1981

Surgical approach:	Vaginal hyst. (n=568)		Abd. hyst. (n=1283)		RR
Complications:					
Febrile morbidity:	15.3		32.3		2.1
Source unidentified		7.2		16.8	
Urinary tract infection		3.4		7.0	
Abdominal incision infection		0		5.0	
Vaginal cuff infection		2.1		3.1	
Pelvic infection		1.2		1.3	
Upper respiratory tract infection		0.9		0.4	
Pneumonia		0.4		0.4	
Sepsis		0.4		0.2	
Peritonitis		0.2		0	
Other		0.4		0.5	
Hemorrhage requiring transfusion	8.3		15.4		1.9
Intraoperative transfusion		4.9		10.0	
Postoperative transfusion		3.4		5.4	
Unintended major surgical procedure:	5.1		1.7		0.3
Intraoperative					
to complete hysterectomy		1.1		0	
to repair bowel trauma		0.4		0.3	
to repair bladder trauma		1.4		0.3	
to control bleeding		0.7		0.2	
Postoperative					
To repair ureter trauma		0		0.2	
To repair bowel trauma		0.2		0	
To repair bladder trauma		0.2		0	
To control bleeding or evacuate hematoma		1.2		0.3	
Other		0		0 3	
Life-threatening event	0		0.4		–
Pulmonary embolus/infarct		0		0.2	
Myocardial infarction, cardiac and/or pulmonary arrest		0		0.1	
Anaphylactic reaction		0		0.1	
Disseminated intravascular coagulation		0		0.1	
Rehospitalization	1.8		2.8		1.6
Bleeding		0.7		1.1	
Infection		0.7		0.6	
Pulmonary embolus		0		0.3	
Other		0.4		0.7	
Death	0.2		0.1		0.4
One or more complications	24.5		42.8		1.7

Table 4 Concerned organs

Hysterectomy	Vaginal Hyst.	VaginalHyst.+Colporrhaphy
	8482 cases (%)	11 081 cases (%)
Lesions		
– bowel	0.09	0.23
– bladder lesion	0.90	0.64
– ureter lesion	0.07	0.14
– great vessel	0.07	0
Rehospitalization		
– hemorrhage	0.84	0.97
Requiring transfusion		
– ileus	0.11	0.14
– peritonitis	0.07	0.07
– febrile morbidity (>38°>7 days)	0.80	0.68
– disorder to cicatrize	1.12	1.71
– embolism pulmonary	0.13	0.22
– thrombosis	0.13	0.23
– fistula	0.07/0.18	0.32
Death	0.02	0.07

1981; these data were reported from Dicker and colleagues[11], CREST (Collaborative Review of Sterilization) 1978–1981.

It should be noticed, that the percentage rate of complications for the abdominal hysterectomy is twice as high as the rate for the vaginal hysterectomy.

In 1980 and 1984 Stark[12,13] compared the complications of simple vaginal hysterectomy (8482 cases), to the complications of vaginal hysterectomy and colporrhaphy (11 081 cases); this inquiry was carried out at 85, respectively 101 hospitals. The concerned organs were classified in the following way (Table 4).

This comparison deserves special attention because of the laparoscopic assisted vaginal hysterectomy, which frequently needs colporrhaphy as well. The results of J.A. Deprest and colleagues regarding the complications on 4502 cases of laparoscopical hysterectomy are shown in Table 5; the same results can be compared to abdominal and vaginal hysterectomy (Table 6).

DISCUSSION

The severe complications, as shown in Tables 5 and 6, amount altogether to 3.24 % (146 complications within 4502 cases); most of the complications concern the surgical lesion of the urinary tract, with 1.43 %. The most frequent traumas, are 39 cases with perforation of the bladder; this rate is equal to 0.87%, with 13 lesions of the ureter, that is 0.29%, and with 12 ureter fistoles which is equal to 0.27%.

However, the complications of the laparoscopic approach through the abdominal wall and the rate of mortality are missing.

Following the collective results of J.A. Deprest, Farr Nezaht and colleagues[14] published the frequency and the type of complications which are reported for 361 cases of hysterectomy, carried out in their own Institute, and utilized as well the laparoscopic way. In this last case the frequency of complications, though being numerically higher, namely 11.1%, in fact is even lower for urologic injury (0.58%), if compared with the data reported from R.C. Dicker *et al.*[11] in Table 3.

The data of laparoscopic hysterectomy reported by J.A. Deprest[7] and compared to the results of Dicker[11] concerning abdominal and vaginal hysterectomy, result in a reduced frequency of the complications, in favor of laparoscopic assisted hysterectomy (Table 6).

But all the comparative examinations are only performed with the abdominal hysterectomy, and not with vaginal hysterectomy, since the authors do not believe, that the surgical cases determined for vaginal hysterectomy indication, can be carried out with the LAVH surgical technique.

Also Summit and colleagues[2] are of the same opinion, after having examined the costs and the complications reported about the laparoassisted hysterectomy and compared to the vaginal hysterectomy.

Already in a substantial number of cases, comparing the laparoscopic hysterectomy to the abdominal hysterectomy, we noticed too, the advantage of a short period of hospitalization, and a short period of regeneration. However, based on own experience, there has to be taken into consideration, that because of involution processes, the senile vagina is not suitable for a vaginal hysterectomy or for the vaginal extraction of the uterus in the LAVH.

Anyway, a voluminous uterus, which fills all the pelvis, hinders the access to the endoscopic instruments, and thus makes the control of the complications and of hemostasis difficult.

The wisdom and the principals of our ancestors must not be contradictions in this context, considering that also for the most versatile laparoscopists there always exists the difficulty 'to pass a camel through the eye of a needle', without injuring one or the other. We are not able to make conclusions for the follow-up, and we do not know all the lesions which were already reported from the other authors, which exactly concern the urogenital tract (1.43%) and the vascular lesions (0.78%).

Our experiences of laparoscopic assisted vaginal hysterectomy, (LAVH), gathered over several years and still not published, reported some complications of infectious nature, although we applied intraoperative antibiotic prophylactic treatment. In one case, on the 4th day, before discharging the patient from the hospital, the temperature increased to 39.8 degrees Celsius and more for a whole week, although also in this case we used broad spectrum antibiotics. At the echography examination, concentrated behind the vagina, a fluid sac was discovered of circa 7 cm diameter; this place was very painful on palpation.

Applying a urinary bladder catheter (10 Charrier) which was introduced through the suture of the vaginal cup, we were able to drain a liquid accumulation of about 100 ml, which did not contain coagulum and was putrid and deep black. The problem of pelvic pain, and the difficulty of urine spontaneously passing (dysuria and the retention of urine), was resolved in a short period (within the first 24 hours). The high temperature also returned to its normal value within 48 hours. As already mentioned, our cases and surely many others, are still not published, while it has to be stated, that an imprecise number of operations could not be completed, and the frequency of the complications cannot be estimated and will probably be higher.

CONCLUSIONS

The exact rate of complications is not really known, and is derived from the papers already published.

In this connection, the frequency of the complications obtained on the basis of data received from the international literature and registered on MEDLINE until 1995, in the field of laparoscopic assisted vaginal hysterectomy, do not represent objectively convincing results, because this surgical technique is relatively new and is not uniformly standardized[15].

In fact, altogether the number of LAVH obtained until now from the international literature, is very small considering the total number of hysterectomies, carried out in the USA, approximately 600 000 yearly and increasing. Besides, these statistical results mean, that today 72% of the hysterectomies, which are in fact 432 000 abdominal hysterectomies, are carried out using the abdominal technique, and this is a very high rate when compared to European values.

But there has to be taken into consideration, that many of the authors do not like to communicate publicly the number of complications in their reports describing the clinical cases. This would reflect their own negative experience and thus, could compromise their own professional reputation, but especially they do not want to be involved with medical–legal proceedings.

In Germany, except for malignant gynecologic pathologies, the percenage rate of abdominal hysterectomy is lower, compared to the USA results; the frequency varies and is subordinate to the hospital centers, it is in the range of 35% to 70%, an average of 52.5%. The Public Health Service in the USA and the insurance system, in this context, also play a determining role.

We preferred the laparoscopic resection of the vesico-uterine peritoneum and to complete the suture of uterine vessels on both sides using the vaginal method; this technique, known from the vaginal hysterectomy, presents a low rate of complications for the bladder and for the ureter lesions. The binding of the uterine vessels using the laparoscopical method with LAVH[7], that was calculated as 76.1%, was executed with the stapler or with electrodesiccation.

This technique requires particular experience and surgical skill to get the identification of the uterine arteries exactly at the point where the vessel crosses the ureter in front. But, the application of electrical energy with high frequency and the electrodesiccation of uterine vessels, can involve the ureters with two simultaneous injurious mechanisms:

Table 5   Complication of observational studies on total laparoscopic hysterectomies

Primary author, year	TypeLH[3]	Number of cases	Operation time** (min)	Uterine weight (g)	Length of hospital stay (day)
Reich 1989	IV	1	180	NR	4
Nezhat 1990	III	1	90	NR	NR
Magos, 1991	II	6	NR	NR	NR
Minelli, 1991	I, II, III	7	90-180	NR	NR
Maher, 1992	III	17	160	NR	3.1
Langebrekke, 1992	II, III	10	145	90-120	2.3
Mage, 1992	III, IV	44	75-90	141	5.2
Lang, 1992	III	4	165	160	7
Lee, 1993	III	82	152	NR	2.6
Wilke, 1993	III	31	NR	NR	>4
Davis, 1993	NR*	46	191	191	1.25
Daniell, 1993	III or IV	68	136	NR	2.6
Hunter, 1993	III	54	(146++)	NR	4
Smith, 1993	NR	15	169	81	2.6
Reich, 1993	I- IV	107	180	216	2
Hourcabie, 1993	III, IV	103	NR	NR	4 22.6 39
Liu, 1993	III, IV	395	102.35	162.72	1.19
Carter, 1993	III	37	151	120	2.7
Ostrzenski, 1993	III	10	205	187-515	1
Canis, 1993	III, 1V	33	149	162	4.8
Phipps, 1993	1, II	114	65/82	NR	2.0
Bishop, 1993	II, III, IV	25	122	NR	1.44
Saye, 1993	II	167	59	141	< 1
Kadar, 1994	N R	24	192	384	3,3
Wood, 1994	I, II, III	141	NR (>120)	NR	<3
Johns, 1994	I, IV	103	79	122-123	2,5
Galen, 1994	III	50	NR	NR	< 1,0
Ou, 1994	I, IV	839	97	NR	1,7
Chapron, 1994	IV	31	171	NR	4,0
Richardson, 1995	NR	75	131	NR	3,2
Jones, 1995	NR	100/250	123/NR	153/NR	3,3/NR
BELCOH YST, 1995 (Belgian Collaborative Study Group on Laparoscopy)	II, III, IV	935	117.5	163	4,01

onversions %) of ases)[12]	Hemorrhagic event % of cases	Major Complications (% ca.)	Nature of major complications
	0	0	
	0	0	
	0	0	
	0	0	
	0	0	
	0	20	1 near ureter injury (pig tail), 1 reintervention for hemorrhage
,7	7	9	1 bladder lesion, 1 obstructive ileus, 2 infections causing readmission
	0	0	
4	0	2.4	2 bladder injuries
	0	3	1 ureter lesion
	4.3	4.3	1 ureter stented, 1 bowel perforation
8	2.9	0	
8	0	3.8	1 ureter lesion, 1 vesico- vaginal fistula (stapler)
R	40	7	1 bladder lesion
9	0	6	1 bladder lesion, 1 bowel lesion, 2 fistulas, 1 pulmonary embolism, 1 incisional hernia
R	0	4	2 bladder lesions, 1 ureter, 1 fistula
7	0.25	2.7	5 bladder lesions, 1 fistula, 1 bowel lesion 1 incisional hernia, 1 obstructive ileus, reinterventions for hemorrhage
	0	3	1 readmission for ileus; spontaneous resolution
	0	10	1 bladder lesion
.3	0	6	1 readmission lesion
5	0	1.75	1 ureter, 1 reintervention for abcess and colostomy
4	4	4	1 bladder lesion
	0	0	
	NR	0	
	4,9	7,8	3 pulmonary emboli, 4 hemorrhages, 2 vesicovaginal fistula, 2 bladder injuries
	0	0,9	1 bladder lesion
	12	2	1 bladder lesion
9	0,5	1,9	8 bladder lesions, 3 hemorrhagic events
2	0	0	4 incissional hernias, 1 pulmonary embolism
7	NR	NR	1 bladder lesion
0,4	NR/0,4%	6,4	3 ureter lesions (one including bladder), 1 fistula, 3 isolated bladder lesions, 1 incissional hernia, 1 obstruction, 5 hemorrhages, 2 neuropraxis, pulmonary embolism
	NR	3,2	2 ureter injuries, 1 fistual, 7 bladder lesions, 13 hemorrhages, 3 obstructive ileus, 2 neuropraxis, 1 pulmonary embolus, 1 unanticipated ovarian cancer

Table 6   Major complication for laparoscopic hysterectomy compared to larger series of abdominal and vaginal hysterectomies

Nature of complication	Abdominal hysterectomy (%)	Vaginal hysterectomy (%)	Laparoscopic hysterectomy n (%)
Urinary tract trauma requiring surgery			64 (1.43%)
Bladder injury	0.3–0.4	1.5–18	39 (0.87%)
Fistula (urinary)	0.32	0.07/0,18	12** (0.27%)
Ureter injury	0.2–0.1	0.0–0.1	13** (0.29%)
Reintervention for hemorragien	0.3	1.2%	35 (0.78%)
Gastro-intestinal complication	0.3–0.9	0.9%	17 (0.38%)
Bowel perforation	0.3/0.23	0.4/0.23	8 (0.18%)
Ileus	0.25/0.26	0.11/0.14	9 (0.20%)
Postoperative hernia/wound dehiscence	0.2	*	9 (0.20%)
Readmission	0.6	0.7	8 (0.18%)
Infectious complication	4.44/4.58	1.92/2.39	7 (0.16%)
Others			1 (0.02%)
Thrombo-embolic events	0.5–0.71	0.0–0.38	7 (0.16%)
Neurologic complication	0.2	0	5 (0.11%)
*Miscellaneous****			1 (0.11%)

(1)   Termic conduction;
(2)   Electric conduction.

You must remember that the ureter transports the urine, that it is a second class electric conductor; the consequence is a fistule caused by burns and/or necrosis. Until today, we did not apply the stapler, but instead suture, loops and electrodesiccation with high frequency[8,9].

We propose a straw-guide on both the ureters; just like in surgical oncology. Before starting Wertheim or Te Linde, we carry out a preventive treatment of the ureter with catheter to kidney calix, for better identification.

REFERENCES

1.   Wingo PA, Huezo CM, Rubin GL, *et al.* The mortality risk associated with hysterectomy. *Am J Obstet Gynecol* 1985;152:803
2.   Summit R.L., Stovall T.G., Lipscomb G.H., Ling F.W. Randomized Comparison of Laparoscopy-Assisted Vaginal Hysterectomy with standard vaginal hysterectomy in an outpatient setting. Obstet. Gynecol 80 (1992) 895-901
3.   Richardsons R.E., Bournas N, Magos A.L. Is laparoscopic hysterectomy a waste of time? Lancet 345 (1995) 36-41

4. Johns AD, Diamond MP. Laparoscopically Assisted Vaginal Hysterectomy. J Reprod Med. 39 (1994). 424-428
5. Munro M., Parker W. Classification of Laparoscopic Hysterectomy. Obstet. Gynecol. 82 (1993) 624-629
6. Garry R., Reich H., Liu CY. Laparoscopy hysterectomy-definition and indications. Gynecol. Endosc. 3 (1994)1-3
7. J.A. Deprest, M.G. Munro, P.R. Koninckx. Review on laparoscopic hysterectomy. Zentralblatt fur Gynakologie 117 (1995) 641-651
8. Scarfi A. Text-Atlas of Gynecological Laparoscopy (Italian language text) Edizioni internazionali CIC. Via Spallanzani 11, Roma (1994)
9. Scarfi A. LAVH (Laparoscopic Assisted Vaginal Hysterectomy) with my own suture. Folgaria, International Symposium Alpen-Adria March 1998
10. Sonderausgabe zur neuen Weiterbildungsordnung (WBO) der Landesarztekammer Baden-Wurttemberg vom 17 Marz 1995; Artzeblatt Baden Wurttemberg, Gentner Verlag Stuttgart 4/95
11. R.C. Dicker, J.R. Greenspan, L.T. Strauss, M.R. Cowart, M.J Scally, H.B. Peterson, F. Destefano, G.L. Rubin, H.W. Ory. Complications of abdominal and vaginal hysterectomy among women of reproductive age in the United States. Am. J. Obstet. Gynecol. December 1, 1982
12. Stark, G. Ergebnisse der Erhebungen postoperativer Komplikationen. In Stark, G. Problematik der Qualitatssicherung in der Gynakologie. Nurnberger Symposium. Demeter, Grafelfing 1980
13. Stark, G. Qualitatssicherung in der operativen Gynakologie, in Stark, G. Umstrittene Probleme in der Geburtshilfe und Gynakologie. Nurnberger Symposium. Demeter, Grafelfing 1984
14. Farr Nezhat, M.D., F.A.C.S., Ceana H. Nezhat, M.D., Dahlia Admon, M.D., Stephen Gordon, M.D., Camran Nezhat, M.D., F.A.C.S.: Complications and results of 361 Hysterectomies performed at laparoscopy. Journal of the American College of Surgeons. March 1995. Volume 180
15. Ronald O. Schwartz. Complications of Laparoscopic Hysterectomy Obst. and Gynecol. 1993? 81: 1022-1024
16. R. Pokras, V.G. Hufnagel. Hysterectomy in the United States 1965-1984. AJPH July 1988, Vol. 78 No 7

LAPAROSCOPIC TREATMENT OF ECTOPIC PREGNANCY

M.G. Porpora, M. Natili and E.V. Cosmi.

2nd Institute of Obstetrics and Gynaecology, "La Sapienza" University of Rome- Italy

INTRODUCTION

The incidence of ectopic pregnancy (EP) has increased more than fourfold over the last 20 years (1). This phenomenon is probably related to the increase of risk factors such as pelvic inflammatory disease (P.I.D.), intrauterine devices (IUD) use, abdominal and pelvic surgery and the frequent use of assisted reproduction techniques. The mortality rate of this pathology, however, has been reduced of 90% in the same period of time, even if EP is still responsible for 13% of all the deaths related with pregnancy and it is the most frequent cause of maternal mortality in the first trimester of gestation (1). Serum β-hCG and progesterone measurements and transvaginal ultrasounds usually permit the diagnosis of an ectopic pregnancy, as early as 5 weeks of amenorrhea, even before symptoms occur. Depending on the patient's condition, the status of the ectopic pregnancy and the patient's desire for further childbearing, treatment may be expectant, medical or surgical, either conservative or radical.

A conservative treatment medical, particularly with systemic or topic administration of Methotrexate (MTX) or expectant. Expectant management has been suggested when the patient is asymptomatic and β -hCG level has a decreasing trend, especially if it is less than 1000 mIU/ml at the time of diagnosis (2; 3). Nevertheless, although this management may be effective in selected patients, it requires a prolonged monitoring, can cause a useless delay of the treatment and may be followed by tubal obstruction or chronic ectopic pregnancy (4). Although conservative therapy generally offers a higher percentage of intrauterine pregnancies (5; 6) some authors do not report a significant difference between conservative and radical treatment (7; 8). In fact numerous factors, such as tubal status before pregnancy, prior pelvic surgery and the age of the patient, play an important role in the reproductive prognosis of these women (9). Therefore, the choice of treatment is still controversial.

The aim of our study was to assess the efficacy, the safety and the subsequent reproductive outcome of different laparoscopic treatments of tubal pregnancy.

PATIENTS AND METHODS

From June 1993 to October 1997, 41 women with tubal pregnancy underwent laparoscopy. The mean age was 30,2 years (range 17-42). The gestational age varied from 4 to 11 weeks (mean 7 weeks). At transvaginal ultrasound examination the major diameter of the pregnancy ranged from 10 to 50 mm (mean 25 mm). The initial serum level of β-hCG ranged from 80 to 9200 mUI/ml (mean 1652 mUI/ml) and in all cases was increasing. All patients gave written informed consent and underwent laparoscopic surgery. At laparoscopy location of ectopic pregnancy was ampullary in 79,3% of cases, isthmic in 19,7% and fimbrial in 1%. In 31 women a conservative treatment was performed because of the presence of selection criteria for this therapy: stable hemodinamic conditions, tubal wall integrity, the highest diameter <50 mm, patient's desire of further childbearing. Antimesenteric linear salpingostomy, with extraction of trophoblastic tissue from the abdominal cavity through a laparoscopic endobag, was performed in 21 cases, intramniotic injection of 20-50 mg of methotrexate (MTX), through a 19 gauge spinal needle, in 9 patients, and tubal milking in one. A salpingectomy was performed in 10 patients. In 3 cases, because of the presence of uncontrolled bleeding after an attempt of salpingostomy, in 5 because the affected tube was extremely damaged whereas the contralateral was normal, in 2 because the tube had been previously treated conservatively for an EP and the patients preferred to undergo subsequent IVF.

Salpingectomy was performed with application of an endoloop at the proximal part of the tube, its excision with scissors and further coagulation of the fallopian stump. In all cases peritoneal washing was performed in order to remove blood clots and residual trophoblastic tissue, if present. The effectiveness of treatment, after conservative surgery, was evaluated by measuring serum β-hCG levels after 24-48 hours and then weekly until its complete disappearance. In case of abnormal trend of β-hCG values and ultrasonographic abnormalities the patient underwent further surgical treatment.

RESULTS

The results of treatments are illustrated on the table 1.

No intra-operative or post-operative complications occurred. Mean duration of surgery ranged from 30 minutes for local injection of MTX to 90 for salpingectomy. Mean hospital stay was 1,7 days. In 29 patients conservative treatment was effective; β-hCG disappearance occurred within 3 weeks from linear salpingostomy and 4 from MTX injection. In 2 cases we observed a persistence of disease and a second laparoscopy with salpingectomy was performed.

Twenty patients, 8 who have received a local injection of MTX, 7 who underwent linear salpingostomy, 4 who had a salpingectomy and 1 in whom a tubal milking was performed, wished to have further pregnancy. After MTX, 7 patients had a term pregnancy and one an ectopic pregnancy. After linear salpingostomy 4 patients achieved a spontaneous intrauterine pregnancy, whereas the other 3 were submitted to IVF. The only patient who underwent tubal milking had a spontaneous term

TABLE 1.

CHARACTERISTICS AND RESULTS OF TREATMENT

Type of operation	Mean duration (min)	Success (%)	Mean hospital stay (days)	IUP(%)	EP (%)
Intramniotic MTX	30	9 (90)	2	4 (57)	1(14,2)
Linear salpingostomy	70	20 (95,2)	1.5	7 (70)	0
Salpingectomy	90	10 (100)	1.2	3 (42,8)	1 (14,2)
Milking	50	1 (100)	1	1(100)	0
Total	70	39 (95,1)	1.7	15(57,7)	2 (7,7)

pregnancy. In the group treated with salpingectomy, 2 patients had a term pregnancy and one an ectopic pregnancy in the contralateral tube.

DISCUSSION AND CONCLUSIONS

The increasing incidence of ectopic pregnancy has induced the gynaecologists to make a great effort to obtain an early diagnosis and to perform a prompt, safe, and effective treatment of this condition. The combination of serum β-hCG and progesterone measurements with transvaginal ultrasounds generally permits a rapid diagnosis. Medical and surgical treatments have been proposed. In our experience medical therapy with local injection of MTX under laparoscopic control has shown to be easy to perform and effective (10). In fact the mean duration time of this procedure has been 30 minutes, it has been successful in 90% of cases with no immediate or long term side effects. Moreover an intrauterine term pregnancy was achieved in 57% of cases. However, this treatment requires a careful selection of the patients (hemodinamic stability, no evidence of active bleeding, unruptured tubal wall). Linear salpingostomy is very effective in terms of resolution of the disease (95,2%) and subsequent fertility (70% of intrauterine pregnancies), and it can be performed on a larger group of patients but requires surgical expertise. Salpingectomy is easy and effective, however, the subsequent pregnancy rate is significantly lower than after conservative management and do not preserve from a further ectopic pregnancy. Therefore this radical treatment should be performed only in case of an extremely damaged tube, after tubal sterilization or when the patient does not desire to preserve her reproductive potential.

In conclusion, as Gomel has recently observed, surgery remains the best choice of treatment of tubal pregnancy (11). In fact it permits confirmation of the diagnosis, evaluation of the affected and the contralateral tube and the whole pelvis and to perform an immediate and effective treatment, irrespective of the size of the gestation, tubal rupture and presence of hemoperitoneum (11). In the past two decades laparoscopy has largely replaced laparotomy for the treatment of ectopic pregnancy because it offers several advantages compared with laparotomy (lower morbidity, shorter hospital stay, quicker recovery times and higher patient's compliance).

The therapeutic choice between radical or conservative treatments is still controversial. However, in young women who desire future pregnancies, the best choice is still a conservative treatment, whereas in patients, who do not want further childbearing or to take a risk of a recurrent ectopic pregnancy, salpingectomy is the best surgical approach. In all cases, it is necessary that the patient is carefully informed on the characteristics and the risks of the treatment proposed and aware of the possibility to switch a laparoscopy to a laparotomy.

REFERENCES

1. Goldner TE, Lawson HW, Xia Z, Atrash HK. Surveillance for ectopic pregnancy - United States, 1970-1989. MMWR 1993; 42 (SS6): 73-85.

2. Garcia AJ, Aubert JM, Sama J, Josimovich JB. Expectant management of presumed ectopic pregnancies. Fertil Steril 1987; 48(3): 395-400.

3. Trio D, Strobelt N, Picciolo C, et al. Prognostic factors for successful expectant management of ectopic pregnancy. Fertil Steril 1995; 63(3): 469-72.

4. Porpora M G, Alò P L, Cosmi E V. Unsuspected chronic ectopic pregnancy in a patient with chronic pelvic pain. Int J Gynecol Obstet 1998 (in press).

5. Yao M and Tulandi T. Current status of surgical and non surgical management of ectopic pregnancy. Fertil Steril 1997; 67: 421-433.

6. Largebrekke A, Sornes T, Urnes A. Fertility outcome after treatment of tubal pregnancy by laparoscopic laser surgery. Acta Obstet Gynecol Scand 1993; 72: 547-549.

7. Maymon R, Shulman A. Controversies and problems in the current management of tubal pregnancy. Human Reprod Update 1996; 2: 541-555.

8. Oelsner G, Goldenberg M, Admon D, et al. Salpingectomy by operative laparoscopy and subsequent reproductive performance. Human Reprod 1994; 9 (1): 83-86.

9. Job-Spirs N, Bouyer J, Pouly JL, et al. Fertility after ectopic prgnancy. First results of a population- based cohort study in France. Hum Reprod 1996; 11 (1): 99-104.

10. Porpora MG, Montanino - Oliva M, De Cristofaro A, et al. Comparison of local injection of methotrexate and linear salpingostomy in the conservative laparoscopic treatment of ectopic pregnancy. J Am Ass Gynecol Laparosc 1996; 3: 271-276.

11. Gomel V. For tubal pregnancy, surgical treatment is usually best. Clin Obstet Gynecol 1995; 38: 353- 61.

THE VAGINAL ROUTE: AN ALTERNATIVE FOR HRT

*Donati Sarti C, *Mincigrucci M., Becorpi A., Baldi S., Di Marco L., Ottanelli S.
*Menopause Clinic Department of Obstetrics and Gynecology of Perugia, Italy.

Department of Obstetrics and Gynecology, University of Florence, Italy.

Vaginal application of medication has for many years been wrongly considered exclusively as a topical treatment for feminine urogenital pathology. In reality, the vaginal method can be considered a systemic administration method which exploits the absorbing powers of the malpighian epithelium; absorption that is also demonstrated by the possible pharmacodynamic and toxic effects provoked by the application in this site of some substances which can be analogous or greater than oral or parenteral administration of the same substances.

The absorption capacity of the vagina is not uniform because influenced by various factors including the characteristics of the substance, the vehicle in which it is dissolved, by its coefficient of diffusion and distribution that varies according to the vaginal pH. The vaginal epithelium is particularly adapt for absorption because it lacks the barrier effect of the horny layer. The substances, in particular steroids and above all estrogens, after having rapidly saturated the epithelium, quickly flows into circulation through the perivaginal venous plexus that through the internal iliac veins is a tributary of the vena cava inferior. Thus the substances absorbed through the vagina have the characteristic of avoiding "hepatic first pass" and the consequential rapid metabolization or inactivation, so much so that some authors think that the topical therapeutic effect of some substances, in particular estrogens, is tied to a tissue redistribution after their passage in circulation.

The vaginal application of drugs can thus consent the use of smaller doses with a better metabolic clearance, it avoids the influence of meals and other physiopathic conditions and excludes gastric-type side effects (13).

This application method can be used during hormone replacement therapy in menopause for natural progesterone. In fact, it is known that if this substance is administered per os in its crystalline state, it is inactivated at the intestinal level; for which it can be administered orally in micronized form alone. On the other hand, this formulation is also metabolized hepatically after only 6 hours, making several administrations necessary in the course of the day (100 mg/die three times a day) to obtain efficient levels of circulating hormones (26, 8) and what is more, active

239

metabolites would form, having a sedative hypnotic effect (1). Intramuscular administration of this substance would not only be inconvenient and very painful for the patient, but can also cause even serious problems at the injection site and requires high dosages. This method can therefore be an alternative to a systemic method allowing a more constant and uniform absorption, even the grade of estrogenization of the vaginal mucous positively influences the absorption of the steroid because estrogens increase the number of receptors for progesterone (12).

With this method lower hematic rates and greater uterine concentrations are obtained than with other methods. In fact, with 200 mg of vaginally administered micronized progesterone there are hematic hormones rates equal to 5 ng/ml compared to the 12-20 ng/ml parenterally, and a uterine concentration of 10 ng/ml compared to levels under 3 ng/ml obtained in the luteal phase (19). The same results are confirmed by various studies including one by Miles (24) that compares vaginal to intramuscular administration of progesterone in 20 women without gonads during assisted artificial fecundation. In a recent study by Cicinelli *et al.* (6), a greater hematic concentration is reported in the uterine artery than in the radial artery after vaginal administration of progesterone. From this we can hypothesize that for the gel formulation there is a uterine first pass, demonstrated by Bulletti *et al.* (2), directly from the vagina with a cell-to-cell passage from or through microvascular connections between the vagina and endometrium that allows this first uterine passage. Therefore the by-pass of the enterohepatic system with a consequentially longer duration in circulation of the active hormone (35), and the hypothesized uterine first-pass enable the progesterone administered with this method to induce a secretory transformation in the endometrium (10) with the least metabolic impact (23, 16).

For this property of determining secretory transformation of the endometrium with lower doses in respect to the intramuscular method, the vaginal method has long been studied and used for sterility and in particular in the field of assisted reproduction, both for the preparation of the endometrium and to support and maintain the initial phase of pregnancy. The oral use of progestinics is not indicated also because they could have a teratogenic effect on the fetus (24,35, 17).

In the search for therapeutic schemes where progestinic is used at the minimal endometrial protective dose, and for preparations with a minor metabolic impact capable of inducing secretory transformation of the endometrium during hormonal replacement therapy in menopause, the vaginal application of natural progesterone can be a valid alternative, especially in obese, hypertense or diabetic patients, or those with disorders of the hepatic functions, where synthetic progestinics, especially of androgenic derivation, can determine negative metabolic repercussions.

The limitations of this type of administration, particularly for therapies that can also be very long as in menopause, is patient compliance. For this reason different formulations aimed at improving compliance are being sold and studied.

The first to be used in therapy were galenic suppositories with exipients of either fatty acids or polyethylene glycol. The latter provides a significant residual of progesterone, 8.8+/-0.9 ng/ml, 24 hours after administration as opposed to what is obtainable with suppositories that contain fatty acids (kbase 7.9+/-3.9 ng/ml and Fbase 4.7+/-1.1 ng/ml (22).

The creme formulation uses polyethylene glycol and is absorbed rather slowly so as to obtain adequate hematic levels of progesterone with a single daily administration (9). In addition, 90% of the active principal in the creme is micronized in particles of 10 microns in diameter (the smallest micronization obtained), allowing a good absorption as the periferic hormonal levels are proportional to the state of micronization of the compound which, the greater the micronization, the greater the absorption (12).

Many problems raised by these systems of transvaginal administration can be overcome through the use of micronized vaginal progesterone of non-immunogenic polycarbophil in a bioadherent gel, well-tolerated and able to adhere to the mucin and the cells of the vaginal epithelium through hydrogenous bonds, while hydrophobic interactions increase the stability of the bond (30). It is insoluble in water and adheres for about three days to the vaginal epithelium, equal to its turn-over, allowing for a constant and controlled release of progesterone inside the vagina, absorbed in the watery phase and continuously replaced by the reserve dissolved in the lipid phase. Two types of formulations containing micronized progesterone exist in concentrations of 4% (45 mg) or 8% (90 mg).

The possibility of reducing the number of applications, in fact, in the case of administration on alternate days the quantities of progesterone released during the period between 24 and 48 hours are equal to those released in the first 24 hours (29), allows the bioadherent gel to improve compliance especially in long-term treatment such as hormonal replacement therapy.

The effects on the endometrium have been evaluated during hormonal replacement therapy with E_2 per os in association with progesterone in bioadherent gel at a dose of 45 mcg and 90 mcg on alternate days for 6 administrations.

Ultra-sound evaluation of the endometrial rima and of the mitotic index, together with morphometric and histological analysis have evidenced a secretory transformation with both dosages (4). Such observations have been confirmed by Ross *et al.*, (31), with the association of natural oral conjugated estrogens and progesterone gel at a dosage of 45-90 mg administered according to the above-described scheme.

The bleeding pattern in the sequential regime has demonstrated to be regular, superimposable to that obtained with synthetic progestinics and independent of the dosage of progesterone (11).

Treatment according to the combined continued scheme has determined amenorrhea in 75% of the cases independently of the concentration used (11, 3).

The use of vaginally administered estrogens allows us to obtain plasmatic concentrations capable of determining systemic effects on the target-organs.

The estrogens administrated include 17-beta estradiol, estriol, conjugated equine estrogens and promestriene in various formulations of administration: rings, vaginal creme, vaginal compresses and suppositories.

The first experiences with ring devices were as contraceptive devices, using a vaginal ring medicated with levonorgestrel or combined with E_2 (18). In particular, a ring device with a diameter of 55.6 mm and a section of 9.5 mm was used giving off 20 mcr/die of levonorgestrel alone or else combined with E_2 50 or 100 mcg. The patients were subdivided into three groups: the first treated with the vaginal ring alone, the second and third with the addition of patch estradiol at a dosage of 50 or 100 mg/die.

After three months of therapy only a few interindividual differences relative to the plasmatic levels of LNG independent of the dosage of estradiol administered emerge from our study. E_2 increases ovarian suppression dose-dependently without diminishing the number or duration of bleeding. Successively, Weissberg *et al.* (37) used a combined ring with Ethynyl-Estradiol 20 mcr/die + Norethisterone acetate 1 mg/die for 6 months.

Stumpf *et al.* (33), with the aim of obtaining physiological levels of E_2 in hypoestrogenic women, used a ring device of polysyloxan, already used as a trilaminar-type contraceptive releasing E_2 in different dosages, respectively 100, 200, 400 mcg.

The results demonstrated levels of plasmatic E_2 respectively corresponding to the specific phases of a normal menstrual cycle.

Presently, there are different types of rings available:

Trilaminar: with a section of 9.5 mm, diameter of 54 mm, containing 100-200-400 mg of E_2 in the intermediate portion, no steroids in the most external portion, while in the innermost portion there can, again, be E_2 .

Monolaminar: where E_2 is homogeneously distributed throughout the whole device at a dose of 400 mg. It has a section of 49 mmq with 22 mmq of surface. Once assembled, the ring must be inserted after 3-5 days.

Monolaminar (34): with a diameter of 60 mm in which crystalline E_2 is dissolved in the polymer at a dosage of 53 mg, it is homogeneously given off at an initial dosage of 0.4 mg/die, after 20 days 0.2 mg/die, after 50 days 0.1 mg/die.

Monolaminar (32) with a thickness of 9 mm and a diameter of 55 mm containing 2 mg of homogeneously dispersed E_2 which in vitro releases 5-10 mcg/die. With this the plasmatic levels of E_2 during therapy are 100-200 pmol/l.

The ring where E_2 is homogeneously dispersed and without interfacing between the different portions guarantees adequate and constant quantities of E_2 circulating, equivalent to, as Stumpf's study in 1986 (33) demonstrated, 45-55 pg/ml for the rings containing 100 mg of E_2, 70-100 pg/ml for 200 mg of E_2, 120-150 pg/ml for 300 mg of E_2. In fact, the trilaminar ring provides an increasing minimal quantity of E_2 that returns to basal levels after 2-3 months; indeed, FSH and LH are not greatly suppressed in these three months.

There can be spotting in less than 1% of the cases. The vaginal pH is analogous to that found during the fertile age. As for vaginal dispareunia and atrophy there is a notable reduction in symptomatology.

Post-menopause application of the vaginal ring releasing E_2 (53 mg) is motivated in the control of climacteric and urogenital symptomatology. Schiff (37) and then Stumpf (33) studied and compared the plasmatic concentrations obtained with these preparations using the classical administration and vaginal administration with the application of vaginal rings. The transvaginal echographic control revealed that endometrial thickness in Smithís work was 3-4 mm with spotting <1% (32).

Vartianen *et al.* (38) report the post treatment endometrial histology with 6 cases of proliferative endometrium, 4 cases with a pronounced estrogenic effect, 4 cases with atrophic endometrium, 3 cases with moderated estrogenic effects, 2 cases with slight effects. Also, Henriksson (39) reports neither the appearance of bleeding nor endometrial proliferation.

The effect on the vaginal mucosa consists of significant reduction of the petechiae, of inelasticity and vaginal friability with a clear improvement in vaginal lubrication and reduction in the quantity of urination.

Conjugated equine estrogens can be administered in vaginal creme at a dosage of 0.625 mg/die.

Nachtigall in a study in 1995(41), compared the systemic effects for three months of treatment determined by ECE administered in vaginal creme at a dosage of 0.625 mg/die with those obtained with the use of vaginal rings releasing E2 at a dosage of 7.5 mcg/die.

The result has evidence the greater capacity for endometrial and mammary stimulation of ECEs in respect to the use of E2 (out of 129 patients with a vaginal ring, 2 presented endometrial hyperplasia against the three cases of hyperplasia found among the 67 patients in therapy with vaginal creme). These results confirm the thesis on the systemic efficiency of vaginal administration evidencing that with the use of ECE monotherapy is not sufficient.

17-β-estradiol can also be administered under the form of vaginal compresses consisting of a matrix of hydroxipropyl methylcellulose mixed with carbon which allows a controlled release of the active ingredient, dispersion that is independent of vaginal pH levels. The novelty in respect to other forms of vaginal administration lies, in fact, in the gelatinous matrix that guarantees the gradual and homogeneous distribution of the estrogenic preparation. Given the elevated affinity of 17-β-estradiol for the receptors lying in various areas of the genito-urinary apparatus the local effect measurable in clinical, metabolic and cytological terms is superimposable on the effect obtained using the traditional administration methods (40). From Holst (40), already after three months of treatment using 25mcg/die of 17-β-estradiol there emerges a clear reduction of the symptomatology that characterizes the genito-urinary atrophy typical of post-menopause. In fact, in the same study, out of 23 cases of moderate and severe atrophy, there remained only one case of moderate atrophy with partial resolution of all the severe forms after three months of treatment. The effects of this therapy on the vaginal cytology can be studied through the modification of the rapport between parabasal cells, intermediate cells and superficial cells that constitute the vaginal epithelium (Maturation Index). The vaginal and urethral epithelial cells represent, in fact, one of the main targets of estrogens, they, indeed, possess dose-dependent cellular receptors. The activation of receptors for estrogens promotes the proliferation and vacuolization of the epithelial cells. Vaginal pH is reduced and there is a stabilization of the bacterial flora. Holds (40) showed in a double-blind study the modifications of the vaginal environment through pH evaluation that already after 3-5 days of therapy with 25 mcg of estradiol was reduced because of the increase in lactic acid due, in turn, to the increase in the production of glycogen.

The evaluation of the karyokinetic index effectuated at 3,9,16,22 weeks of treatment by Mattsson (25) with 2 different doses of estradiol, respectively 25 and 50 mcg/die, does not show a significant difference. Therefore, the stimulation on the vaginal mucosa can be considered dose-independent, despite Nilssonís data (28) which emphasize the therapeutic inefficiency of 10 mcg of estradiol on the symptomatology from vaginal atrophy despite apparent clinical improvement. Still according to Nilsson (28), the absorption of vaginal estradiol is initially dose-dependent and then becomes dose-independent after 14 days. Finally, the levels of estrone circulating and of gonadotropin remain unmodified.

According to Matsson (25), endometrial response to the topical administration of estradiol is dose-dependent. In fact, among the patients who were administered 17-β-estradiol at a dose of 50 mcg/die there appears a situation of proliferative endometrium.

In addition, the use of this formulation seems interesting in the three weeks that precede colporrhaphy, whether to increase tissue elasticity, or to reduce the number of recurring cysts (14).

Estriol administered vaginally deserves further reflection for its biological peculiarities.

This is a natural estrogen, considered for some time now a weak estrogen in the different estrogenic actions in respect to E2. In fact, estriol determines some structural modifications of the receptor complex that condition a brief nuclear retention time of about 1-4 hours, against the 6-24 hours of nuclear retention of E_2 (7). Thus, E3 is able to determine estrogenic effects that develop rapidly after the receptoral stimulation, represented by vasodilatation with an increase of tissue vascularization, from imbibition and consequential increase of the energetic substrata.

On the contrary, slight activity is demonstrated in the processes that require a more prolonged stimulation, such as cellular multiplication with activation of mitosis in the target tissues.

E_2 can be administered in creme form or vaginal suppositories at a dosage of 0.5-1 mg in daily administration in strongly symptomatic patients, on alternate days or in bi-weekly administrations in the remaining clinical situations. Therapeutic treatment with E_3 at a dosage of 1 mg/die also shows an improvement of the bone density measured with Dexa with a course similar to that obtained in subjects of equal age treated with E_2 transdermically, with significantly higher values in comparison to untreated patients (15).

Melis, in a study of 1996 (23), compared the effects of the administration of intravaginal E3 associated calcitonin in spray-form on the neurovegetative symptomatology and on the evolution of the process of bone demineralization. From the study it emerges that E_3 alone is able to improve climacteric symptomatology with measurable results already after a year of treatment. After a year of therapy with E_3 and Ca the reduction of BMD is equal to -1+/-0.4%, while with calcium therapy alone the reduction of BMD is -2.4%+/-0.3%.

Relatively to the protective effects on the cardiovascular system, E_3 does not prove to be influenced by the simultaneous use of progestinics (21).

REFERENCES

1. Arafat E.S., Hargrove J.T., Maxon W.B., Desiderio D.M., Wentz A.C., Anderson M.I.Sedative and hypnotic effects of oral administration of micrinized progesterone my be mediated through its metabolites. Am J. Obstet Gynecol 1988; 159:1203-9.

2. Bulletti C., De Ziegler D., Giacomucci E., Bolelli G.F., Franceschetti F., Polli V, Rossi S., Flamigni C. Demostration d'un premier passage uterin. Symposium

the first uterine pass effect a new options in progesterone therapy.Abstract from Montpellier September 21, 1995.

3. Bulletti C., *et al.*, The vaginal progesterone gel, Crinone in menopause : 2 terapeutic opthions for improving the control of vaginal bleeding. Abs. 3 rd International Symposium Women ës Health and Menopause, Florence Italy.

4. Casanas-Rouk F, Nisolle M, Marbaix E *et al.* Morphometric, immunohistological and three-dimensional evaluation of the endometrium of menopausal women treated by oestrogen and Crinone, a new slow release vaginal progesterone.Human Repr., 1996; 11: 367-70

5. Cicinelli E., Sabatelli S., Petruzzi D., Stragapede S. Assorbimento per via vaginale di una soluzione oleosa di progesterone (Gestone) in donne in età fertile.Minerva Ginecol. 1995; 47:99-102.

6. Cicinelli *et al.*Plasma concentrations of progesterone are higher in the uterine artery than in the radial artery after vaginal administration of micronized progesterone in an oil-based solution to postmenopausal women.Fertil Ster., 1998; 69, 3: 471-73

7. Clark J.H., Paszko Z., Peck E.J.J.R., Nuclear binding and retention of receptor estrogen complex : relation to the agonist and antagonist properties of estriol. Endocrinology 1997;100:91-96.

8. Devroey P., Palermo G., Borgain C., Van Waesberghe L., Smitz J., Van Steirteghem A.C. progesterone administration in patients with absent ovaries. int. j. Fertil. 1989; 34:188-93.

9. Dei M., Verni A., Rosati D., Perini R. Profili farmacologici e clinici di progesterone e progestinici.Rivista di Ostetricia e Ginecologia 1990. Vol 3^ n.1: 3-10.

10. De Ziegler D., Scidler L., Scharer E., Bouchard P. Administration non orale de la progesterone: Experiences et avenir del la voie transvaginale. Rev. Med. Suisse Ramande (Switzerland) 1994,; 114/9:811-817.

11. De Ziegler D., *et al.*, Estrogen and vaginal progesterone in menopause. Poster presented at the 43 rd Annual Meeting of the Society for Gynecologic Investigation Abs 166, March 20-23, 1996

12. Di Carlo F., Racca S., Gallo E., Conti G., Russo A., Mondo F., Francalanci S. Estrogen and progesterone receptors in human vagina. J. Endocrinal Invest 1985; 8:131-134.

13. Esposito G. Assorbimento e aspetti cinetici dei farmaci somministrati per via vaginale . Giorn. It. Ost. Gin. n. 3-1992.

14. Felding C, Mikkelsen Al, Clausen Hlle V, Loft A, Larsen L. Grupe Preoperative treatment with oestradiol in woman scheduled for vaginal operation for genital prolapse. A randomized, double-blind trial.Maturitas, 1992; 15: 241-249

15. Genazzani A.R., Zichella l. La terapia ormonale in climaterio e postmenopausa. Documento di consenso, I Conferenza Nazionale di Consenso in Scienze Ginecologoche ed Ostetriche, Madonna di Campiglio, 17-24/marzo 1996. Milano:Churchill Livingston 1996.

16. Giacomini G., Naldi S., Polli V. Effetti metabolici del progesterone naturale somministrato per via vaginale,LXVI Congresso SIGO Sorrento 23-27 Ottobre 1989.

17. Gibbons W.E. Protocol cal 1620-007 US. Integrated Study Report Symposis and Integrated Statistical and Clinical Study Report. Evaluation of an intravaginal progesterone preparation (Cal 1620) in a donor oocyte program.October 1996

18. Landgren B.M., Aedo A.R., Yohannisson E., Cekan S.Z. Studies on a vaginal ring releasing levonorgestrel at an initial rate of 27 mcg-24h when used alone or in combination with transdermal systems releasing estradiol.Contraception, 1994; 50: 87-100

19. Lobo R.A.. Vaginal Route Paradox: a direct transport to the uterus. Abstract from Montpellier, September 21, 1995.

20. Melis G.B., Gambacciani M., Paoletti A.M., Spinetti A., Cagnacci A., Giusti G., Fioretti P. effetti clinici ed endocrini della somministrazione di una crema vaginale contenente estriolo in donne in postmenoausa. In : Fioretti P., Melis GB., eds. Aggiornamenti in Scienze Ginecologiche ed Ostetriche. Roma : CIC Ed. Int. 1988.

21. Melis G.B., Cagnacci A., Paoletti A.M., Gambacciani M., Soldani R., Spinetti A., Fioretti P., Nella terapia ormonale sostitutiva del climaterio femminile 3° Congresso della Socità It. Menopausa Bologna 16-19 novembre 1988

22. Maddocks S., Hakh P., Moller F., Reid R. A double- blind placebo controlled trial of progesterone vaginal suppositories in the treatment of premenstrual syndrome. Am J. Obstet Gynecol 1986; 154:573-81.

23. Melis G.B., Cagnacci A., Bruni V., Falsetti L., Jasonni V.M., Nappi C., Polatti F., Volpe A. Salmon calcitonin plus intravaginal estriol : an effective treatment for the menopause. Maturitas 1996; 24: 83-90

24. Miles R.A., Pothon R.J., Lobo R.A., et al.Phramacokinetics and endometrial tissue levels of progesterone after administration by intramuscolar and vaginal routes: a comparative study. Fertil Steril, 1994; 62: 485-90

25. Mattsson L.A., Cullberg G., Eriksson O., Knutsson F. Vaginal administration of low dose estradiol effects on the endometrium and vaginal cytology.Maturitas, 1989; 11: 217-222

26. Maxon W.B., Hargrove J.T. Bioavailability of oral micronized progesterone. Fertil. Steril. 1985; 44:622-6.

27. Nilsson C.G., Haukkamaam, Vierolah, Luukkainen T. Tissue concentrations of levonorgestrel in women using a levonorgestrel-releasing IUD. Clin Endocrinol, 1992; 17: 529-36

28. Nilsson K., Heimer G. Low dose estradiol in the treatment of urogenital estrogen deficiency. A pharmacokinetic and pharmacodinamyc study.Maturitas, 1992; 15: 121-127

29. Kisicki J. Protocol 321-01, Clinical Report: Pharmacokinetic study of three dosage strngths of Cal-1620 with natural progesterone. September, 1993 Maturitas, 1994; 18: 239-44

30. Robinson J.R., Leng J-H.S., Park H. Mechanism of adhesion of swelling unsoluble polymers to mucin-epithelia sufaces Proceeding of the 12th Internation Symposium on Controlled Release of Bioactive Materials, 1985; 12

31. Ross D., Pryse-Davies J., Collins W.P. et al Randomised double-blind endometrial study of a vaginal progesterone gel in Oestrogen Treated postmenopausal women

(Abstr P 290). 8th International Congress on the Menopause. Sidney. Australia,November, 3-7, 1990

32. Smith P., Heimer G., Lindskog M., Ulmsten U. Estradiol releasing vaginal ring for treatment of postmenopausal urogenital atrophy. Maturitas, 1993; 16: 145-154

33. Stumpf P.G. Selective costant serum estradiol levels achived by vaginal rings. Obstet. Gynecol., 1986; 67: 91-94

34. Villanueve B., Casper R.F., Yen S.S.C. Intravaginal administration of progestrone: enhaced after estrogen treatment. Fertil. Steril. 1981; 35:433-7.

35. Fanchin R. *et al.*, uterine contraction (UT) at the time of embryo transfer (ET) alter IVF out come. American Society for reproductive Medicine.53rd Annual meeting.Abs ., October 1997 .

36. Schiff I., Wentwork , Koos B, Rian K.J., Tulkinschi D. Effect of estriol administration on the hyphogonadal uman. Fertil Steril 1978 ; 30:278-82.

37. Weissberger A.J., Ho K.K.Y., Lazarus L. Contrasting effects of oral and transdermal routes of estrogen replacement therapy on 24h growth hormone (gh) secretion, insulin-like growth factor I, and gh-binding protein in postmenopausal women, J Clin.Endocrinol. Metab. 1991; 72: 374-381.

38. Vartiainen J., Wahlstrom T., C-G Nilsson. Effects and accettability of a new 17-beta oestradiol releasing vaginal ring in the treatment of post-menopausal compliance. Maturitas 1993; 17: 129-137.

39. Henrikssonon L., Stjernquist M., Boquist L., *et al.* A comparative multicentre study of the effects of continous low dose estradiol released from a new vaginal ring versus estriol vaginal pessaries in postmenpausal women sintomps and sings of urogenital atrophy .Am. J. Obstet. Gynecol 1994; 171 (3): 624-631

40. Holst J., Grondahl J., Von Shoultz B. Vaginal cytologiy and plasma hormones follwing local treatment of postmenopausal women with oestradiol and dieno estrol.University Hospital, Department of Obstetrics and Gynecology, S-901 85 Umea, Sweden

41. Nachtigall Lila E. Clinical trial of the estradiol vaginal ring in the U.S.Maturitas 22 Suppl.(1995)S43-S47

Endocrinology of Menopause

G. Spera, P. Martini, A. Cornoldi, S. Falcone, C. Lubrano

Università degli Studi di Roma "La Sapienza", Dipartimento di Fisiopatologia Medica, Policlinico Umberto I, Viale del Policlinico, 00161 Roma, Italy

Menopause is defined as the permanent cessation of menstruation due to loss of ovarian follicular activity. The diagnosis could be established only retrospectively, after a period of 12 months spontaneous amenorrhea in women with elevated levels of FSH, because it is not possible to characterise a predictive hormonal pattern. The menopausal transition represents a period of marked variability in hormonal levels; this period - classified as "pre-menopause"- is around 10 years and represents a progressive reduction of fertility despite the ovulation which can be verified until the last cycle. The demonstration of the age-dependent loss of fertility can be proved by data obtained with artificial insemination; in fact, the rate of success declines with the women's age[1]. The age of the onset of the menopause ranges between 44 and 56 years, with an average of 50.4 years[2]. This is the natural consequence of the numerical collapse of the follicular ovarian cells, which , at birth are equal to more than 2 million and then decrease to fewer than 5000, at the menopause[3].

ENDOCRINOLOGY OF MENOPAUSE

The hormonal modifications are characterised by an increase in the gonadotropin levels together with a reduction of the estrogen levels (Figure 1). The increase of FSH and of LH is slow and gradual and requires from 6 to 12 months to reach stable levels; the FSH levels increase more than the LH and this is probably due to a reduction of the estrogens and of the inhibin concentrations[4]. The reduction of the follicular aromatase induces the decrease of the Estradiol (E2) and so Estrone (E1) becomes the major circulating estrogen. Estrone is produced almost exclusively in the fat tissue from the aromatisation of the Androstenedione (A) of surrenal origin. While the circulating levels of Prolattina (PRL), hormone of the growth (GH), TSH, ACTH and Cortisolo do not change significantly[5], the androgens suffer a light but important lowering of about 15%[6]. This decrease is accompanied by an analogous reduction of the circulating SHBG, maintaining the same relationship as between the free

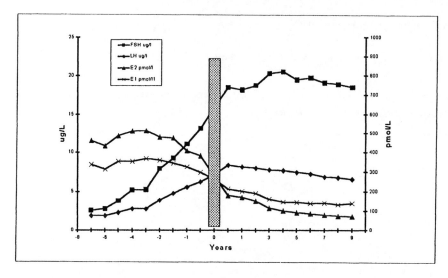

Figure 1 Mean serum levels of FSH,LH, estradiol and estrone during
the perimenopausal transition
Modificated from: Rannevik G et al. *Mauritas* 1995; 21:103

and bound quotas of these steroids[7]. The ovary, therefore, preserves its own steroidogenetical activity
and the hormones mainly produced become A and Testosterone (T)[8] (Table 1). In relative terms, the
ovarian daily contribution of A decreases from around 50% around to anything from 5% to 20% and
T increases from around 25% to 40 %[9]. The circulating A and T become the respective precursors of
E1 and E2 in that they convert from the aromatase which is in the subcutaneous fat and which in the
perimenopausal period, shows an increase in quantity and in its activity. For this reason there is a
strong positive correlation between A and E1 and between estrogens and BMI (Body Mass Index)[10].
Therefore in the menopause the estrogen levels become dependent on both the serum levels of T and
A and the quantity of subcutaneous fat.

Table 1 Concentrations of steroids (pg/ml) in ovarian and peripheral blood

Vein	Testosterone	Androstenedione	Estradiol	Estrone
Ovarian	3033±1046	3455±1330	31.1±6.3	71.5±13.3
Peripheral	198±27	754±174	14.6±2.9	30.3±3.4

From Judd HL et al. *J Clin Endocrinol Metab* 1974; 39:1020

THE CLIMACTERIC SYNDROME

During the premenopausal period, certain disturbances can arise which will trouble the woman
throughout her climatery[11] (Table 2). The major clinical symptoms in the climacteric and

Table 2 Manifestations of the gradual decrease and final cessation of the ovarian function in the climacteric and postmenopausal periods

Main Groups of Symptoms	Common Manifestation
Endocrine Symptoms	Bleeding irregularities
	"Menopausal syndrome" (principally vasomotor disturbance as hot flashes)
	Local regressive changes in the urogenital tract
Nervous System Disturbances	Insomnia
	Nervousness
	Headache
	Irritability
	Fluctuation in mood
	Depression
Metabolic Changes	Osteoporosis
	Alterated lipid and carbohydrate metabolism
	Atherosclerosis

From Zador G. *Acta Obstet Gynecol Scand* 1977; 65: 19 – 26

postmenopausal periods are: menstrual irregularity, cefalea, modification of the mood and the so-called "hot flushes". The last of these is, undoubtedly, the one patients complain about mostly.

The mechanisms involved in the determination of the hot flushes remain controversial. It has been now ascertained that the estrogenic decrease has a fundamental role to play. At the beginning of each hot flush there is a peak of LH; this increase is not the cause, but the reflex of a hypothalamic mechanism that instigates the hot flush. This has been confirmed by the fact that in the surgical menopause this symptom precedes the increase of gonadotropine[12], and by the observation that women with a deficit of GnRH do not present that symptom, which appears instead following the administration of GnRH agonist[13]. Other mechanisms participate in the occurrence of the hot flush; for instance, a reduction in the endogenous opioids, α-adrenergic and serotoninergic mechanisms, but everything seems to refer back to an original decrease in the circulating estrogenis[14] (Figure 2). An

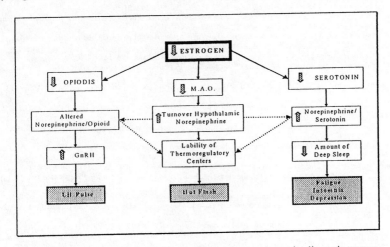

Figure 2 Possible mechanism of central nervous system change in climateric women. From Hammond CB. *Ostet Gynecol* 1996; 87: 2S

inverse correlation exists between the levels of circulating E_2 and the occurrence of the vasomotor symptoms, which are less frequent or less severe in obese women[15]. The hot flushes are removed with the substituted estrogenic therapy[16], which even prevent the demineralisation of the bones.

Instead, there is no correlation between hormonal parameters and sexuality, which is influenced by personal attitudes and from the psychological comfort in the sexual sphere.

The only positive hormone correlated with "sexual comfort" is the DHEA[17].

MENOPAUSE AND THYROID

Already during the premenopause there is a physiological diminution of the thyroid function in partnership with an increase of the BMI[18]; the correlation between TSH and BMI, positive in this phase, becomes negative in the postmenopause[19]. A screening for thyroid illness in the menopause has shown that more than 10% of women have serum levels of thyroid altered hormones: 0.6% were found to be hyperthyroid, 1,6% of the results were overtly hypothyroid, 2.4% presented a subclinical hypothyroidism, while the remaining group showed positive antibody titles higher than those of the control group with hormonal values within the limits of the norm[20]. Besides influencing the BMI, the thyroid hormones modify the BMD (Bone Mineral Density). The so-called subclinic hypertyroidsm, which is obtained with suppressive doses of L-tiroxina, is able to reduce the bone mass by means of its improved action on both the osteoclastics and on the osteoblastics. This accelerated osteoporosis justifies particular attention to the opotherapy of the thyroid[21]. If administered in late menopause, the same therapy does not modify the bone metabolism[22].

REFERENCES

1. Schwartz D, Mayaux MJ. Female fecundity as a function of age. *N Engl J Med* 1982; 306: 404-406
2. Whelan EA et al. Menstrual and reproductive characteristics and age at natural menopause. *Am J Epidemiol* 1990; 131: 625-632
3. Richardson SJ in The biological basis of the menopause. *Bailliere's Clin Endocrinol Metab.* 1993; 7:1
4. Buckler HM, Evans CA, Mamtora H, Burger HG, Anderson BC. Gonadotropin, steroid, and inhibin levels in women with incipient ovarian failure during anovulatory and ovulatory rebound cycles. *J Clin Endocrinol Metab* 1991; 72: 116-124
5. Yen SSC. The biology of menopause. 1977 *J Reprod Med* 18: 287-296
6. Longscope C. Hormone dynamics at the Menopause. *Ann N Y Acad Sci* 1990; 592: 21-30
7. Ranevik G et al. A longitudinal study of the perimenopausal transition: altered profiles of steroids and pituitary hormones, SHBG and bone mineral density. *Maturitas* 1995; 21: 103-113
8. Judd HL et al. Endocrine function of the postmenopausal ovary: concentrations of androgens and estrogens in ovarian and peripheral vein blood. *J Clin Endocrinol Metab* 1974; 39: 1020-1024
9. Adashi EJ. The climacteric ovary: a viable endocrine organ. *Semin Reprod Endocrinol* 1991; 9: 200-205
10. Kaye SA et al. Associations of body mass and fat distribution with sex hormone concentrations in postmenopausal women. *Int J Epidemiol* 1991; 20: 151-156
11. Zador G. The pathophysiologyand methods of treatment of climacteric disorders. *Acta Obstet Gynecol Scand* 1977; 65: 19-26
12. Casper RJ, Yen SSC, Wilhem MM. Menopausal flushes: a neuroendocrine link with pulsatile LH secretion. *Science* 1989; 205: 823-825
13. De Fazio J et al. Induction of hot flushes in premenopausal women treated with a long-acting GnRH agonist. *J Clin Endocrinol Metab* 1983; 56: 445-448
14. Hammond CB. Menopause and hormone replacement therapy: an overview. *Obstet Gynecol* 1996; 87: 2S-15S
15. Erlik Y et al. Estrogen levels in postmenopausal women with hot flushes. *Obstet Gynecol* 1982; 59: 403-407
16. Steingold KA. Treatment of hot flushes with estradiol administration. *J Clin Endocrinol Metab*, 1985; 61: 627-632
17. Cawood EH, Bancroft J. Steroid Hormones, the menopause, sexuality and well-being of women. *Psychol Med* 1996; 26(5): 925-936
18. De Aloysio D et al. Premenopause-dependent changes. *Gynecol Obstet Invest* 1996; 42(2): 120-127
19. Kirchengast S. Body dimensions and thyroid hormone levels in premenopausal and postmenopausal women from Austria. *Am J Phys. Anthropol;* 1994(4): 487-497
20. Faughnan M et al. Screening for thyroid disease at the menopausal clinic. *Clin Invest Med* 1995; 18(1): 11-18
21. Ongphiphadhanakul B, Puavilai G, Rajatanavin R. Effect of TSH-suppressive doses of levothyroxine on bone mineral density in Thai women. *J Med Assoc Thai* 1996; 79(9): 563-567
22. Fujiyama K et al. Suppressive doses of thyroxine do not accelerate age-related bone loss in late

ESTROGENS AND NITRIC OXIDE: A CARDIOVASCULAR DUET.

F.Facchinetti, F. Piccinini, A. Cagnacci, A. Volpe.

Dipartimento di Scienze Ginecologiche Ostetriche e Pediatriche,

Università di Modena e Reggio Emilia, Italy.

Cardiovascular disease is one of the most important cause of illness and death in women, namely over the sixth decade. The difference in the incidence between premenopausal women and men of the same age for such disorder, suggests that endogenous sex hormones may have a primary role. This is supported by evidence that estrogen replacement therapy (ERT) in postmenpausal women decreases the risk of cardiovascular events although the cardioprotective mechanism remains unclear (1).

The beneficial effects of estrogens may be related to the positive balance in HDL/LDL cholesterol: thus limiting the uptake of cholesterol ester into the arterial wall. However not all the cardiovascular benefit can account to the lipidic profile (2). Recent studies demonstrate that both long and short term estrogen administration improves "in vivo" the endothelium-dependent vasodilation in coronary arteries of ovariectomized animals, suggesting that other mechanism are involved. One of such mechanism is that estrogen can induce cardioprotection through L-arginine (L-ARG)-nitric oxide (NO) pathway. Several observations support this hypothesis: NO infact have many cardiovascular actions, e.g. vasodilation, inhibition of platelet aggregation and vascular smooth muscle cell growth. Hayashi et al. demonstrated that aortic rings from female rabbits release

NO according to estradiol levels (3). Hishikawa et al. treated human endothelial cells wtih 17-βestradiol and noted that it stimulates constitutive NO synthase activity (4). Other authors demonstrate that circulating levels of NO increased with follicular developement and correlated with 17 β estradiol levels. Van Buren et al. affirm that the pharmacological blockade of NO synthase attenuates estradiol-induced vasodilation of the uterine circulation (5).

For all these reasons our purpose was to investigate the effect of long term ERT on NO and on blood pressure in postmenopausal women.

MATERIALS AND METHODS

Subjects and Protocol

Twentyfive healthy, normotensive, postmenopausal women in spontaneous menopause from at least one year were enrolled in the study. Menopause status was confirmed by values of FSH >40 IU/L and estradiol <25 pg/ml. Normotension was initially diagnosed by office blood pressure measuring, using a mercury sphygmomanometer according to the recomendations of the American Society of Hypertension (6). A preliminary 24-hour blood pressure monitoring (ABP Monitor Spacelabs Medical, Inc Redmand, Washington) was utilized to confirm the conventional diagnosis of normal blood pressure. All subjects were counseled about the nature of the study and signed the consent to partecipate to the research, previously approved by the local ethical committee. All women are free from hormone or antihypertensive medications. Those showing abnormal changes of lipid and glucose metabolism as well as those presenting with thyroid illness were excluded from the study.

Thus, in a double-blind fashion each woman was randomized to receive a treatment for two months with patches rated to deliver either 50 µg/day of 17 βestradiol (Dermestril 50; Rotta Research Laboratorium S.p.A.) or placebo. At the end of the two months each subject was switched to the alternate treatment for the next two months.

Blood samples were collected after overnight fasting on baseline conditions, and at the end of each treatment course. Blood pressure was monitored for 24-h at the end of each 2-months treatment period. Blood pressure was sampled every 30 minutes throughout the 24-h period and analyzed as the 24-h mean, the daytime mean (08:00-20:00 h), and the nighttime mean (20:00-08:00 h). Three women dropped out for lack of compliance and three for change of address.

Assays

Blood was soon centrifuged after collection and serum stored at -20°C, until assay. One ml of serum was added to 30 mg sulphosalicilic acid powder (Sigma, St. Louis, MO), vortexed and centrifuged at 2000 g for 20 minutes. A fraction of clear supernatant was mixed with an equal volume of o-phtaldialdeide for 1 minute. Such fluorescent derivative was then injected into an High Performance Liquide Chromatography apparatus (Waters, MN) equipped with a RP C-18 column. Flow rate was adjusted to 1 ml/min. Mobile phase was constituted by a mixture of 0.012 M Phosphate buffer with Acetonitrile and Methanol (91:4:5), pH 5.9. Citrulline (Cit) and Arginine (Arg) show a retention time of 6.8 and 10.5 minutes, respectively.

A pool of serum from postmenopausal women served as external standard. Cit levels were 30.7 µM and Arg levels were 92.1 µM. As internal standard was used L-Metionine sulfone. Intra-assay coefficient of variation were 4.7% and 5.9% for Cit and Arg, respectively.

Statistical analyses

The data are reported as means ± SD. Comparisons before and after ERT were based on t-test.for paired sample. Correlations were established using Pearson equation.

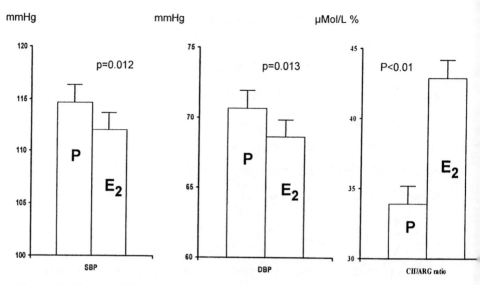

Figure 1 Mean (±SD) of systolic and diastolic nighttime blood pressure with placebo (P) or estradiol (E$_2$). Mean (±SD) of CIT/ARG ratio in the same two groups.

RESULTS

The mean age of the 19 women who definitely complete the study was 53 ± 4 years (range 48-64) and the months since menopause were 34.5 ± 24.5 (range 6-98). Mean baseline concentrations of ARG and CIT were 134.7 ± 55.1 and 48.7 ± 21.2 μMol/L respectively, and nitrites levels were 6.5 ± 2.9 μMol/L. No significant differences in nitrite levels were found between estradiol and placebo treatment. ARG levels significally decreased from 143.9 ± 57.2 (P) to 119.3 ± 36.8 (ERT) μMol/L (P<0.05) while CIT levels did not change (from 42 ± 16.8 (P) to 45.8 ± 17.4 (ERT) μMol/L). We also calculated the CIT/ARG ratio between P and ERT treatment as an expression of in vivo NO synthase activity. The evaluation of CIT/ARG ratio (%) in the two different treatments demonstrated a significant increase from P (33.9 ± 18.5 μMol/L) to ERT (42.9 ± 21.6 μMol/L) (P<0.01) (Fig. 1). No correlations were found between CIT/ARG ratio and age, time since menopause nor with baseline ARG and CIT levels.

During transdermal estradiol a tendency towards lower levels was observed for 24-h systolic (SBP), diastolic (DBP) and mean blood pressure (MBP). At daytime values of SBP ($p<0.06$) and heart rate (HR) tended to be lower during ERT, while DBP and MBP were virtually unmodified. At night a significant decrease ($p<0.012$) was observed for SBP, DBP, MBP, HR (Fig.1). No correlations existed between changes in blood pressure upon treatment and changes in CIT/ARG ratio. A positive correlation was found between changes in CIT/ARG ratio and menopausal duration ($r=0.53$, $p<0.05$).

CONCLUSIONS

These data demonstrate that transdermal estradiol replacement in postmenopausal women is able to stimulate NO production through the metabolism of endogenous L-Arg. Such an effect seems specific since the CIT/ARG ratio, an expression of "in vivo" NO synthase changes, increases only during estradiol treatment while it remains unaffected during placebo. The ability of estradiol in reducing Arg levels and increasing CIT/ARG ratio is further sustained by the observation that the design of this study was a cross-over and hence both placebo and estrogen responses were observed in the same subjects.

The data dealing with blood pressure indicate that the main effect of estradiol is exerted on SBP, while the effect, is minimal, if any, on HR. The effect on blood pressure is less evident during the day than at night. Either the effect of estradiol is counteracted at day, or it is enhanced at night. Although statistical definite correlations were not demonstrated in this report it seems evident that the nocturnal decrease of BP upon estradiol is associated with an enhancement of NO synthase activity, as supported by the increased values of CIT/ARG ratio. That NO synthase activity could be stimulated by estradiol was already reported both by Cicinelli et al. (7) and Imthurn et al. (8). The data of this study indicate that such NO release could contribute to the cardiovascular benefit exerted by estradiol in postmenopausal women.

REFERENCES

1. Stampfer MJ, Colditz GA, Willett WC,Manson JE, Rosner B, Speizer FE, et al. Postmenopausal estrogen therapy and cardiovascular disease. Ten-year follow-up from the Nurses'Healthy Study. N Engl J Med. 1991;325:756-62.

2. Walsh BW,Schiff I, Rosner B,Greenberg L,Ravnikal V, Sacks FM. Effects of postmenopausal estrogen replacement on the cconcentration and metabolism of plasma lipoproteins. N Engl J Med. 1991;325:1196-1204.

3. Hayashi T, Fukuto JM,Ignarro LJ, Chaudhuri G, Basal release of nitric oxide from aortic rings is grater in female rabbits than in male rabbits:implications for atherosclerosis. Proc Natl Acad Sci USA 1992;89:11259-63.

4. Hishikawa K,Nakaki T, Marumo T, Suzuki H, Kato R, Saruta T. Induction of constitutive nitric oxide synthase by estradiol in human endothelial cells. Hypertension. 1994;24:386. Abstract.

5. Van- Buren GA, Yang DS, Clark KE. Estrogen-induced uterine vasodilation is antagonized by L-nitroarginine methyl ester, an inhibitor of nitric oxide synthesis. Am J J Obstet Gynecol. 1992;167:828-833.

6. American Society of Hypertension. Reccomendations for routine blood pressure measurement by indirect sphygmomanometry. Am J Hypertens. 1992;5:207-209.

7. Cicinelli E, Ignarro LJ, Lograno M, Matteo G, Falco N, Schonauer L. Acute effects of transdermal estradiol administration on plasma levels of nitric oxide in postmenopausal women Fertil Steril. 1997;67:63-66.

8. Imthurn B, Rosselli M, Jaeger AW, Keller PJ, Dubey RK. Differential effects of hormone-replacement therapy on endogenous nitric oxide (nitrite/nitrate) levels in postmenopausal women substituted with 17ß-estradiol valerate and cyproterone acetate or medroxyprogesterone acetate. J Clin Endocrin Metab. 1997;82:388-394.

ENDOPROSTHETICS IN HIP AND KNEE JOINTS

AFFECTED BY OSTEOPOROSIS

W. Thomas*, F. Bove** - Rome

* Pres. Comit. Scient. AILA (Fondazione per la lotta all'artrosi e osteoporosi) ** Pres. AILA

Because of the continuous increase of the average life expectation, political economy and health policy of necessity had to turn their main interests to the problem of osteoporosis which is one of the major complication of post-menopausal women (Melton et al. 1992; Hans et al. 1996). The obviously most crucial skeletal part with respect to the development of an osteoporosis process is the proximal femur extremity. Orthopaedic surgeons are confronted with this problem for the following two aspects:

1. the necessity of treating pathological femur neck fractures due to osteoporosis, and

2. the endoprosthetic treatment of degenerative alterations of hip joints affected by severe osteoporoses of proximal femur bones.

If in such cases an indication for the application of an endoprosthesis is undoubtedly set, many surgeons adopt the concept of using bone cement for the fixation of endoprostheses. We consider such a procedure as questionable particularly in the presence of an osteoporosis and want to present our own considerations in this regard as well as our concept of cementless fixation.

Problems concerning the use of cement with osteoporosis

1. When preparing a femur bone affected by osteoporosis for the insertion of an endoprosthesis, yellow marrow and porotic spongiosa are removed. In most cases only a relatively smooth coating

of the interior femur cortex remains. Thus, the applied cement plombage does not meet sufficient structures for toothing, for which reason the primary stability becomes problematic.

2. The polymerization temperature after the insertion of cement is normally higher than the denaturation limit of proteins and causes a further biological damage to the already weakened anchorage bedding (Iida et al. 1974).

3. In advanced age and especially in the presence of an osteoporosis, the periosteal arterial blood supply system is virtually completely depleted, while only the endosteal blood supply of the bone remains effective. By inserting a cement filling, this endosteal blood supply is considerably disturbed.

As a consequence of the above circumstances, an insufficient and not durable primary stability as well as above all a necrotic alteration of the anchoring bone within the proximal femur can frequently be observed, with the risk of micro and macrofractures and the consequence of an early loosening (Morray, Kavanagh 1992).

The concept of cementless endoprosthetics with osteoporosis

If the above mentioned problems linked with the cement fixation in cases of osteoporosis of the bones to be treated are to be prevented, it is necessary to envisage a cementless treatment with sophisticated features of the implant parts. In this case, three requirements have to be met:

1. high primary stability (mechanical fixation);
2. secondary stability through bone ingrowth (biological fixation);
3. continuity of endosteal blood supply.

Point 1. In order to obtain a high primary stability, the shaping and structuring of the endoprosthesis surface according to modern biomechanical and biological notions is of the utmost importance. The endoprosthesis must have an anatomical shape, in order to assure a possibly optimal contact between surface and bone and the total filling of the marrow space prepared by using instruments ("fit and fill" - Horne 1992). Thus, an anatomical antetorsion of the proximal part of the endoprosthesis is obtained at the same time. This contributes in its turn to increasing the rotational primary stability (Henssge et al. 1985; Krueger et al. 1985). The surface structure of the endoprosthesis should be sufficiently rough to assure at first a mechanical toothing within the anchorage bedding. For the physiological force induction into the proximal intertrochanteric part of the femur bone, a structure should be applied to the endoprosthesis only within its proximal area. (Oh, I.; Harris, W.H. 1978; Burgkart et al. 1993).

Thanks to such shaping features of the endoprosthesis, one should obtain that micromotions between the endoprosthesis and the anchorage bedding have a dimension as reduced as possible (high primary stability), in order that bone substance may easily grow in. Experimental studies demonstrated that the critical range in view of obtaining bone ingrowth is appr. 150 micron (Cameron et al. 1973; Pilliar et al. 1986). Endoprostheses having a lower primary stability can only be supposed to assure a connective tissue fixation. Burgkart and colleagues were able to demonstrate in 1993 that the partially structured anatomical Eska hip endoprosthesis used by ourselves with maximal micromotions of 35 micron in the proximal and 60 micron in the distal area guarantees a high primary stability.

Point 2. If an endoprosthesis theoretically allows a safe bone ingrowth thanks to its biomechanical feature and its primary stability, this must be guaranteed by the quality of the surface structure. Galante and colleagues showed that only porous structures are able to induce a real bone ingrowth (Galante et al. 1971). Several publications demonstrated that increased sizes of surface netting structures (pore size) improve the stability and vitality of ingrowing bone trabeculae. These works show that pore sizes below 100 micron allow only connective tissue contact, while structures with pore sizes above 500 micron enable the ingrowth of well vascularized bone trabeculae (Hulbert et al. 1970, Bobyn et al. 1980; Ploetz, Meßmer 1996). The spongiosa-metal surface structure of the endoprosthesis (produced by Eska-Implants, Lübeck, Germany) used by ourselves has a tridimensional interconnecting mesh structure imitating the architecture of normal bones as to shape and dimensions (Gradinger et al.). The production technique of this structure, technically improved in 1991, allows realizing a high-stability metallic trabecular structure on the endoprosthesis surface in a single cast. A further advantage of these precisely reproducible structures is that they can be produced with different construction heights, so that it is possible to adapt them optimally to different anatomical conditions (big bone trabeculae - big structures; little bone trabeculae - little structures). In many experimental and clinical studies it was demonstrated that such structures allow a safe deep and vital bone ingrowth (Thomas 1992; Wicke-Wittenius 1992; Dufek 1993; Sprick, Dufek 1993).

Point 3. One among the most important requirements for a durable stable endoprosthesis fixation, especially in cases of osteoporosis, is the guaranty of endosteal blood supply. The macrostructures of spongiosa-metal assure the continuity of endosteal blood supply, so that within the contact zone and the ingrowth area vital trabeculae with a central blood vessel supply may develop. Dufek, in his relevant publications, also demonstrated that these trabeculae grow deeply behind the metal bridges (bone-ingrowth interlocking) (Dufek 1993; Sprick, Dufek 1993) (Fig. 1).

According to these theoretical biomechanical and biological considerations, the Eska endoprosthesis* used by us consists of the following parts: the metal acetabulum base has a hemispheric shape like the natural acetabulum and is made up by a rigid metal body guaranteeing a high primary stability through its spongiosa-metal surface and peripheral anchoring elements. The inside cone allows receiving various joint elements for which, according to the biomechanical concept adopted, polyethylene, ceramic, metal or ceramic-polyethylene compound (Eska Keram) are available. The endoprosthesis pedicle was developed through a moulding process of the femur bone inside shape and has an anatomic form with proximal antetorsion and an asymmetric partial coating of spongiosa-metal on the proximal part (Fig. 2). On the cone of the endoprosthesis neck it is possible to apply endoprosthetic spheres in metal or ceramic with different diameters and neck lengths.

Cases

As concerns osteoporosis, we analyzed our total cases in two regards:

1. Femur neck fractures due to osteoporosis:

70 of our femur neck fractures treated with cementless Eska endoprostheses were followed up during a period up to 10 years (minimum 6 months, maximum 10 years, average 6.30), of whom 60 (86%) were female and 10 (14%) male. Distribution by age was between 55 and 98 years, 77.5 on the average. In 37 cases the right side was affected, in 31 cases the left side. With the same rehabilitation program as for our normal arthrosis operations, during the first months we observed an equally fast increase of the function score according to Harris. Between the third and 12th month the improvement of the rehabilitation was slower, while between the first and the second observation year a definite increase towards the final score could be registered. The latter showed no difference with respect to that of primary implants.

---

* Produced by Eska-Implants (Lübeck, Germany).

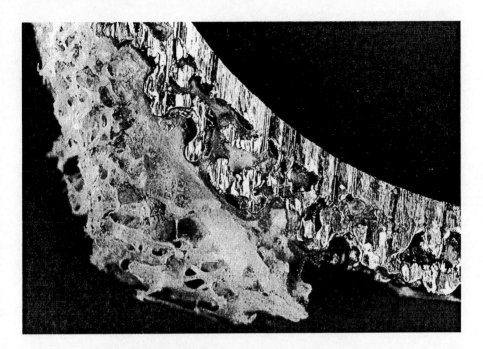

Fig. 1: ESKA hip prosthesis – bone ingrowth

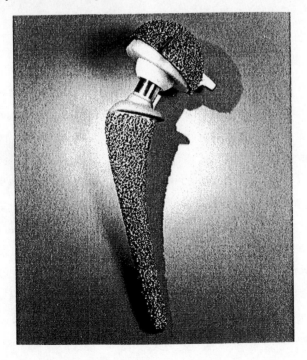

Fig. 2: ESKA hip prosthesis – Spongiosa metal

2. Arthrosis treatment with osteoporosis:

In this study we observed separately the cases of coxarthrosis with concomitant osteoporosis of high degree treated by ourselves. For this purpose we adopted the classification according to Singh and colleagues of 1970 and followed up particularly the classes of severe osteoporosis of degrees II and III as well as the lighter osteoporoses of degrees IV in a longitudinal study. In the course it came out that, as for the femoral neck fractures, during the initial stage of the first months a delay of the functional rehabilitation was observed and that, as it was expected, osteoporoses of higher degree showed the maximum delay. After the first observation year there was no longer a difference between the osteoporosis groups also in comparison with the total group of primary treatments of coxarthroses.

This documentation shows that the treatment of a bone affected by an osteoporosis of high degree with a cementless endoprosthesis allows to obtain fair functional results, provided it has appropriate features. Such an endoprosthesis must guarantee a high primary stability and have a surface structure allowing a good secondary stability through bone ingrowths (macroporous structure) and at the same time permitting a continuous endosteal blood supply of the anchoring bone. This is of particular importance for otherwise healthy postmenopausal women often affected by osteoporosis (Cosmi E.V. et. al.1997).

Knee arthroplasty

With the knee endoprostheses (Eska knee endoprosthesis system) used by ourselves we observed the same biological effect of deep bone ingrowth in spongiosa-metal structures of knee endoprostheses (explants after infection or ligament relaxation). Formerly we availed ourselves of a sledge endoprosthesis for gonarthroses with stable ligaments and of a partially coupled gliding axis endoprosthesis, but recently we combined the experiences of both systems in a modular system allowing coverage of all the indications. At the knee joint we meet the problem of osteoporosis in a particularly severe way in cases of revision surgery of cemented implants with a beginning or advanced osteolysis. In such cases we adopt the solution of cementless implants and observe a very fast reconstruction of the anchorage bedding either by a treatment implying stabilization through a centromedullar pegging or especially through a reconstruction of the bone bedding with transplants. We observed 64 revision surgery cases during a period of 10 years and were able to work out 90% (58) of these cases. Three patients died in the meantime and three could not be contacted. In the

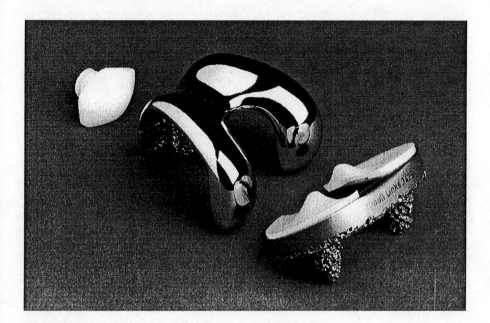

Fig. 3: ESKA knee prosthesis – Spongiosa metal

course of these revision operations, the observation of the functional score (HSS-Score) showed a lightly delayed rehabilitation in comparison with the primary treatment cases in the first year, but afterwards a durable stability with an average score below primary treatment cases by 10 points. We recently developed an anchoring concept consisting of an increase in primary stability by means of a further intraspongious or intracortical screwing, in order to obtain a fast and safe secondary stability through bone ingrowth. This concept proves effective especially in cases of osteoporosis of high degree, because by this system we implement a mere surface treatment, avoiding a further weakening of the marrow space caused by openings (Eska - resurfacing knee system) (Fig. 3).

Thanks to the availability of modern computerized analysis methods, we recently started checking all our patients, especially those affected by osteoporosis, by the densitometric procedure (DPXA-Hologic). In this way, apart from the functional score through clinical analyses, walking analyses and radiological findings, we are able to observe very exactly the remodelling of the anchoring bone. In our studies up to now we observed among others that densitometric images confirm the biomechanical concept of the endoprosthesis used by us: in comparison with the opposite side, the proximal area shows a high bone density with the periendoprosthetic anchorage bedding, while no increases of bone density appear in the pedicle point area (no pedicle point hyperostosis - no stress shielding).

Summary

Arthroplasty with endoprostheses at hip and knee joints with concomitant osteoporosis of high degree represents a particular challenge for orthopedic surgery. In such cases we consider the principle of cement anchoring as critical because cement assures only an insufficient anchoring, since the high polymerization temperature may cause further damages to the anchorage bedding and cement fillings may disturb the endosteal vascularization. Therefore, in such cases we favour, with much clinical success, the principle of cementless anchoring by means of an endoprosthesis which must meet the following requirements:

1. high mechanical stability through an anatomical shaping and a biomechanically fair structural coating in the proximal area;

2. open-cell tridimensional interconnecting surface structure enabling the ingrowth of stable, well vascularized bone trabeculae;

3. guarantee of an endosteal, transendoprosthetic blood supply to feed the bone in the contact area with the endoprosthesis.

REFERENCES

1) Bobyn, J.D.; Pilliar, R.M.; Cameron, H.V.; Weatherly, G.C.; Kent, A.M.:
The effect of porous surface configurations on the tensile strength of fixation of implants by bone ingrowth
Clin. Orthop. 1980, 149:291

2) Burgkart, R.H.; Glisson, R.R.; Koellig, A.; Ascherl, R.; Ploetz, W.:
Micromotion in fully versus semi-porous-coated femoral components
3rd Conference of the EORS, Paris, 19-20/4/1993

3) Burgkart, R.H.; Glisson, R.R.; Saeber, A.V.; Fulgham, C.S.:

Strain pattern in fully versus semi-porous-coated femoral components

3rd Conference of the EORS, Paris, 19-20/4/1993

4) Cosmi, E.V.; Minozzi, M.; Riosa, B.; et al.:

Bone mass density in post-menopausal women

Intern. J. Gynecol. Obstr. (1997) 58: 287-291

5) Dufek, P.:

Knocheneinwuchs in Metallimplantate mit spongiöser Struktur der Oberfläche

Jahrbuch der Orthopädie, Verlag Biermann, Zülpich 1993

6) Galante, J.; Rostocker, W.; Lueck, R.; Ray, R.D.:

Sintered fiber metal composites as a basis of attachment of implants to bone

J. Bone Jt Surg. 1971, 53-A: 101-14

7) Gradinger, R.; Mittelmeier, W.; Koellig, A.; Ploetz, W.; Grundei, H.:

Zementlose Hüftgelenkendoprothese mit dreidimensionaler offenzelliger interkonnektierender Oberflächenstruktur - Entwicklung und Ergebnisse

W. Zuckerschwerdt, München, Bern, Wien, New York (forthcoming)

8) Hans, D.; Dargent-Molina, P.; Schott, A.M.; Sebern, J.L.; Cormier, C.; Kotzki, P.O.; Delmas, P.D.; Pouilles, J.M.; Breart, G.; Meunier, P.J.:

Ultrasonographic heel measurements to predict hip fracture in elderly women:

The EPIDOS prospective study

Lancet 1996, 348: 511-14

9) Henssge, E.J.; Grundei, H.; Etspueler, R.; Koeller, W.; Fink, K.:

Die anatomisch angepaßte Endoprothese des proximalen Femurendes

Z. Orthop. 1985, 123:821

10) Horne G.:

Fit and fill, fashionable fact or fantasy?

J. Bone Jt Surg. 1992, 74-B: 4-5

11) Hulbert, S.F.; Young, F.A.; Matthews, R.S.; Klawitter, J.J.; Talbert, C.D.; Stelling, F.H.:

Potential of ceramic materials as permanently implantable skeletal prosthesis

J. Biomed Mater Res 1970, 4: 433

12) Iida, M.; Furuya, K.; Kawachi, S.; Masuhara, E.; Tarumi, J.:

New improved bone cement (MMA-TBB)

Clin. orthop. 1974, 100:279

13) Krueger, M.; Henssge, E.J.; Sellin, D.:

Gegossene spongiösmetallische Implantate im Tierversuch

Z. Orthop. 1985, 123:962-5

14) Melton, L.J.; Chrischilles, E.A.; Cooper, C.; Lane, A.W.; Riggs, B.L.:

Perspective: now many women have osteoporosis?

J. Bone Miner. Res 1992, 7: 1005-10

15) Morrey, B.F.; Kavanagh, B.F.:

Complications with the femoral component of total hip arthroplasty. Comparison between cemented and uncemented techniques

Journal of Arthroplasty 1992, 7: 71-9

16) Oh, J.; Harris, W.H.:

Proximal strain distribution in the loaded femur

J. Bone Jt Surg. 1978, 60-A: 75-85

17) Pilliar, R.M.; Lee, J.M.; Maniatopoulos, C.:

Observations on the effect of movement on bone ingrowth into porous-surfaced implants

Clin. orthop. 1986, 208: 108-13

18) Ploetz, W.; Meßmer, C.:

Osteointegration von Endoprothesenschäften.

Anwerdentagung Hüftendoprothetik

Lübeck 1996

19) Sprick, O.; Dufek, P.:

Biologische Fixation und klinische Ergebnisse der zementfreien Lübecker Totalendoprothese aus

Spongiosametall

Z. Orthop. 1993, 131: 524-31

20) Wicke-Wittenius, S.:

Experimentelle Untersuchungen zum zementfreien Hüftgelenkersatz beim Hund unter besonderer

Berücksichtigung der Spongiosametalloberfläche

Thesis, Technical University, München 1992

PHARMACOLOGICAL CHARACTERISTICS OF TRANSDERMAL HORMONE REPLACEMENT THERAPY

GC Monza [1], SG Cella [2], GL Parenti [3], EE Müller [2]

[1] Medical Dept, Novartis Farma SpA
[2] Department of Medical Pharmacology, University of Milan
[3] Centre for Menopause, General Hospital, Mariano Comense, Italy

INTRODUCTION

The short and long term clinical benefits of hormone replacement therapy (HRT) in postmenopausal women are well established [1] and a wide variety of HRT preparations are currently available. As HRT is a replacement therapy, the optimal pharmacological profile of any preparation would be obtained with the delivery of the physiological hormone, 17β oestradiol, at low dose, avoidance of first pass metabolism and provision of a hormonal environment closely mirroring that seen prior to menopause. The latter would be characterised by relatively constant blood levels of oestradiol (E2), in the pre-menopausal range, and a ratio of circulating E2 to oestrone (E1) ≥ 1. In addition, blood levels of E2 must be sufficient to alleviate menopausal symptoms, prevent osteoporosis and provide cardioprotection.

Oestrogens may be administered as oral or transdermal regimens, vaginal creams, intramuscular injections, subcutaneous pellets, buccal oestrogens, and gel-based preparations to be rubbed on the skin. In clinical practice, HRT is most commonly administered by the oral or transdermal route. Both oral and transdermally administered oestrogens are highly effective in preventing the sequelae of oestrogen deficiency although the pharmacological profile varies markedly with these two routes of administration [2,3].

The main pharmacological differences between oral and transdermal administration arise from the use of non-physiological oestrogens in most oral preparations and the extensive first pass metabolism of oestrogens given by mouth, which requires relatively high doses to be administered. Overall the daily administration of oral E2 exposes patients to concentrations of E2 and E1 12 and 9 times higher respectively than those elicited by transdermal delivery [4]. Transdermal therapeutic systems deliver the lowest effective dose of E2 through the skin by a patch or plaster, directly into the systemic circulation. The first pass effect is avoided, and the continuous day and night hormone delivery closely resembles physiological oestrogen production.

PHARMACOKINETICS

Oral vs. Transdermal administration

The oral route requires high doses of oestrogen to be administered as 30% is inactivated within the intestinal mucosa and liver before reaching the systemic circulation (i.e. first pass metabolism) [5]. The once daily administration of high doses of oestrogens by mouth results in marked variations between peak and trough plasma levels of E2 and E1 [6] (Figure 1a). Mean levels of E2 are well above those seen during the pre-follicular phase pre-menopause e.g. 115 pg/mL

Figure 1a   Typical plasma levels of E2 and E1 after oral administration of 2 mg oestradiol valerate

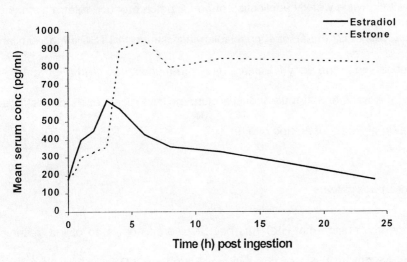

Figure 1b   Typical plasma E2 levels after transdermal administration of 50μg oestradiol per day from a reservoir system [10]

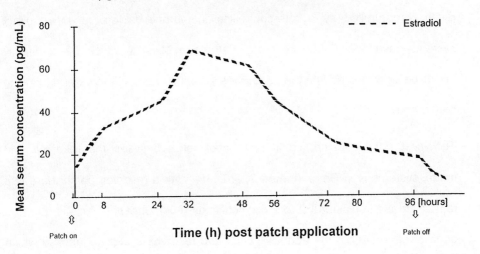

following 2mg/day micronised oestradiol [7]. During first pass metabolism, up to 90% of E2 is metabolised to E1 and the inactive conjugates, oestrone sulphate and oestrone glucuronide. This results in an E2/E1 ratio significantly <1, more typical of the postmenopausal rather than pre-menopausal state [8].

This is in contrast with transdermally administered oestrogen. Low doses delivered via twice weekly application of an E2 patch produce relatively constant plasma levels of E2 (mean of 40pg/ml following Estraderm TTS® 50µg), similar to those observed in the early follicular phase pre-menopause [7,9] (Figure 1b). In addition the transdermal route induces more 'physiological' levels of oestrogens with a ratio of E2/E1 of around one [9].

Transdermal systems

Until recently transdermal HRT has been delivered from a so called 'reservoir' delivery system. In the reservoir system (Estraderm TTS®), E2 is dissolved in ethanol within a discrete drug reservoir and the rate of drug delivery from the patch is controlled by a rate-controlling membrane. More recently, matrix systems have been introduced (e.g. Estraderm Mx®) in which E2 is directly dissolved or dispersed into the adhesive layer without any ethanol or rate-limiting membrane.

The most notable difference in pharmacokinetics between the reservoir and matrix systems is in Cmax (Figure 2) [10,11]. With a reservoir patch there is a rapid increase in plasma E2 to a distinct Cmax (80-100pg/mL). This is due to a burst of ethanol from the adhesive when the reservoir system is applied which carries a substantial amount of E2 into the skin and results in a peak during the first day. The matrix patch (Estraderm Mx®) shows a somewhat more steady release pattern with an indistinct and lower Cmax (60-85pg/mL).

Several matrix patches are now available and all those intended for twice weekly

Figure 2 **Mean plasma concentrations of E2 with a reservoir system (Estraderm TTS® 50) and a matrix system (Estraderm MX® 50) [10]**

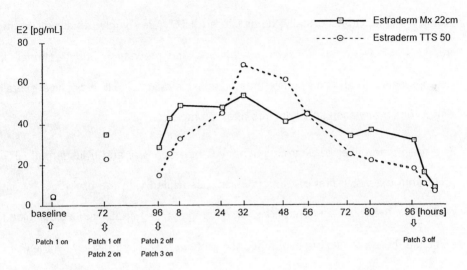

application show similar plasma concentration-time curves with relatively constant levels of E2 and a lower and indistinct Cmax compared with the reservoir [11, 12]. In addition to a different concentration-time profile, the variability in E2 levels between patients is higher with a matrix patch compared to the reservoir. This higher variability appears to be mainly due to some individuals (~10%) who absorb more E2 from the matrix system which has no rate-controlling membrane [10,11]. Despite the differences, some matrix systems (e.g. Estraderm MX®) have been shown to be bioequivalent to the reservoir system (Estraderm TTS®) for extent of absorption as measured by AUC [10].

PHARMACODYNAMICS

Oral vs. Transdermal administration

Both oral and transdermally administered HRT are highly effective in the treatment of oestrogen deficiency symptoms and prevention and treatment of osteoporosis. In addition both routes of administration result in positive overall effects on cardiovascular risk factors after the menopause.

The main differences in pharmacodynamics between oral and transdermal HRT arise from extensive first pass metabolism associated with the oral route. With oral HRT, the high concentrations of oestrogens in hepatic sinusoidal blood stimulate the synthesis of several hepatic proteins. The increase in synthesis of some clotting factors, sex-hormone-binding globulin, cortisol-binding globulin and renin substrates associated with oral HRT are considered undesirable [13]. Possible complications resulting from these hepatic effects are intravascular coagulation, cholelithiases, and high blood pressure [14, 15] Women with a history of clotting problems, gallbladder disease or hypertension should therefore be advised to avoid oral HRT. Oral oestrogens also increase serum triglyceride concentrations [16] which is a risk factor for heart disease in postmenopausal women [17]. In contrast, transdermal E2 causes no change in clotting factor synthesis or renin substrate [18,19] and lowers plasma triglycerides [16].

Transdermal systems

HRT delivered by the transdermal route (in the form of Estraderm TTS®) is well established to be highly effective at relieving menopausal symptoms and to have measurable effects on vaginal cytology, as well as preventing and treating postmenopausal bone loss and having positive effects on cardiovascular risk factors [18,19,20,21]. In keeping with their bioequivalence, comparable efficacy has been demonstrated for some matrix systems and Estraderm TTS® [22,23,24].

SUMMARY

HRT may be administered by a variety of routes, of which oral and transdermal are the most common. The pharmacological profile varies with the route of administration and transdermal E2 results in a more physiological profile than oral administration.

There are now 2 main types of delivery system for transdermal administration of E2, reservoir and matrix systems. These two systems results in different pharmacokinetic profiles, with more constant blood levels seen with matrix E2 patches but with higher inter-subject variability than reservoir patches. Estraderm TTS® and Estraderm MX® represent established examples of a reservoir and matrix patch and are bioequivalent for extent of absorption.

The pharmacodynamic characteristics of transdermal HRT are similar to oral but without the impact of first pass effect with its associated increase in the synthesis of various unwanted proteins. The pharmacodynamics of Estraderm TTS® and Estraderm Mx® are comparable, in keeping with their bioequivalence.

The pharmacological profile associated with the transdermal administration of low doses of 17β-oestradiol directly into the systemic circulation is markedly different to that of oral HRT, but both routes of administrations result in positive overall effects on cardiovascular risk factors after menopause.

REFERENCES

1   Sagraves R. Estrogen therapy for postmenopausal symptoms and prevention of osteoporosis. J Clin Pharmacol 1995;35:2S-10S.

2   Corson SL. A decade of experience with transdermal estrogen replacement therapy: overview of key pharmacologic and clinical findings. Int J Fertil 1993;38:79-91

3   Rozenbaum H. Advantages and disadvantages of estrogen treatment by transdermal or oral administration. Eur J Obstet Gynaecol 1996;65:33-37

4   Setnikar I, Rovati LC, Vens Cappell B, Holgenstock C. Transdermal vs oral estradiol: pharmacokinetics on repeated doses. Arzneimittel-Forsch 1996; 46:766-773

5   Lievertz RW. Pharmacology and pharmacokinetics of estrogens. Am J Obstet Gynecol 1987;156:1289-1293

6   O'Connell MB. Pharmacokinetic and pharmacologic variation between different estrogen products. J Clin Pharmacol 1995;35:18S-24S

7   Scott RT, Ross B, Anderson C et al. Pharmacokinetics of percutaneous estradiol: a crossover study using a gel and a transdermal system in comparison with oral micronized estradiol. Obstet Gynecol 1991;77:758-764

8   Kuhl H. Pharmacokinetics of estrogens and progestogens. Maturitas 1990;12:171-197

9   Powers MS, Schenkel L, Darley P et al. Pharmacokinetics and

pharmacodynamics of transdermal dosage forms of 17β-estradiol: comparison with conventional oral estrogens used for hormone replacement. Am J Obstet Gynecol 1985;152:1099-1106

10   Mueller P, Botta L, Ezzet F. Bioavailability of estradiol from a new matyrix and a conventional reservoir-type transdermal therapeutic system. Eur J. Pharmacol 1996;51:327-330.

11   Le Roux Y, Borg ML, Sibille M et al. Bioavailability study of Menorest®, a new estrogen transdermal delivery system, compared with a transdermal reservoir system Clin Drug Invest 1995;10:172-178

12   Blacker C, Brion N, Caulin F et al. Plasma concentration of estradiol after transdermal administration of Systen® 50 (Erorel®) or Menorest® 50. Clin Drug Invest 1996;11:339-346

13   Belchetz PE. Hormonal treatment of postmenopausal women. N Engl J Med 1994;330:1062-1071

14   Van Erpecum KJ, Van Berge Henegouwen GP. Oestrogen replacement therapy and risk of hepatobiliary disease in postmenopausal women. Br J Clin Pract 1996;Suppl 86:9-13

15   Foidart J-M. Use of transdermal oestradiol (Estraderm TTS) in hypertensive postmenopausal women. Br J Clin Pract 1996,Suppl 86:14-16

16   Crook D, Cust MP, Gangar KF, Worthington M, Hillard TC, Stevenson JC, Whitehead MI, Wynn V. Comparison of transdermal and oral estrogen-

progestin replacement therapy: effects on serum lipids and lipoproteins. Am J Obstet Gynecol 1992;166:950-955

17   Castelli WP. The triglyceride issue: a view from the Framingham. Am Heart J 1986;112:432-437

18   Balfour JA, Heel RC. Transdermal estradiol. A review of its pharmacodynamic and pharmacokinetic properties and therapeutic efficacy in the treatment of menopausal complaints. Drugs 1990;40:561-582

19   Balfour JA, McTavish D. Transdermal estradiol. A review of its pharmacological profile, and therapeutic potential in the prevention of postmenopausal osteoporosis. Drugs and Ageing 1992;2:487-507

20   Mattson LA, Samsioe G, von Schoultz Bo, Wiklund MUI. Transdermally administered oestradiol combined with oral medroxyprogesterone acetate: the effects on lipoprotein metabolism in postmenopausal women. Br J Obstet Gynecol 1993;450-453

21   Hillard TC, Bourne TH, Whitehead MI et al. Differential effects of transdermal estradiol and sequential progestogens on impedance to flow within the uterine arteries of postmenopausal women. Fertil Steril 1992;58:959-63

22   Bacchi Modena A, Bolis P, Campagnoli C et al. Efficacy and tolerability of Estraderm MX, a new estradiol matrix patch. Maturitas 1997;27:285-292

23   Data on file. Novartis Pharma Ltd, Basle, Switzerland

24   Data on file. Novartis Pharma Ltd, Basle, Switzerland

Fatty acid synthase predictive's strength in early breast carcinoma patients.

Authors' names: Piero L. Alo', Giorgio Trombetta, Simona Monaco, Daniele Eleuteri Serpieri.

Academic Institution: Dipartimento di Medicina Sperimentale e Patologia, Università di Roma "La Sapienza", Rome, Italy.

Address for correspondence: Piero L. Alo' Dipartimento di Medicina Sperimentale e Patologia (Anatomia Patologica) Università di Roma "La Sapienza" viale Regina Elena 324, Rome, Italy

Abstract

Fatty Acid Synthase (FAS) is the major enzyme required for endogenous fatty acid biosynthesis. FAS is expressed at low levels in many normally proliferating human tissues. Recently FAS has been also demonstrated to be strongly expressed in neoplastic tissues with a poor prognosis. Aim of this study is to evaluate associations between FAS and common markers of relapse in breast carcinoma patients. Fifty-one patients with node negative breast carcinomas were followed up for more than ten years. Immunohistochemical expression of FAS was statistically associated with clinical data of the patients and with histological subtype of the tumor, tumor grading, inflammation, perineural and peritumoral vascular and lymphatic vessel invasion and with estrogen and progesterone receptor status. Chi-square test revealed associations between FAS and peritumoral lympatic vessel invasion ($P=0.001$). Statistical analysis revealed that FAS predicted recurrence ($P=0.0001$) as peritumoral lymphatic vessel invasion (0.002), estrogen ($P=0.008$) and progesterone ($P=0.007$) receptor status. In conclusion the combination of FAS with morphological and immunohistochemical features may be useful to select patients at risk of recurrence.

Introduction

Mammographic screening is becoming the major tool for the detection of small node negative breast carcinomas (1) . Early diagnosis however is not followed by good prognosticators of recurrence (2). Morphological features and immunohistochemical hormonal receptor status have been extensively evaluated but with controversial results (3). Identification of new markers therefore may be useful for prognostic improvement. Recent studies have demonstrated that certain breast cancers express Fatty Acid Synthase (FAS) (4) . FAS is a multi-enzyme protein required for the conversion of acetyl-CoA and malonyl-CoA to palmitate (5). FAS is expressed at low levels in most normal human tissues due to down-regulation by dietary lipids (6) and at high levels in some human neoplasms where it is used to synthesize endogenous fatty acids for membrane biosynthesis and also to export large amounts of lipids. The goal of the present study is to assess if FAS may be statistically associated with common markers of relapse in breast tumors.

Materials and Methods

Fifty-one Stage I female breast cancer patients at the University of Rome "La Sapienza" from 1980 to 1985 were studied. Clinical informations were extracted from patient charts. No patient received adjuvant therapy. Date and site of first recurrence, new primary cancer diagnosis and patient current status (alive or deceased) were all recorded. The status of disease at death was determined by autopsy. Histopathological data included tumor size, histological subtype and grading, inflammation, necrosis, perivascular blood vessel invasion (PBVI), peritumoral lymphatic vessel invasion (PLVI), desmoplastic reaction, involvement of perineural spaces and pathology of the remaining breast. The histological appearance of recurrence was also recorded. Patients were followed postoperatively for more than 10 years until December 1998. Disease free survival (DFS) was calculated as the period from surgery to the date of first recurrence.

Recurrence was defined as the first documented evidence of new disease manifestation(s). Any new involvement was accurately assessed by clinical, radiological, and, when feasible, histologic examination of the relapse. Immunohistochemical studies were performed on 2μ sections of formalin fixed, paraffin embedded tissue with the use of the indirect avidin-biotin complex (ABC) immunoperoxidase assay (7) using a commercially available Vectastain ABC kit (Vector Lab, Burlingame, CA). Primary antibodies used in this study were as follows : estrogen and progesterone receptors (Ortho Diagnostic System, Inc., Raritan, NJ), monoclonal antibody to FAS (ChekTec Corporation, Baltimore, MD). Negative controls consisted of tissue sections incubated with non relevant monoclonals (mAbs) of the some isotype. Survival curves were drawn by the Kaplan-Meier method and the univariate relationship between prognostic indicators and DFS was assessed (8). Differences between the curves were analyzed by the log-rank test (9).

Results

At the time of this report, the median follow-up was more than 10 years. Patients ranged in age from 44 to 80 years (mean, 64 years). The mean age at surgery was 56 years. Expression of FAS was seen in 19 primary tumors (37%) whereas 32 were negative (62%). In 13 patients with recurrence, FAS expression was positive in 11 patients and in 3 primary tumors of 4 patients who died for carcinoma. Estrogen receptor positivity was detected in 25 patients (49%) and in 10 primary tumors of 13 patients with neoplastic recurrence. Progesterone receptor positivity was expressed in 16 patients (31%) and in 7 patients with neoplastic recurrence. Statistical analysis revealed a significant association only between FAS and PLVI (P=0.001) (Table 1) and with progesterone receptor status (P=0.02). FAS significantly predicted DFS (P=0.0001) and was significantly associated with a higher risk of recurrence. In addition to FAS, other prognostic factors found to be significantly associated with DFS were PLVI (P=0.002), ER (P=0.008), PgR status (P=0.007) (Table 2). Bivariate analysis revealed that FAS was a further prognostic discriminant within all of the subsets characterized by different ER, PgR and PLVI.

Discussion

Although there is a growing understanding of the predictive significance of individual prognostic factors in breast carcinomas the topic of how to use them in concert is still largely unexplored (10). This study revealed FAS to be an independent powerful prognostic marker of relapse in early breast cancers. Before FAS other markers have been considered predictors of relapse in breast carcinomas.   The relevance of estrogen and progesterone receptor status in predicting recurrence has been thoroughly studied in breast carcinomas with conflicting data (11). Positive ER and PgR status however   in early breast cancers seem to be good prognosticators for recurrence and may be associated with longer DFS (12). The statistical association of FAS and PgR status is not surprising as some breast cancers have progestin-induced FAS (13) . Moreover FAS expression seems to play a role in cellular proliferation and differentiation in response to estrogen and progesterone stimulation. Peritumoral lymphatic vessel invasion (PLVI) is known to be an adverse prognostic indicator (14) . It is an independent prognostic indicator of recurrence and it is useful in selecting of high risk node negative breast carcinoma patients who may be eligible to receive adjuvant therapies . Recent studies have shown that FAS may be a reliable prognostic factor in cancers other than breast carcinoma. High levels of FAS have been found in adenocarcinoma of the colon (15), prostate (16) , endometrium (17) and ovary (18) and have been associated with adverse outcome. Our paper demonstrated that the immunohistochemical determination of FAS may be

Table 1. Statistical relationship between FAS and other variables in 51 T1cN0M0 breast carcinomas

Parameter	FAS negative (n=32)	FAS positive (n=19)	P value
Menopausal status			
Pre-	7	4	0.94
Post-	25	15	
DNA-ploidy			
Diploid	23	13	0.79
Aneuploid	9	6	
PLVI			
Absent	24	5	0.001
Present	8	14	
ER status			
Positive	14	11	0.32
Negative	18	8	
PgR status			
Positive	6	10	0.02
Negative	26	9	
C-erbB-2			
Negative	24	13	0.61
Positive	8	6	
Cathepsin D			
Negative	16	12	0.36
Positive	16	7	

PLVI: peritumoral lymphatic vessel invasion

ER: estrogen receptor

PgR: progesterone receptor

Table 2. Log-rank analysis of markers predicting DFS in 51 T1cN0M0 breast carcinomas

Variable	No	Log-rank $\chi 2$	P value
Menopausal status			
Premenopausal *	11	0.69	0.40
Postmenopausal	40		
FAS status			
Negative	32	16.72	0.0001
Positive *	19		
DNA-ploidy			
Diploid	38	0.80	0.36
Aneuploid *	13		
PLVI			
Absent	29	10.01	0.002
Present *	22		
ER status			
Positive	25	7.36	0.008
Negative *	26		
PgR status			
Positive	38	7.50	0.007
Negative *	13		
c-erbB-2			
Negative	37	0.07	0.79
Positive *	14		
Cathepsin D			
Negative	28	0.124	0.72
Positive *	23		

* Refers to the unfavorable prognostic category

a reliable prognostic factor in early breast cancers; moreover its association with PLVI can be an important tool to screen patients at risk of relapse.

References

1. Feig S.A.: Mammographic screening of women aged 40-44 years. Benefit, risk and cost consideration. Cancer 15 (supp 10);2097-106:1995.
2. Gasparini G., Pozza F., Harris A.C.: Evaluating the potential useful and predictive indicators in node-negative breast cancer patients. J. Natl. Cancer Inst. 85;1206-1219:1993.
3. Osborne C.K., Prognostic factors for breast cancer; have the met their promis? J. Clin. Oncol. 10;679-682:1992.
4. Kuhajda F.P., Katumuluwa A.I., Pasternack G.R.: Expression of haptoglobin related protein and its potential role as a tumor antigen. Proc. Natl. Acad. Sci. USA 86 ;1188-1192 :1989.
5. Mc Carthy A.D., Hardie D.G.: Fatty acid synthase: an example of protein evolution by gene fusion. Trend. Biochem. Sci. 9 ;60-63 : 1984
6. Paulauskis J.D., Sul H.S.: Hormonal regulation of mouse fatty acid synthase gene trascription in liver. J. Biol. Chem. 264 ;574-577 :1989.
7. Hsu S.M., Raine L., Fanger H.: The use of avidin-biotin peroxidase complex (ABC) in immunoperoxidase technique: a comparision between ABC and unlabelled antibody (PAP) procedures. J. Histochem. Cytochem. 29 ;577-580 :1981.
8. Bennet S.: Log logistic regression models for survival data. Appl. Stat. 32 ;165-171 :1983.
9. Dixon W.J.: (ed). BMDP Statistical Software Berkeley: University of California Press ;1985
10. Mansour E.G., Ravdin P.M., Dressler L.: Prognostic factor in early breast carcinoma. Cancer 74/1 ;381-400 :1994
11. Cooke T., Shields R., George D., Maynard P., Griffith S.K.: Oestrogen receptors and prognosis in early breast cancer. Lancet 1 ; 995-997 :1979.
12. Helin H.J., Helle M.J., Helin M.L., Isola J.J.: Immunocytochemical detection of estrogen and progesterone receptors in 124 human breast cancers. Am. J. Clin. Pathol. 90 ;137-142 :1988
13. Chalbos D., Joyeux C., Escot T., Galter F., Rochefort H.: Progestin-induced fatty acid synthetase in breast cancer. Ann. N.Y. Acad. Sci. 595 ;67-73 :1990.
14. Clemente C.G, Boracchi P., Andreola S., Del Vecchio M., Veronesi U., Rilke F.O.: Peritumoral lymphatic invasion in patients with node negative mammary duct carcinoma. Cancer 69;1396-1403:1992

15. Rashid A., Pizer E.S., Moga M., Milgraum L.Z., Zahurak M., Pasternak G.R., Kuhajda F.P.: Expression of fatty acid synthase in colorectal cancer. Am. J. Pathol. 150 ;201-208 :1997.

16. Epstein J.I, Carmichael M., and Partin A.W.: OA519 (Fatty acid synthase) as an independent predictor of pathologic stage in adenocarcinoma of the prostate. Urology 45 ;81-86 :1995.

17. Pizer E.S., Wood F.D., Pasternack G.R., Kuhajda F.P.: Altered fatty acid biosynthesis in endometrial carcinoma. Mod Pathol 8 ;95A :1995

18. Hardman W., Gansler T., Schaffel S., Henningar R.A.: OA-519 immunostaining portends poor prognosis in ovarian cancer. Mod. Pathol. 8 ;90A :1995.

CLINICAL VALUE OF SERUM C-ERBB-2 VIS-A'-VIS 3D ECHOGRAPHY IN PATIENTS WITH BREAST CANCER

E.V. Cosmi, E. Cosmi, Jr., A. Alberini, M. Grasso, R. Vigna and A. Barbati*

Second Institute of Obstetrics and Gynecology, University 'La Sapienza' Rome; *Institute of Gynecology and Obstetrics, University of Perugia, Italy

INTRODUCTION

Cancer of the breast is the most common malignancy in women and the leading cause of death due to cancer among them. It is estimated that one of every nine women will get this pathology in her lifetime. At present, mammography is a sensitive tool for early detection of clinically occult breast cancer; but the specificity and the positive predictive value remain limited owing to the overlap in the appearance of benign and malignant masses. In fact, approximately 75% of breast masses detected by mammography in which surgical biopsy is performed ultimately prove to be benign. Even with the recent advances in mammographic imaging, 10%-30% of breast cancers may be missed (often obscured by radiographically dense fibroglandular breast tissue), and other cancers are not detected early enough to make a cure possible. Furthermore, the clinical behaviour of breast cancer shows striking differences between women affected by this pathology, even among patients with an identical clinical stage or with a given lymph-node status, which are considered as the most reliable prognostic indicators; thus, a multivariate study of these parameters cannot predict the outcome in some patients, particularly those without nodal involvement: 25% of them will have a recurrence within 10 years. For these reasons, the primary strategy for reducing mortality remains: 1) an improvement of diagnostic techniques; and 2) the identification of new parameters useful to select patients with a high risk of recurrence.

When fibroglandular tissue partly or completely obscures the masses on mammography, ultrasound (US) may be used with real time linear array probe of 7 Mhz to 10 Mhz. Recently, power Doppler or color Doppler have been used to study the vascularization of breast lesions which gives useful diagnostic information concerning the characteristic of the type of the lesion[1]. Three dimensional ultrasound (3D-US) represents the most recent evolution of ultrasound diagnostic methods.

An other field largely investigated, concerns the oncogenes[2], since they have been shown to play a role in the pathogenesis of breast cancer, it was hypothesized that their overexpression might be associated with specific risk factors for breast cancer. Of all oncogenes found amplified in breast tumors, c-erbB-2 oncogene amplification has been shown to be most frequently present, i.e., in 17-30% of all breast tumors. This oncogene, also known as HER-2 or neu, first identified in carcinogen-induced rat neuroblastoma, it is located in chromosome 17 (locus 17q21); it encodes a 185 kda transmembrane protein that shows extensive homology to the receptor for the epidermal growth factor. Amplification and overexpression of c-erbB-2 measured directly from the tumor tissue, has been correlated with a negative prognosis and high probability of relapse. Recent data[3] indicate that the external domain of c-erbB-2 is a soluble fragment that may be released from cell surface and become detectable in the serum of patients with breast cancer. This raises the possibility of using serum c-erbB-2 antigen as a diagnostic marker for patients with breast cancer. In the present study, we pay particular attention to these new techniques including biophysical (3D-US) and biochemical (oncogene markers) methods.

MATERIAL AND METHOD

3D-US was performed using a Combison 530 Kreztechnik, Austria apparatus with a transducer of 7-10 Mhz. Serum levels of c-erbB-2 oncoprotein were quantified by using an immunoenzymatic assay (Triton diagnostics) in patients with primary benign ($No=35$) or malignant breast tumors ($No=52$), in post-operative recurrent ($No=21$) and non-recurrent patients ($No=23$) and, finally in a group of apparently healthy controls in order to establish a cut-off value.

RESULTS

3D-US offers some advantages for early diagnosis of certain breast pathologies. These include: measurement of the dimension and volume of the cyst, and better assessment of septa and inner vegetations. In our experience, 3D-US may provide additional information to routine ultrasound study, particularly in case of cystic dysplasia. In fact, 3D-US, by storing the image, allows a later evaluation of suspected lesions.

The cut-off value for c-erbB-2 positivity was defined as 20 U/ml (calculated as the mean plus two times the standard deviation observed in the control group). Using this value, serum concentrations of c-erbB-2 in the healthy group were below 20 U/ml. Conversely, increased levels were observed in 25% of patients with breast cancer and in 47% of patients with recurrent malignancy; c-erbB-2 levels were significantly higher in patients with advanced breast cancer (stage III/IV) and in those with recurrent malignancy compared to patients with early stage cancer (stage I/II). In patients with benign breast disease, increased levels of the oncoprotein were observed in a small percentage of cases (figure 1). Furthermore, c-erbB-2 serum levels were seen to change in response to the state of disease during the follow-up of four patients. In two of them, elevated c-erbB-2 levels occurred before clinical appearance of metastasis, in one the elevation occurred

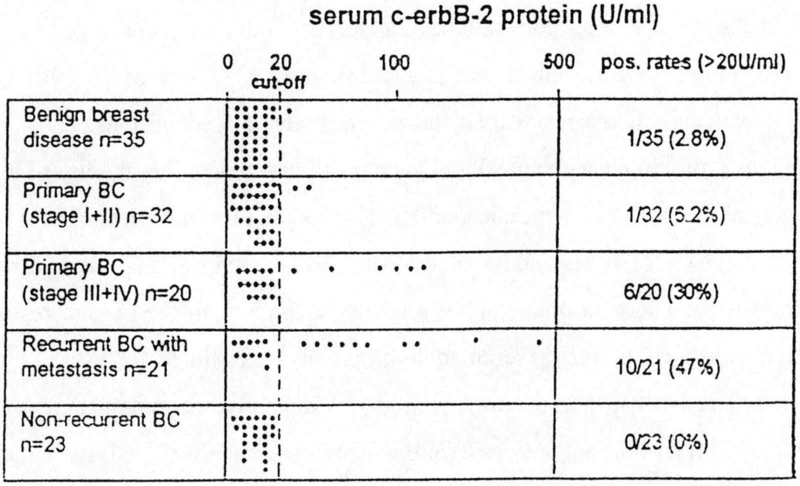

serum c-erbB-2 protein (U/ml)

	0 20 100 500	pos. rates (>20U/ml)
Benign breast disease n=35	cut-off	1/35 (2.8%)
Primary BC (stage I+II) n=32		1/32 (5.2%)
Primary BC (stage III+IV) n=20		6/20 (30%)
Recurrent BC with metastasis n=21		10/21 (47%)
Non-recurrent BC n=23		0/23 (0%)

Figure 1. Distribution of serum c-erbB-2 levels in patients with benign breast disease or with breast cancer.

simultaneously, and in the other a decrease in serum c-erbB-2 levels was seen after successful treatment.

CONCLUSION

In an attempt to predict more accurately if a lesion is benign or malignant, breast ultrasound has been found to be helpful. Sonographic features such as margins, echotexture, through-transmission of sound, and orientation relative to the chest wall are used to determine a benign versus malignant nature of a mass.

According to our experience, the tridimensional volumetric investigation in the study of nodular lesions of the breast seems to have the following advantages in the contrast to conventional bidimensional ultrasound: a) the possibility of a more complete study of the echostructure characteristics of the lesion in three plane of space, in a special way in the transverse plane parallel to the cutaneous plane, which isn't possible with conventional echography. Thus, 3-D seems more accurate for the study of borders of both nodular cystic lesions; b) the possibility of investigation in each space plane in the volume studied similar to a CT scan with close scanning planes (about 0.8 mm); c) the possibility in case of nodular lesions to obtain 3-D space section for a more accurate investigation of borders and internal structure of the lesion; d) the possibility to memorize the volumetric informations on a magnetic external support in order to allow a repeat of the investigation in any movement and place through transmission of data. We believe that it may be particularly advantageous in the study of cystic lesions.

Previous immunohistochemical and genetic studies concerning the use of c-erbB-2 oncogene in breast cancer management, showed that its amplification was related to the presence of lymph nodes metastasis, disease relapse, and survival and, as such, was considered a predictor of clinical outcome[4,5]. In the present report, the data obtained by c-erbB-2 serum determination, to evaluate its value as tumor marker, suggest that the oncoprotein might be indicative of malignancies and the assay could be useful not only as a routine test in preoperative analysis, but also as a diagnostic tool in monitoring patients with breast cancer, in which the oncoprotein is overexpressed. At present, only integrated and/or complementary methodology may improve the management of breast cancer. A sensitive prognostic test, useful for an early diagnosis and to select patients with a high risk of recurrence, is currently being sought. The availability of a system which uses Tc99 and gamma rays to detect the lesion seems a promising method.

Supported by the Italian Research Council (CNR) Italy, Target Program PF ACRO.

BIBLIOGRAPHY

1. Raza S., Baum JK. Solid breast lesions: evaluation with power Doppler US. Radiology 1997; 203: 164 – 168.

2. Slamon DJ, Godolphin W, Jones LA et al. Studies of the HER-2/neu proto-oncogene in human breast and ovarian cancer. Science 1989;244:707-712.

3. Fontana X, Ferrari P, Namen M, et al. C-erbB-2 gene amplification and serum level of c-erbB-2 oncoprotein at primary breast cancer diagnosis. Anticancer Res 1994;14/5B:2099-2104.

4. Barbati A, Cosmi EV, Sidoni A et al. Value of c-erbB-2 and p53 oncoprotein co-overexpression in human breast cancer. Anticancer Res 1997;17:401-406.

5. Wright C, Angus B, Nicholson S et al. Expression of c-erbB-2 oncoprotein: a prognostic indicator in human breast cancer. Cancer Res 1989;49:2087-90.

Free Communications and Posters

Doppler blood flow velocimetry of maternal intrarenal arteries during pregnancy

Ginda W.J., Markwitz W., Ropacka M., Ruszkiewicz Z., Bręborowicz G.H.

Department of Perinatology and Gynecology
Medical School
Poznań, ul. Polna 33
60-535 Poznań

Summary

The color Doppler method has enabled examination of even smaller vessels. In our study we hypothesized that Doppler velocimetry in segmental and interlobar arteries is sensitive enough to detect the increased vascular resistance in hypertension complicated pregnancy.

We obtained that for patients with pregnancy induced hypertension (PIH), PI values calculated from interlobar kidney arteries are more useful than those obtained from segmental arteries ($p<0.05$). Doppler velocimetry based RI values calculated for both arteries are similar in both groups are similar.

Based on our results, intrarenal artery Doppler indices, especially PI in interlobar artery, might be of use as a promising guide to clinical decisions.

Introduction

Pregnancy leads to substantial physiologic and hemodynamic alterations in the maternal urinary tract, including increased renal blood flow, increased glomerular filtration rate, progressive decrease in urine flow, and ureteral thickening (Dunlop, 1981). It seems possible that such changes would be reflected in altered Doppler indices of blood flow. Doppler velocimetry of intrarenal arteries allows noninvasive assessment of renal vascular resistance and perfusion. This method is currently used in the evaluation of such problems as obstruction, renal artery stenosis, renal vein thrombosis, acute tubular necrosis, hemolytic-uremic syndrome, and chronic renal diseases affecting the tubulointerstitial or vascular compartments of the kidney (Fitzgerald and Drumm, 1977; Krumme et al., 1996). Renal dysfunction during pregnancy, whether the result of chronic renal disease or pregnancy induced hypertension, is associated with a substantial decrement in renal blood flow. Doppler blood flow velocimetry seems to be a noninvasive method of serial assessment of the renal vasculature during pregnancy. It may be useful in predicting or quantifying renal deterioration and assessing response to treatment.

Therefore the main goal of this study was to analyze the waveforms of intrarenal segmental and interlobar arteries and to evaluate whether the Doppler velocimetry of these vessels is altered in pregnant women with mild hypertension.

Materials and methods

Doppler velocimetry of segmental renal, umbilical and uterine arteries was performed in 40 women with uncomplicated pregnancies, after informed consent was obtained. For consistency, the left kidney was chosen for insonation. All had normotension and nonproteinuria with no personal or family history of renal disease. Gestational age varied between the 18-42 week of gestation, and was calculated by the last menstrual period and confirmed by ultrasonic fetal biometry done in 1 trimester.

As the second group we evaluated 20 pregnant women which manifest mild hypertension (PIH).

Doppler waveforms were obtained from the right and left uterine artery with the women in the left and right lateral decubitus position, respectively. The left kidney, in the right lateral decubitus position of the patients, was insonated in a longitudinal plane and was first examined in real time to exclude gross anomalies. After the color flow mapping was superimposed to visualize intrarenal arteries. The Doppler gate was placed over the segmental (SA) or interlobar (IA) arteries and a spectral trace of the velocity waveforms was recorded over 3 to 5 cardiac cycles during a period of suspended maternal respiration. The insonation angle was maintained below 30°. The Doppler gate length was 2-5 mm. The resistive (RI), as well as pulsative (PI) values were calculated for each vessels. The procedure was repeated for both uterine arteries and umbilical artery. The analysis of the flow velocity waveforms of uterine and/or umbilical arteries was used to exclude the patients with any signs of abnormal flow from control group (as the refference see Harrington et al., 1995; Kaninopetros et al., 1991). The duration of examination varied 15 and 30 minutes.

All ultrasonographic images were obtained with Acuson 128 XP equipped with color Doppler facility, using a 3.5 MHz abdominal transducer.

Regression analysis was used to evaluate relationships between Doppler indices and gestational age. We compared the slopes by T-test by means Statistica program.

Results

The values of pulsality index calculated for interlobar arteries PI (IA) show a slight but not significant increase with advancing gestational age (a= 0.0007; r = 0.64) whereas in PIH the regression was described by equation y=-0.002x+0.92; (r=-0.60) (Fig.1). Comparison between these groups reveals that the difference between slopes is statistically significant at p<0.005

In opposite the difference doesn't exists between the pulsality indices calculated for segmental artery PI (SA) (a= - 0.008, r= - 0.40; a= - 0.001, r= - 0.59) respectively.

Resistive indices calculated for both groups shows a week linear regression (a= 0.00009,r=0.15; a= 0.004, r=- 0.39 respectively) but unlike the IA no difference has been found between the groups (a= - 0.0005, r=0.75; a=-0.003, r=0.16 respectively).

Discussion

Alterations in renal hemodynamics during pregnancy reflect changes in blood flow in intrarenal arteries. The evaluation of them have an important role in high-risk fetuses (like PI index in renal artery calculated for hypotrophic fetuses) (Vyas et al., 1989). In our study we analyzed PI and RI indices in intrarenal arteries. We obtained that for

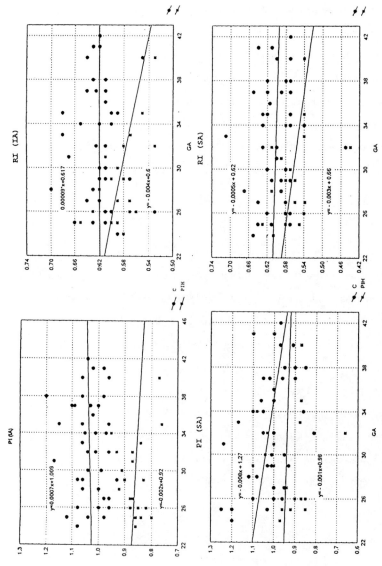

Figure 1 Time-dependent effects of PIH and uncomplicated pregnancy on the blood flow in interlobar artery and segmental arteries expressed as PIs and RIs. Filled circle represents measurements done on women with uncomplicated pregnancy. The filled squares represent measurements done on women with PIH. The equations correspond to the linear regression lines respectively.

patients with PIH, PI values calculated from interlobar kidney arteries are more useful than those obtained from segmental arteries. These differences do not concern RI values calculated for interlobar and segmental arteries which are similar in both complicated and uncomplicated pregnancy groups. In opposite to study done by Liberati probably according to stronger selection parameters (no pathological finding in uterine and/or umbilical artery in course of pregnancy) we have find statistically significant difference in PI (IA) (Liberati et al., 1994).

It is very well known that pregnancy induced hypertension is associated with glomeruloendotheliosis which is characterized by endothelial and mesangial cell proliferation. It causes the constricted vascular bed of the kidney reflecting in diminished renal plasma flow and glomerular filtration rate (Gaber et al., 1994). Some authors found significantly increased renal artery Doppler indices suggesting the increased downstream resistance (Sohn and Fendel, 1988). However other studies could not confirm these findings (Levine et al., 1992; Horrigan et al., 1996). It may suggest that the renal artery is not sensitive enough to show the alterations in intrarenal flow. Our results suggest that the mechanisms of intrarenal autoregulation might be altered in mild hypertension, leaving the glomeruli unprotected from vasoactive peptides.

Based on our results intrarenal artery Doppler indices, especially PI in interlobar artery, might be of use as a promising guide to clinical decisions.

References

Dunlop W.: Serial changes in renal hemodynamics during normal human pregnancy. Br J Obstet Gynecol 1981; 88:1

Fitzgerald D.E., Drumm J.E.: Non-invasive measurement of humanfetal circulation using ultrasound: a new method. Obstet Gynecol 1964; 23:637

Gaber L.W., Spargo B.H., Lindheimer M.D.: Renal pathology in pre-eclampsia. Baillieres Clin Obstet Gynaecol, 1994; 8: 443

Harrington K., Carpenter R.G., Nguyen M., Campbell S.: Changes observed in Doppler studies of the fetal circulation in pregnancies complicated by preeclampsia or the delivery of small-for-gestational age baby. I. Cross-sectional analysis. Ultrasound Obstet Gynecol, 1995; 6:19

Horrigan T.J., Reese C.S., Pares J.A., Clarke H.S., Desmond A., Kropp K.A.: A study of resistive indices in the arcuate arteries of the kidney over the course of gestation. J. Perinatol, 1996; 16:467

Kaminopetros P., Higueras M.T., Nicolaides K.H.: Doppler study of uterine artery blood flow: comparison findings in the first and second trimesters of pregnancy. Fetal Diagn Ther, 1991; 6:58

Krumme B., Blum U., Schwertfeger E., Fluegel P., Hoellstin F., Schollmeyer P., Rump L.C.: Diagnosis of renovascular disease by intra and extrarenal Doppler scanning. Kidney Int 1996; 50:1288

Levine A.B., Lockwood C.J., Chitkara U., Berkowitz R.: maternal renal artery Doppler velocimetry in normotensive pregnancies and pregnancies complicated by hypertensive disorders. Obstet Gynecol 1992; 79:264

Liberati M., Rotmensch S., Zannoli P., Bellati S.: Doppler velocimetry of maternal renal interlobar arteries in pregnancy induced hypertension. Int J Gynecol 1994; 44:129

Sohn C., Fendel H.: Arterielle renale und uterine Durchblutung in normalen und gestotischen Schwangerschaften. Z Gebutsh u Perinat 1992; 192:43

Vyas S., Nicolaides K.H., Campbell S.: Renal flow velocitiy waveform in normal and hypoxemic fetuses. Am. J. Obstet Gynecol 1989; 161:168

NEW APPROACH IN THE EVALUATION OF HYDROSALPINX: Scanning Electron Microscopy after NaOH Maceration.

[1-2]E. VIZZA, [1]S. CORRER, [1]R. HEYN, [2]V. VITTORI, [2]C. SBIROLI and. [1]P.M. MOTTA

[1]Department of Anatomy, University of Rome "La Sapienza, via Borelli 50, 00161 Rome, Italy;
[2]Department of Gynaecology "San Carlo di Nancy-IDI Sanità" Hospital, via Aurelia 275, 00165 Rome, Italy.

INTRODUCTION

Hydrosalpinx is the result of a degenerative process caused by a salpingitis or a pelvic inflammatory disease (PID) and it is characterised by destruction of the mucosal folds with its microvasculature and occlusion of the fimbriae (1). This degenerative process induces significant and irreversible alteration of the extracellular matrix organisation of the tube (2). The recent development of selective maceration techniques for scanning electron microscopy (SEM) opened a new era in the study of the microanatomy of cell and tissues (2-8).

In the present study, this technique is used to elaborate a three-dimensional (3D) model of the extracellular fibrillar matrix skeleton of the Fallopian tube in normality and in hydrosalpinx in order to better elucidate the etiopathogenesis of hydrosalpinx as well as its physiopathologic impact on tubal function.

MATERIAL AND METHOD

Ten normal tubes were used as control and ten tubes affected by hydrosalpinx. Normal tubes were obtained during hysterectomy in fertile women for metrorrhagia or fibroids whereas the hydrosalpinxes were obtained from laparoscopic or abdominal adnexectomy. All the specimens were obtained by previous informed consent of the patients to collaborate to the study. The tubes were fixed by immersion in 2.5% glutaraldehyde in PBS. For details in tissues preparation, these have been described previously (2, 7, 8).

RESULTS.

NORMAL TUBE.

After 2N NaOH maceration of cells and amorphous ground substance, the general morphology of the tube is preserved since it was possible to recognise the different histological layers composing the tube wall (Fig. 1). The myosalpinx appeared in cross section as a continuous irregular honeycomb skeleton (Fig. 2). At high magnification, it consisted of a soft network of fibrils organised in thin sheaths anastomosed each other and delimiting delicate tunnel-like spaces (Fig. 2). In fact, the collagen fibrils of the EM formed a sort of continuous perimysium that housed the smooth muscle cells (SMC) bundles (Fig. 2) which were selectively macerated. This fine connective framework delimited and, at the same time, connected the ramifications of the muscular network.

At the level of the mucosa, the collagen component formed a well organised "*skeleton*" whose architecture varied in the different areas of the tube. In the isthmus, the mucosa

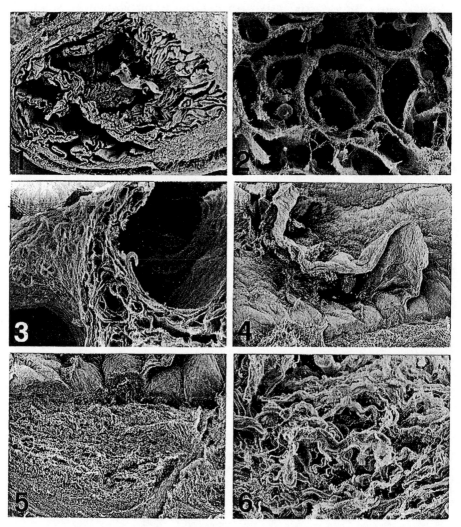

Fig. 1. Human ampulla, normal tube. Overview of a cross section. The lumen is filled up by a large number of thin and ramified mucosal folds. SEM 15X. **Fig. 2.** Human ampulla, myosalpinx. The typical honeycomb organisation of the collagen skeleton that generates a scaffold supporting the SMC bundles is evident. SEM 2.500X. **Fig. 3.** Human ampulla, mucosal folds. The collagen skeleton of the mucosal folds of the ampulla consists in a delicate network of thin and interwoven bundles of fibrils and single free fibrils. SEM 500X. **Fig. 4.** Hydrosalpinx. Compare with fig. 1. Note the high decrease in number and ramification of the mucosal folds. SEM 18X. **Fig. 5.** Hydrosalpinx. Cross section of the Fallopian tube wall. The tipical compartmentalisation in mucosa and myosalpinx of the collagen skeleton is lost. The

contained thick collagen bundles with a woven course whereas in the ampulla the collagen consisted in thin bundles stabilised by a network of free single fibrils forming a soft framework (Figs. 1 and 3).

HYDROSALPINX.
The general morphology of either the tubal lumen and wall is distorted in hydrosalpinx (Fig. 4). In fact, here the mucosal folds almost disappeared and those few, still present, were fibrotic and not ramified (Figs. 4 and 5). In the cross-sectioned tubal wall the spatial organisation and the compartmentalisation into mucosa and myosalpinx was no more evident (Fig. 5). The collagen skeleton of the tubal wall showed the same continuous random and fibrotic appearance but was not possible to identify the passage from myosalpinx to the mucosa. At higher magnification, a significant alteration of the extracellular collagen fibrillar matrix was observed. The organisation in small woven bundles stabilised by a reticular network of single fibrils typical of the normal tube collagen skeleton disappeared (Fig. 6). Instead, the extracellular fibrillar matrix of the tube is characterised by a random and abundant deposition of fibrils often connected to form irregular thick bundles (Fig. 6).

DISCUSSION
Anatomical, Functional and Clinical Considerations.
These results suggest that in normal tube the *myosalpinx* and its collagen *skeleton* are coupled in a unique morphofunctional system that allows the muscular forces to be transmitted in those sites of the tubal wall where the SMC were usually not present (i.e. mucosal folds). The healthy and normal interaction of these two morphofunctional components of the tube can insure the complete functionality of this organ (2, 3, 7). Moreover, the differences in quantity and architecture of collagen fibrils and SMC bundles of the isthmus and ampulla suggest that the biomechanical properties of these tubal segments are different. Therefore, according to the diverse organisation of the microvasculature and the smooth muscle bundles of the myosalpinx, each tubal segment is likely to play a different specific role in the tubal transport of gametes and embryo including its development (2, 3).

The hydrosalpinx is characterised by the complete loss of both the architecture of the collagen skeleton and the integration between the collagen skeleton and the myosalpinx. Therefore, these significant changes of the inner microanatomy of the collagen fibrillar skeleton of the tube cause an irreversible alteration of the morphofunctional integrity of the tube.

The question whether salpingectomy should be performed or not in case of hydrosalpinx is still a debated topic. Recent studies have suggested that the presence of hydrosalpinx has a negative effect on *in vitro* fertilization (IVF) outcome, with markedly diminished implantation and pregnancy rates, and increased early pregnancy loss (9-11). In addition, hydrosalpinx is considered by some authors as associated to a higher risk of ectopic pregnancy (10). The present observations suggest that a conservative treatment of hydrosalpinx is not advantageous in all cases but the treatment should be individualised according to the local pelvic situation and the degree of hydrosalpinx degeneration of the tube.

Our study points out that in hydrosalpinx, even if the tubes are open, their functionality is completely lost. The alterations of the extracellular fibrillar skeleton in hydrosalpinx are irreversible and consist in the loss of the internal microanatomy of the tube. Therefore, at the light of these detailed micro-anatomical results and according to other recent clinical evidences (10, 11), salpingectomy should be always performed in case of evident hydrosalpinx at laparoscopy.

In conclusion the present study demonstrated the validity of maceration techniques and SEM in the study of microanatomy of the tube in normal and pathologic conditions. In fact, these techniques allow to develop a complementary 3D approach that help to better understand the etiopathogenesis and the physiopathology of the Fallopian tube.

REFERENCES

1. Robbins S.L. and Contran R.S. Pathologic Basis of Disease. W.B. Saunders Co., Philadelphia, London, Toronto. 1996 p. 1246
2. Vizza E, Heyn R, Magos LA, Muglia U, Sbiroli C, Motta PM. Smooth muscle cells and extracellular fibrillar matrix of the human myometrium amd myosalpinx studied by scanning electron microscopy after alkali maceration. In Motta PM (ed) *Recent Advances in Microscopy of Cells, Tissues and Organs* Rome: Delfino Publ. 1997; 527-34
3. Goranova V, Vizza E, Correr S, Heyn R, Motta PM. Collagen fibrillar skeleton in pregnant rabbit endometrium at term: A SEM study after NaOH maceration. *Arch Histol Cytol* 1996; 59: 127-35
4. Ohtani O. Three-dimensional organization of the connective tissue fibers of the human pancreas: A scanning electron microscopic study of NaOH treated tissue. *Arch Histol Jap* 1987; 50: 557-66
5. Ohtani O. The maceration technique in scanning electron microscopy of collagen fibers frameworks: Its application in the study of human livers. *Arch Histol Cytol* 1992; Suppl 55: 225-32
6. Takahashi-Iwanaga H, Fujita T. Application of an NaOH maceration method to a scanning electron microscopic observation of Ito cells in the rat liver. *Arch Histol Jap* 1986; 49: 349-57
7. Vizza E, Correr S, Muglia U, Marchiolli F, Motta PM. The three-dimensional organization of the smooth musculature in the ampulla of the human Fallopian tube: a new morpho-functional model. *Hum Reprod* 1995; 226: 2400-5
8. Vizza E, Correr S, Goranova V, Heyn R, Angelucci PA, Forleo R, Motta PM. The collagen skeleton of the human umbilical cord at term. A scanning electron microscopic study after 2N-NaOH maceration. *Reprod Fertil Devel* 1996; 8: 1-10
9. Sharara FI, Scott RT Jr, Marut EL, Queenan JT. In-vitro fertilization outcome in women with hydrosalpinx. *Hum-Reprod* 1996; 11(3): 526-30
10. Puttermans P, Brosens IA. Salpingectomy improves in-vitro fertilization outcome in patients with a hydrosalpinx: blind victimization of the fallopian tube? *Hum Reprod* 1996; 11(10): 2079-81
11. Bergh C, Hamberger L. Salpingectomy improves pregnancy rate in patients with hydrosalpinx. *Hum Reprod* 1996; 11(9): 2068-9

Acknowledgements
Funds for this study were provided by M.U.R.S.T. 1995-97, Italy.

Use of a New Intrauterine Contraceptive Device "GyneFix". Comparative Study.

Bastianelli C., Lippa A., Dionisi B., Farris M., Cerenzia G. e Valente A.
I Institute of Obstetric and Gynaecology
Centre of Gynaecological Endocrinology and Family Planning
University "La Sapienza", Rome, Italy.

INTRODUCTION

The intrauterine devices (IUDs) used world-wide for several years have been modified in their shape, dimension and components to improve efficacy and to reduce side effects. To date, there are three different kinds of IUD: inert (not available in Italy); copper IUD and progestin IUD, all characterised by a plastic frame with different design. Since geometrical factors are considered responsible of the most frequently reported side effects such, as bleeding and pain, an attempt to minimise these problems has been conceivedin a new frameless device.

The GyneFix, also known as Cu-Fix or Flexigard, consists of a non-biodegradable suture thread made of surgical 00 monofilament polypropylene, on which are threaded 6 copper sleeves, each 5 mm in length and 2.2 mm in diameter, providing a total surface area of 330 mm^2. The upper and the lower sleeve are crimped onto the thread, whose end is provided with a single knot which serves as a small retention body, when inserted in the myometrium of the uterine fundus, by means of a specially designed inserter that allows a predetermined penetration depth of 1 cm, protecting from uterine perforations.

The aim of the study was to evaluate the efficacy, but moreover the tolerance of this device, comparing it to traditional copper IUDs.

MATERIALS AND METHODS

Forty healthy informed women, requesting intrauterine contraception were enrolled in this study, by the Centre of Family Planning of the I Institute of Obstetric and Gynaecology, University of Rome, Italy. The volunteers were randomly allocated into two groups: during the menstrual flow, to group A had inserted the GyneFix, and to the group B a traditional copper IUD (Nova T, Shering; Multiload Cu 375, Organon). Follow-ups had been performed after the 1st cycle and every six months for five years.

At the 1st follow-up all the subjects underwent a pelvic ultrasound scan.

To every women was given a menstrual diary to report menstrual cycles patterns and eventual side effects. Age, parity, menstrual patterns, hysterometry, hematocrite before insertion and subsequent and eventual previous intrauterine contraception had been recorded for all the subjects.

RESULTS

The total of cycles observed was 840 for the group A (GyneFix) and 1058 for the group B. Age at insertion was between 24 and 43 years (mean age 36,7) for the group A and between 26and 45 years (mean 37,2 for group B).

The mean menstrual flow , before insertion, was 4 days in the GyneFix group and 4.4 days in the control group. The mean hysterometry was 7.4 and 7.5 for the group A and B, respectively.

The mean hematocrite value at insertion was 41,2% in the group A and 41,7% in group B; during the study no significant variation has been observed in the follow-ups.

Within the first six months four devices were expelled, all of them in the GineFix group: respectively 1 at 1st cycle, 1 at 4th, 1 at 5th and 1 at 6th.

After 12 months, 16 women in group A, were still under treatment. One women at 26th cycle, for medical reasons (spotting); four for personal reasons, respectively 2 at 27th, 1 at 36th and 1 at 48th cycle, requested anticipated removal. Eleven women completed the study. One pregnancy recorded, during the study in the GineFix group at 6th cycle resulted in a spontaneous abortion. No ectopic pregnancy was observed.

In the control group (group B), no expulsion was observed. After 12 months, 19 women were still on treatment. Anticipated removal was requested by four women

Menstrual flow duration (days)

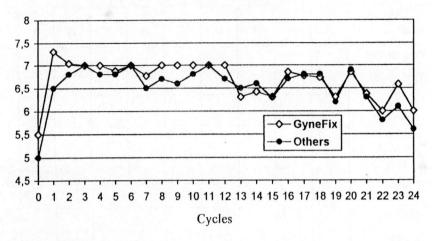

Cycles

for medical reasons (spotting, bleeding, pain), respectively at 12th, 26th, 36th and 49th cycle, and by one women for personal reasons. 15 women completed the study. No pregnancy nor ectopic pregnancy occurred during the study.

COMMENT

The number of women we evaluated and the results we found are too few to be significant, but enough to express some remarks: all the expulsions observed were due to insertion failure for the difficulties encountered with the Flexigard insertion technique, that requests a special training. Extraction instead, was easy and not painful in all the subjects. Acceptance (tolerability), by patients judice, most of them with a previous experience of traditional IUDs, was reported good. Concerning frequence of irregular bleedings, the results didn't show significant advantages in respect to traditional IUDs, while incidence of pelvic pain was reduced.

CONCLUSION

IUDs are one of the most effective contraceptive method, but their use is limited by some contraindication, as nulliparity and uterine cavity dimensions, or by side effects, as pelvic pain and irregular bleedings. In attempt to minimise both the contraindication and the side effects, the IUDs have been modified during the years both in their shape and dimensions.

Table I

Year	1		2		3		4		5	
Kind of IUD*	A	B	A	B	A	B	A	B	A	B
Pregnancies	1	-	-	-	-	-	-	-	-	-
Expulsions	4	-	-	-	-	-	-	-	-	-
Medical removals	-	1	-	-	1	2	-	-	-	1
Personal reasons removals	-	-	-	-	3	1	1	-	-	-
PID	-	-	-	-	-	-	-	-	-	-
Pain	1	4	-	2	-	-	1	-	-	-
Spotting	1	6	-	3	-	2	-	-	-	-
Bleeding	1	4	-	1	-	-	-	-	-	-

* A: GyneFix, B: Traditional IUDs

The Gynefix since frameless and flexible should account for the absence of the major side effects due to the traditional IUDs plastic frame, and could be a good option for contraception for those women with very small or very big uteri, considering the anchoring mechanism, for whom traditional IUDs should be contraindicated.

REFERENCES

1. Batar I.: One-year Clinical Experience with Flexigard. Contraception 46:307-312; 1992.
2. Van Kets H., Van der Pas H., Thiery M., Wildemeersch D., et all.: The GyneFix implant systems for interval, postabortal and postpartum contraception: a significative advance in long-term reversible contraception. Eu. J. Contrac. Reprod. H. Care. 2: 1-13; 1997.
3. UNDP, UNFPA and WHO Special Programme of Research, Development and Research Training in Human Reproduction, World Bank: IUD Research Group.: The Tcu 380A IUD and Frameless IUD "the FlexiGard": Interim Three-Year Data from an International Multicenter Trial. Contraception, 52: 77-83; 1995.

4. Van Kets H., Wildemeersch D., Van der Pas H., Vrijens M., et all.: IUD Expulsion Solved with Implant Technology. Contraception 51: 87-92; 1995.

5. Wildemeersch D., Van Kets H., Van der Pas H., Vrijens M., et all: IUD Tollerance in Nulligravid and Parous Women: Optimal Acceptance with the Frameless CuFix implant System (GyneFix). Long-term Results with a new inserter. Brit. J Fam. Plan. 20: 2-5; 1994.

6. Van Kets H., Thiery M., Wildemeersch D., Delbarge W. Et all: Intrauterine copper contraceptive implants. Contracept. Fertil. Sex. 24: 908-11; 1996.

NORMAL AND ABNORMAL CORPUS LUTEUM FUNCTION

Sanja Kupesic and Asim Kurjak

Department of Obstetrics and Gynecology, Medical School University of Zagreb,

Sveti Duh Hospital, Zagreb, Croatia

INTRODUCTION

The clinical importance of the corpus luteum for a successful establishment of pregnancy is strongly supported by many lines of investigation[1]. A luteal phase defect has been defined as a deficit of more than 2 days in histological development of the endometrium with reference to the day of the cycle. Although a luteal phase defect is often a direct result of hormone production by the corpus luteum, the underlying causes of this dysfunction can be multiple. Decreased levels of follicle stimulating hormone (FSH) in the follicular phase of the cycle, abnormal patterns of luteinizing hormone (LH) secretion, decreased levels of LH and FSH at the time of the ovulatory surge, or decreased response of the endometrium to progesterone have all been implicated.

MORPHOLOGICAL AND BIOCHEMICAL CHARACTERISTICS OF THE CORPUS LUTEUM

The formation of corpus luteum is an important event in reproductive cycle and one of the crucial factors in early pregnancy support. After ovulation, blood vessels of the theca layer invade the cavity of the ruptured follicle starting the formation of the corpus luteum. Once formed, corpus luteum consists of several cell types: K-cells, large luteal cells and small luteal cells. Large luteal cells originate from granulosa, whereas small luteal cells originate from theca cells. Large luteal cells (LLCs) produce more progesterone than small luteal cells (SLCs), but

313

the latter seem to be more responsive to stimulation by luteinizing hormone (LH) or chorionic gonadotropin. In addition to that, SLCs are thought to produce the so called "corpus luteum angiogenic factor" responsible for the neovascularization of the luteal tissue. Possibly, this function of SLCs is totally independent from its steroidogenic function. It has been shown that human luteal cells in culture produce prostaglandin I2, prostaglandin E2 and prostaglandin F2a. Prostaglandins, the production of which is under control of lypoxigenase products of arachidonic acid such as 5-HETE and not under control of chorionic gonadotropin, have direct impact on progesterone production. Prostaglandins I2 and E2 promote progesterone formation, in contrast to F2a that has a distinct luteolytic effect. Although basically regulated by hypothalamus (GnRH) and hypophysis (FSH, LH), corpus luteum definitely has its own fine-tuning paracrine regulation whose secrets are yet to be discovered. The luteal phase of the cycle begins with ovulation and formation of corpus luteum, and ends with the beginning of menstruation. The first event is a significant FSH and LH surge. After that the formation of corpus luteum takes place. SLCs produce more and more LH receptors and thus amplify the production of progesterone. This chain reaction goes till the so called mid-luteal phase which is characterized by peak values of blood LH, progesterone, and the lowest Resistance Index (RI) in corpus luteum blood vessels as proven by transvaginal color and pulsed Doppler by Kupesic et al[1]. Consequently progesterone suppresses the secretion of gonadotropins, LH and progesterone levels decrease, and RI in the vessels of corpus luteum increases. Whether because of "intrinsic error of mechanism", or because of the interference with external factors (e.g. strenuous exercise, ovulation stimulating drugs), a condition called luteal phase defect (LPD) occurs.

LUTEAL PHASE DEFICIENCY - CONVENTIONAL METHODS OF DIAGNOSIS AND TREATMENT

Various names have been assigned to the disorder: short luteal phase, luteal insufficiency, inadequate luteal phase, luteal defect and luteal phase deficiency (LPD). All these names describe the same condition: lack of progesterone, luteal phase of the cycle shorter than 11 days and, when related to endometrium, an out-of-phase endometrium by 2 or more days.

Zeleznik and Little-Ihrig[2] used rhesus monkeys with sectioned pituitary stalk to establish the role of LH in supporting corpus luteum function. Pulsatile administration of gonadotropin-releasing hormone (GnRH) was able to re-establish gonadotropin secretion. By adjusting the height of GnRH pulses, plasma LH concentrations could be changed according to the experimental design. It was shown that plasma LH levels (determined by bioassay), reduced to 50% of the standard values, still sustained progesterone production during the early luteal phase. These results are consistent with the hypothesis that luteal regression during the nonfertile cycles of primates is due primarily to an alteration in luteal cell responsiveness to LH rather than to the magnitude of the gonadotropin secretion.

Jones[3] states that an imbalance between follicle-stimulation hormone and LH levels are to blame for poor folliculogenesis and inadequate transformation of the granulosa and theca cells into granulosa-lutein and theca-lutein cells of the corpus luteum. Therefore, corpus luteum insufficiency could arise. Corpus luteum defect with normal luteal phase length is concluded to be a result of either inadequate granulosa cell function or of an inadequate LH surge, but a fairly normal LH pulse and theca cell response; a short luteal phase is related to a poor LH surge and absent or poor LH pulsatility. It seems that a critical level of LH secretion preceding ovulation is essential for the morphological and functional transformation of the granulosa and theca cells with induction of enzymes for steroidogenesis, regulatory peptides, and various peptide receptors.

Beitinis et al.[4] examined 28 volunteer university students with a history of normal, regular menstrual cycles who entered a program of strenuous physical exercise of 2 months duration. All participants collected serial overnight urine samples over a period of 3 months: first, one control cycle and then two subsequent training cycles. The urine samples were examined for follicle-stimulating hormone (FSH), LH, estriol and free progesterone. All hormonal values were calculated in relation to creatinine excretion. In 18 of the participants, 20 cycles with luteal phase disturbances were observed. Four women developed inadequate luteal phase (i.e. decreased free progesterone values as well as luteal phase duration of less than 9 days) in the first exercise month. Two inadequate and four short luteal phases were observed during the second month of exercise. Since abnormalities were also observed in subjects with short luteal phase, LH and estriol secretion, it could be presumed that strenuous exercise, combined in 12 cases with a significant weight loss, actually leads to anovulation. Of special interest is the finding that only in two women the luteal phase (or ovulation) disturbances appeared in two consecutive cycles. This indicates that in normal women strenuous exercise, change of living conditions, stress, or other extraneous impacts may result in menstrual disturbances affecting either the entire cycle course or the luteal phase only. However, in the majority of cases these effects are transient. Clinical practice proves that many women observed over a period of several months have sporadic, apparently abnormal cycles, but only in very few the disturbance is persistent.

There is still disagreement whether ovarian stimulation causes LPD. Hecht et al.[5] concluded that LPD is infrequent in clomiphene-stimulated cycles, whereas Reshef et al.[6] found that in 30 women treated with human menopausal gonadotropin and hCG, the incidence of endometrial inadequacy was 27%.

One of the biggest problems for scientists in this field of research, and also for the clinicians, is how to evaluate LPD. One of the methods is histologic dating of endometrial biopsies. It is thought to be accurate because it should reflect the amount of progesterone secreted by corpus luteum and morphological transformation of the endometrium by progesterone in preparation for implantation and early pregnancy. Endometrial biopsies are usually taken against the onset of the next menstrual bleeding, assuming the cycle length of 28 days and luteal phase length of 14 days. But, it is not that simple. The length of luteal phase can vary between 12 and 14 days. The preferable time of endometrial biopsy is also disputed. Early and mid-luteal phase biopsies may give wider variation in histologic dating than late luteal phase biopsies. Endometrial biopsy closer to the next menses will better reflect cumulative progesterone action. According to some studies, biopsies taken on days 25 through to 28 of the cycle give an out-of-phase endometrium in 38.6%, but increased to 53.6% if taken before day 25. That does not mean that biopsy taken in the peri-implantation time, yielding higher prevalence of LPD, is also a better one. There might be a catch-up in the biological effect of progesterone which is then not accounted for. A further disadvantage is an interobserver and intraobserver variance.

Gibson et al.[7] ran recently an interesting study. Twenty-five women had endometrial biopsies within the framework of routine infertility investigation. Each subject underwent two endometrial biopsies on the same occasion, yielding 50 slides of paired biopsies from 25 women. Five evaluators read each slide on two occasions at least 2 weeks apart. The results were puzzling: readings of the same slide by the same evaluator were in exact agreement only in 43.1% of instances and a discordance of 3 or more days was found in 5% of cases. The interevaluator differences were much larger. Evaluators assigned the same date to 25% of examinations only, and readings discordant by more than 2 days were encountered in 22% of observation.

The exact site in the endometrium where biopsy should be performed is not yet established.

Measurement of single or selected multiple serum progesterone levels are also used in assessment of LPD. A minimum progesterone level of 2.5-5.0 ng/ml during the mid-luteal phase has been reported as indicative of ovulation, although a minimum midluteal phase level of 10-15 ng/ml has been considered to reflect normal corpus luteum function.[19] Due to diurnal variation and pulsatile secretion with amplitude of 30% over mean values, a single midluteal phase progesterone is not reflective of the functional capacity of the corpus luteum nor of the true amount of progesterone that the endometrium may be subjected to.

Recently, a placental protein14 has been discovered in the endometrium. It is secreted by endometrial glands and it is rarely detected in blood during the anovulatory cycle.[18] Its reliability when used as a test, has not been established so far.

Dawood[8] suggests that only by combining all the methods and regarding the results with healthy scepticism some relevant conclusions can be drawn.

Current treatment for corpus luteum insufficiency includes optimal recruitment of follicles with clomiphene and hCG or hMG. Response to hCG is dependent on the luteal age of the corpus luteum. Optimum and significant increases in progesterone secretion were obtained when 5000 IU of hCG were given 8 and 12 days after, but only a modest increase occurred when hCG was given 4 days after the LH surge, and no increase if given on the day of LH surge.[20] Based on the recent findings, augmentation of corpus luteum function with hCG should be started at the midluteal phase, about 7-8 days after the LH surge, or 6-7 days after the basal body temperature shift (i.e. 21 day of menstrual cycle, when the cycle is 28).[8] Statistically, an insignificant benefit of treatment with progesterone suppositories or oral dehydrogesterone compared with no treatment was found in randomized, controlled trial, and no significant benefit was found in the three comparative studies.

Insler[9] explains that LPD represents only one of a whole series of disturbances including unbalanced extra- and intraovarian hormonal and peptide interaction, ill-timed follicular development, and flawed ovum maturation. Among the women subjected to various studies there is only a small amount of those who, when treated with "pure" FSH during the early follicular phase corrected the endometrial defect observed in previous cycles.

Another entity should be mentioned here. It is the luteinized unruptured follicle syndrome. The luteinized unruptured follicle is a dysfunctional response of the ovary characterized by a cyclical hormone pattern that is similar to that found in normal ovulatory cycles or LPD. In LUF the preovulatory follicle does not rupture, although it luteinizes. Follicular luteinization can produce normal or impaired progesterone secretion, and thus the postovulatory parameters would not show important abnormalities. Even more, a "false" ovulatory cycle can occur, making it difficult to make a diagnosis of this syndrome. Several possible causes of this syndrome have been proposed: an abnormality of LH peak, the absence of a preovulatory discharge of progesterone, primary abnormality of the oocyte, alterations in prostaglandin synthesis or in the synthesis of other mediators that lead to the rupture of the follicle. This condition was first diagnosed laparoscopically, and later on low concentrations of ovarian steroids in peritoneal fluid were said to be of diagnostic value. Some new data on this rare condition will hopefully be obtained by ultrasonography measurements.

THE ROLE OF ULTRASOUND AND DOPPLER STUDIES IN DETECTION OF THE LUTEAL PHASE DEFECT

It is clear that, so far, none of the techniques used to asses LPD have been absolutely reliable and that a new method must be introduced in order to keep the research going. The new method is ultrasonography. For a better visualization of the corpus luteum transvaginal approach is used. As an addition to B-mode and real time image, sophisticated ultrasound equipment includes color and pulsed Doppler sonography. The research into the corpus luteum, LPD, early pregnancy and early pregnancy failures has already taken a whole new direction.

Until recently, research in this field was carried out mainly using B mode and real time imaging. Glock et al.[10] tried to determine whether the ultrasound appearance size, or change in size of the corpus luteum of early pregnancy correlated with serum progesterone, estradiol E2, or 17-hydroxyprogesterone or were even predictive of pregnancy outcome. Their hypothesis was: corpus luteum volumes of early human pregnancy would correlate with the serum concentration of steroids produced in the corpus luteum; appearance of the corpus luteum, based on the amount of cystic component, would correlate with serum hormone concentration or pregnancy outcome; and a decrease in corpus luteum volume would be associated with pregnancy loss. Disappointingly, the acquired data showed a lack of correlation between corpus luteum size and steroid products, and no correlation between changes in volume and changes in steroid products in early human pregnancy. However, a decreasing corpus luteum volume before 8 weeks' gestation is associated with a higher probability of pregnancy loss. Color flow pulsed

Doppler was only used to determine dominant ovary with corpus luteum, and the contralateral one. Dominant ovary showed low impedance waveform with RI 0.39-0.49, characteristic of the blood flow in early pregnancy. The contralateral ovary in each patient demonstrated a high impedance flow RI 0.69-1.0, characteristic of nondominant ovary. One patient had an RI value of 0.74 in the ovary identified as having a corpus luteum, and RI of 0.79 in the opposite ovary; this high RI in both ovaries was associated with a nonviable outcome.

Kupesic at al.[11] tried to evaluate intraovarian resistance index RI in 47 healthy fertile volunteers with ovulatory cycles and compare them to 28 patients with luteal phase defect (LPD) and four patients with luteinized unruptured follicle (LUF Sy). Serial sonography allowed daily measurement of the mean follicular diameter, visualization of the follicular collapse and demarcation of the hypoechoic structure with an irregular wall, solid or complex structure representing the corpus luteum, as well as observation of the thickened endometrium, and presence of the free fluid in the cul de sac. All these findings were suggestive of ovulation. Doubtful cases (non-visualization of the corpus luteum and/or lack of the serial measurements) were excluded from the current study. LPD was diagnosed by measuring the progesterone levels and performing the endometrial biopsy during the mid-luteal phase of the menstrual cycle. Sonographic and Doppler findings were correlated to hormonal and histopathological data. LUF syndrome was documented by daily ultrasound observations and endocrinological measurements. There was evidence of normal follicular development and normal diameter of the preovulatory follicle in all four cases of LUF. During the period of expected ovulation the follicle remained the same size and maintained its tense appearance. Luteinization of the unruptured follicle was seen as a progressive accumulation of strong echoes located on its periphery.

In the group with regular ovulatory cycles (n=47) different ovarian RI values have been observed. During the stage of the follicular growth and development, moderate to high RI (mean

0.56 ± 0.06) was obtained at the rim of the follicle. Significant decline of the RI (p<0.001) occurred for the day of LH peak (RI 0.44 ± 0.04). The lowest RI values were obtained during the mid-luteal phase (RI 0.42 ± 0.06), with a return to higher vascular resistance of 0.50 ± 0.04 during the late luteal phase. In 15 patients, endometrial biopsy was performed, and normal endometrial dating was detected.

In the LPD group (n=28) no difference (p>0.05) was obtained in terms of intraovarian RI during the follicular phase. However, the mean RI throughout the luteal phase (RI 0.56 ± 0.04) was significantly higher (p>0.001) compared to the normals. Furthermore, it did not show any difference between the early, middle and late luteal phase in LPD group (p>0.05).

In the control group, both follicular and luteal RI was significantly lower (p<0.001) on the dominant side. However, in the LPD group no difference (p>0.05) occurred in terms of intraovarian RI between the sides. Mean P levels were significantly lower (p<0.001) in the LPD group (6.9 ± 2.3 ng/ml) than in the controls (24.1 ± 11.4 ng/ml), while histopathology revealed delayed endometrial pattern in all the patients with LPD. The correlation was observed between P and RI during the mid-luteal phase (r=-0.09, p<0.83).

In the patients (n=4) with LUF Sy, no difference in terms of intraovarian RI was obtained after the LH peak. Similar RI values were obtained during the follicular and luteal phase (0.55 ± 0.04 vs. 0.54 ± 0.06). There was no difference between the sides in terms of intraovarian vascular resistance. The mean progesterone value in this group was 14.1 ± 6.2 ng/ml.

Merce et al.[12] elaborate on all aspects of transvaginal color and pulsed Doppler ultrasonography: its advantages, disadvantages, current possibilities and future directions. In their study of luteal ovarian blood flow they introduce the term "luteal conversion" to describe Doppler findings during the luteal phase: easily obtained Doppler signals, increase in intensity of frequency spectrum, increase in turbulence of the blood flow with extensive dispersion of the maximum frequencies and superposition of multiple waveforms presenting variable maximum systolic velocities and, finally, an increase in the surface and intensity that the color signal occupies in the ovary. The same authors, in their study of LPD, observed that the resistance index (RI) of the dominant ovary drops during the luteal phase with respect to the follicular phase, as also occurs in normal cycles, and no differences were noted in this aspect when comparing with any phase of the normal cycle. No significant correlation was demonstrated between the index values and serum progesterone levels either.

Further on Merce et al.[12] deal with LUF Sy. They did not observe any drop in perifollicular intraovarian resistance after the LH peak. During the four days period following the LH surge, and while the follicle increased in size and its luteinization was set up, the RI rose to values in the upper limit of the normal curve. Later on, and in spite of the fact that the resistance dropped, the index values were close to those of the follicular phase. Meaning, the development of the RI in the LUF syndrome was similar to that of anovulatory cycles, showing a loss in the cyclical rhythm and post-peak LH values similar to those of the follicular growth phase. The other interesting thing is the fact that "luteal conversion" did not take place, indicating that the changes described in the intraovarian and perifollicular microvascularization were either not produced, or were altered in LUF, probably because follicle failed to rupture.

Merce et al.[12] also point out the importance of endometrial and ovarian blood flow regarding implantation. They strongly advocate usage of Doppler techniques in future studies of periimplantatory flow phenomenons and their relations to pregnancy outcome.

Glock and Brumsted[13] correlated ovarian blood flow to values of progesterone throughout the cycle. Mean P levels were significantly lower for LPD patients than for normal women throughout the luteal phase ($P<0.001$). Mean resistance index in LPD patients was significantly higher compared with normal women throughout the follicular and luteal phases ($P=0.02$). Although systolic and diastolic velocities were observed to be lower in LPD patients compared with normal women, these differences were not statistically different ($P=0.54$ and $P=0.11$, respectively). High correlations were observed between P and resistance index within each of the luteal time points, achieving its highest value during the mid-luteal phase (early luteal r=-0.73, P=0.03; mid-luteal r=-0.80, P<0.01; and late luteal r=-0.63, P=0.07). The mean resistance index in the dominant ovary was significantly lower than in the nondominant ovary throughout the cycle in normal women (0.50 versus 0.65, P=0.001), but not in those with LPD (0.60 versus 0.66 P=0.37). In the single anovulatory subject, resistance index values remained high (mean 0.76, range 0.70 to 0.82) in both ovaries.

The whole study showed a correlation between the resistance index of corpus luteum blood flow and plasma P in the natural cycle. The strongest correlation was seen in the mid-luteal phase, the period that corresponds to peak neovascularization of the corpus luteum. Consistent to this finding, the authors showed an increase in blood flow impedance in the late luteal phase, the period associated with the onset of corpus luteum regression. These findings suggest the possibility of using the resistance index of corpus luteum blood flow as an adjunct to plasma P assay, as an index of luteal function.

Tinkanen[14], on the other hand found no difference between the blood flow in the corpus luteum in controls with normal luteal phase and infertility patients with abnormal luteal phase. Short luteal phase, claims the author, is not due to premature vascular regression of the corpus luteum as evaluated by measurement of the vascular resistance.

Strigini et al.[15] observed the change of impedance during the luteal phase of FSH-treated cycles. The uterine pulsatility index during stimulated cycles, both before and after ovulation, was significantly reduced compared with spontaneous cycles. That was explained by the increase of plasma E2. Furthermore, Strigini advocates administration of exogenous P as a supplementation to FSH treated cycles, stating that uterine pulsatility index after administration of P drops even more than in spontaneous or only with FSH treated cycles.

Kupesic et al.[1] correlated Doppler velocimetry, histological and hormonal markers. They presumed that when combined together, ultrasound results, measurement of hormone values and endometrial biopsy could explain more about LPD. They found out that mean progesterone levels were significantly lower in the group with luteal phase defect (10.2 ± 4.3 ng/ml) than in controls (21 ± 4.2 ng/ml) ($p<0.01$). The FSH/LH ratio was significantly lower ($p<0.001$) in the group with a delayed endometrial pattern compared to normal subjects during follicular and periovulatory phases (0.70 vs. 1.24; 0.58 vs. 0.75, respectively). There was a close correlation between estradiol levels and the mean diameter of the dominant follicle from days -5 to -1 relative to the days of sonographically observed ovulation. An increase in follicular diameter and endometrial thickness was noted for both normal and luteal phase defect groups.

Intraovarian blood flow resistance showed no difference ($p>0.05$) between the groups during the proliferative phase. A significant decline of the RI ($p<0.05$) occurred in the control group for the day of the LH peak ($RI=0.45 \pm 0.04$), with a return to the follicular phase level of 0.49 ± 0.02 during the second phase of the menstrual cycle. The mean intraovarian RI for the luteal phase defect group ($RI=0.58 \pm 0.04$) was significantly higher ($p<0.001$) than in the control group throughout the luteal phase. Patients in control group had a significantly lower RI in dominant than in nondominant ovary, whereas LPD patients had the almost same RI in both ovaries. The authors measured blood flow in spiral arteries as well. Spiral arteries in the control group demonstrated an RI of 0.53 ± 0.04 during the periovulatory phase, and RI values of 0.50 ± 0.02 and 0.51 ± 0.04 were obtained during the mid-luteal and late luteal phase, respectively. Higher impedance values during the periovulatory phase ($RI=0.70 \pm 0.06$, $p<0.001$), mid-luteal phase ($RI=0.72 \pm 0.06$, $p<0.001$) and late luteal phase ($RI=0.72 \pm 0.04$, $p<0.001$) were obtained from the spiral arteries in the luteal phase defect group. A close correlation has been found between plasma levels of estradiol and the mean diameter of the follicle. The study demonstrates that patients with normal endometrial development show a similar trend of regression for uterine, radial and spiral artery impedance from the follicular to the luteal phase. In contrast, patients with a delayed endometrial pattern are characterized by increased uterine vascular resistance during the luteal phase. Since the most significant difference in terms of RI is obtained for spiral arteries, it might be expected that endometrial blood flow changes could be used to predict the development of the endometrium and likelihood of pregnancy.

CORPUS LUTEUM BLOOD FLOW IN EARLY PREGNANCY

Salim et al.[16] correlated luteal blood in normal pregnancies to the flow in abnormal pregnancies. Their study proved the hypothesis that an absence of luteal flow cannot coexist with normal pregnancy. Impedance to intraovarian blood flow was significantly higher in patients with abnormal early pregnancy (missed, incomplete, and threatened abortion) than in women with normal pregnancy (P<0.01). However, this was not confirmed in patients with blighted ovum, molar, and ectopic pregnancy. The impedance to luteal blood flow was almost the same as in normal pregnancy. This difference among subgroups of abnormal early pregnancy may relate to a different natural history of the disease. Missed and incomplete abortions are manifested as failed early pregnancy with no prospects for further development. Threatened abortion is a potentially similar condition. Whether decreased corpus luteum blood flow is a potential cause or a consequence of the disease remains unclear. Anembryonic pregnancies, molar or ectopic pregnancies are somewhat different. These pathologic conditions usually are progressive and not self-limited. This can explain why is impedance to luteal blood flow in these women similar to that in women with normally progressing pregnancies.

Alcazar et al.[17] agree only partially on the results Salim et al. obtained. Alcazar's group found out that mean RI in missed abortion was higher than in controls. This increased vascular resistance could be explained by the fact that missed abortion consists of a failure of early pregnancy to develop, in which the production of human chorionic gonadotropin is impaired, which in turn could have a negative effect on luteal function. On the other hand, they found no statistically significant difference in RI of patients with threatened abortion.

The true possibilities of transvaginal color and pulsed Doppler sonography in research into corpus luteum and ovarian blood flow are yet to be discovered. Scientific ideas, supported by new equipment will lead to a better understanding of human reproductive physiology, and also to a better treatment of pathological conditions which are still uncurable.

REFERENCES:

1. Kupesic, S., Kurjak, A., Vujisic, S. and Petrovic, Z. (1997). Luteal phase defect: comparison between Doppler velocimetry, histological and hormonal markers. Ultrasound Obstet. Gynaecol., 9, 1-8

2. Zeleznik, A.J., Little-Ihrig, L.L. (1990). Effect of reduced luteinizing hormone concentrations on corpus luteum function during the menstrual cycle of rhesus monkeys. Endocrinology., 126, 2237-2244.

3. Jones, G.S. (1991) Luteal Phase Defect: A Review of Pathophysiology. Curr. Opin. Obstet. Gynaecol., 3, 641-648.

4. Beitinis, I.Z., McArthur, J.W., Turnbull, B.A., Skrinar, G.S. and Bullen, B.A. (1991). Exercise induces two types of human luteal dysfunction: Confirmation by urinary free progesterone. J. Clin. Endocrinol. Metab., 72, 1350-1358.

5. Hecht, B.R., Bardawil, W.A., Khan-Dawood, F.S., Dawood, M.Y. (1990). Luteal Insufficiency: Correlation Between Endometrial Dating and Integrated Progesterone Output in Clomiphene Citrate-Induced Cycles. Am. J. Obstet. Gynecol., 163, 1986-1991

6. Reshef, E. Segars, J.H., Hill, G.A., Pridham, D.D., Jussman, M.A. and Colston-Wentz, A. (1990). Endometrial inadequacy after treatment with human menopausal gonadotropin/human chorionic gonadotropin. Fertil. Steril. 54, 1012-1016.

7. Gibson, M., Badger, G.J., Byrn, F., Lee K.R., Korson, R. and Trainer, T.D. (1991). Error in histologic dating of secretory endometrium: variance component analysis. Fertil. Steril., 56, 242-247

8. Dawood, M.Y. (1994) Corpus luteal insufficiency. Curr. Opin. Obstet. Gynecol., 6, 121-127

9. Insler, V. (1992) Corpus luteum defects. Curr. Opin. Obstet. Gynecol., 4, 203-211

10. Glock, J.L., Blackman, J.A., Badger, G.J. and Brumsted, J.R. (1995). Prognostic Significance of Morphologic Changes of the Corpus Luteum by Transvaginal Ultrasound in Early Pregnancy Monitoring. Obstet. Gynecol. 85, 37-41

11. Kupesic, S. and Kurjak, A. (1997) The assessment of normal and abnormal luteal function by transvaginal color Doppler sonography. Eur. J. Obstet. Gynecol. Reprod. Biol., 72, 83-87

12. Merce, L.T., Garces, D., De la Fuente, F. (1989). Conversion lutea de la onda de velocidad de fluio ovarica: nuevo parametro ecografico de ovulacion y funcion lutea. Acta Obstet. Gynecol. Scand. (ed. Esp.), 2, 113-4

13. Glock, J.L. and Brumsted, J.R., (1995). Color flow pulsed Doppler ultrasound in diagnosing luteal phase defect. Fertil. Steril., 64, 500-4

14. Tinkanen, H. (1994). The role of vascularization of the corpus luteum in the short luteal phase studied by Doppler ultrasound. Acta. Obstet. Gynecol. Scand., 73, 321-323

15. Strigini, F.A.L., Scida, P.A.M., Parri, C., Visconti, A., Susini, S. and Genazzani, A.R. (1995). Modifications in uterine and intraovarian artery impedance in cycles of treatment with exogenous gonadotropins: effects of luteal phase support. Fertil. Steril., 64, 76-80

16. Salim, A., □alud, I., Farmakides, G., Schulmal H., Kurjak, A. and Latin, V. (1994). Corpus luteum blood flow in normal and abnormal early pregnancy: Evaluation with transvaginal color and pulsed Doppler sonography. J. Ultrasound Med., 13, 971-975

17. Alcazar, J.L., Laparte, C. and Lopez-Garcia, G. (1996). Corpus luteum blood flow in abnormal early pregnancy. J. Ultrasound Med. 15, 645-649

18. Fay, T.N., Jacobs, I.J., Teisner, B., Westergaard, J.G. and Grudzinskas, J.G. (1990). A biochemical test for direct assessment of endometrial function: measurement of the major

secretory endometrial protein PP14 in serum during menstruation in relation to ovulation and luteal function. Hum. Reprod. 5, 382-386

19. McNeely, M.J. and Soules, M.R. (1988). The diagnosis of luteal phase deficiency : A critical review. Fertil. Steril. 50, 1-15

20. Yeko, T.R., Khan-Dawood, F.S., and Dawood, M.Y. (1989). Human corpus luteum: Luteinizing hormone and chorionic gonadotropin receptors during the menstrual cycle. J. Clin. Endocrinol. Metab. 68, 529-534

Decidualization-regulated endometrial hemostasis, menstruation and angiogenesis

C.J. Lockwood M.D.

From: The Department of Obstetrics and Gynecology, NYU Medical Center, New York, NY 10016

Dr. Charles J. Lockwood, The Stanley H. Kaplan Professor and Chairman of the Department of Obstetrics and Gynecology, NYU School of Medicine, 550 First Avenue, New York, NY 10016

INTRODUCTION

Regulation of endometrial growth and differentiation during the menstrual cycle

The concerted effects of the ovarian steroids, estradiol (E2) and progesterone (P4), induces an extensive program of endometrial growth and differentiation during a woman's reproductive years. At the end of the idealized 28 day cycle, a precipitous decline in circulating levels of E2 and P4 (steroid withdrawal) triggers hemorrhage and sloughing of the hormonally-responsive functional layer of the endometrium. The goal of the next cycle is to end this hemorrhage; restore the endometrium and its vasculature in the follicular phase; create a milieu receptive to blastocyst attachment in the mid-luteal phase; and in the event of pregnancy, prevent hemorrhage during implantation and early placentation.

These processes are tightly regulated by circulating ovarian steroids. In the follicular phase, E2 levels increase in the absence of significant P4 levels to stimulate mitosis of the major endometrial cell types. During this phase, the glands are straight, the fibroblast-like endometrial stromal cells (ESCs) are spindle-shaped and surrounded by an interstitial-like extracellular matrix (ECM) dominated by fibrillar collagens. The follicular phase endometrium also displays active angiogenesis, a specific process of endothelial cell growth described in the last part of this talk.

Following ovulation at day 14, circulating levels of (P4) rise sharply together with a second wave of E2. In the luteal phase, P4 acts on the E2-primed endometrium to stop proliferation and induce differentiation. The glands become highly convoluted and secrete products into the uterine lumen that contribute to blastocyst implantation. ESCs undergo decidualization, which involves transformation into cuboidal, epithelioid-like cells expressing high levels of prolactin, IGF-BP1, and proteins that regulate hemostasis. In addition, a basement membrane-like ECM, containing laminin, heparin sulfate proteoglycan, collagen type IV and the glycoprotein BM-40, forms around the decidualized ESCs.

329

<u>Major topics</u>
Two of these derive from our hypothesis that decidualized ESCs are strategically positioned to:

I. Prevent hemorrhage during implantational events prior to placentation by: 1) direct mechanisms involving the elaboration of hemostatic and anti-fibrinolytic proteins; and 2) indirect mechanisms that enhance blood vessel stability by creating a basement membrane (BM)-like ECM via synthesis of new ECM proteins and down-regulation of ECM proteolysis.

II. Promote the hemorrhage and vascular disruption of menstruation that inevitably occurs in the absence of successful implantation by: 1) direct mechanisms involving the down-regulation of hemostatic and anti-fibrinolytic proteins; and 2) indirect mechanisms: including up-regulation of ECM-degrading proteases.

In addition, our laboratory is now actively involved in
III. Studies of angiogenesis with human endometrial endothelial cells (HEEC).

I. Regulation of Hemostasis by Decidualized Human ESCs.
Following implantation and invasion of the endometrium by the blastocyst (around 13 days), syntiotrophoblasts breach endometrial capillaries and venules to establish the primordial circulation. Subsequently, extravillous cytotrophoblasts penetrate the uterine spiral arteries to mediate extensive morphological changes. This process provides the embryo with a vital source of oxygen and nutrients prior to placentation, but risks hemorrhage. Trophoblast invasion of of the vasculature occurs in a matrix of perivascular decidualized ESCs. These decidual cells (DCs) are therefore ideally positioned to prevent hemorrhage by promoting endometrial hemostasis.

A. Direct regulation of hemostasis
1. Studies on tissue factor (TF) expression
To examine the role of decidualization in regulating endometrial hemostasis we focused on the relationship between decidualization and expression of tissue factor (TF), the primary initiator of hemostasis <u>in vivo</u>.
In initial studies, TF immunohistochemical (IH) staining and <u>in situ</u> hybridization (ISH) were carried out on endometrial sections obtained across the menstrual cycle and during pregnancy. Neither TF mRNA or protein were evident throughout the follicular and early luteal phases. Consistent with progestin-dominated changes in luteal phase and pregnant endometrium: 1) positive signals for the TF protein and mRNA were clearly evident in stromal cells around blood vessels and under the glandular epithelium at around day 23 of the menstrual cycle (i.e., sites where decidualization is initiated); 2) intensity and of IH staining and ISH staining increased in decidualized stroma of late luteal phase endometrium; and 3) IH staining intensity was yet greater in DCs of pregnant endometria.
TF regulation was studied directly in monolayers of human ESCs derived from pre-decidualized cycling endometria. Consistent with the differential actions of ovarian steroid <u>in vivo</u> in which E2 primes the endometrium for the decidualizing effects of P4; 1) progestins induce the expression of several decidualization markers in the cultured ESCs; 2) E2 is ineffective alone, but augments the actions of the progestins.

Accordingly, we determined that both P4 and medroxyprogesterone acetate (MPA) dramatically upregulated both 1) TF mRNA levels, as determined by Northern blot analysis; and 2) TF protein levels, as determined by both a specific ELISA and Western blot analysis. Although the cells were refractory to E2 added alone, E2 + progestin further increased TF mRNA and protein levels. Both mifepristone (RU 486) and the more specific antiprogestin onapristone reversed upregulated TF mRNA and protein expression, thereby establishing the progestational specificity of this effect.

2. Studies on tissue type plasminogen activator (tPA) and PAI-1 expression

Hemostasis reflects the net effects of TF, which promotes fibrin formation via thrombin activation and of tPA, the primary fibrinolytic agent, whose activity is controlled by the specific PA inhibitor PAI-1. Table 1 summarizes the results of additional studies with cultured human ESCs. It indicates that tPA mRNA and protein expression is inhibited by progestin treatment of ESCs, while PAI-1 mRNA and protein expression is dramatically upregulaed. Note that Table 1 reveals marked reduction in tPA catalytic activity (as determined by a chromogenic assay), compared with only marginal reduction of tPA protein levels. This preferential inhibition in tPA activity reflects a large molar excess of PAI-1 elicited by progestin treatment. Synergy between decidualized ESC-enhanced TF expression and reduced tPA activity secondary to increased PAI-1 expression,thus provides a powerful local hemostatic signal.

B. Indirect regulation of hemostasis

During decidualization, the interstitial type ECM surrounding human ESCs is transformed to a peri-decidular basement membrane (BM) component-enriched ECM (see Introduction). The latter supports and stabilizes blood vessels arising by angiogenesis, thus preventing bleeeding during endovascular trophoblast invasion. This conversion of the ECM reflects the simultaneous synthesis of new BM-like proteins, and inhibition of proteases that target these new ECM components.

1. Studies on the urokinase-type plaminogen activator (uPA) and matrix metalloproteinases (MMPs)

ECM degradation reflects the concerted actions of uPA, which is responsible for degrading provisional ECM components that undergo rapid turnover, with the MMPs, which degrade the bulk of ECM components. The MMPs are grouped into: 1) collagenases (typified by MMP-1) which degrade interstitial collagens; 2) gelatinases (typified by MMP-2) which degrade BM collagens, and denatured interstitial collagens (gelatins); and 3) stromelysins, (typified by MMP-3), which degrade diverse ECM proteins such as proteoglycans, glycoproteins, fibronectin and laminin, and cleaves interstitial and basement membrane collagen type IV and V.

As was the case with tPA, Table 1 indicates that uPA mRNA and protein expression is inhibited by progestin treatment of ESCs. Since PAI-1 is also a potent uPA inhibitor, the marked up-regulation in PAI-1 expression preferentially inhibits uPA catalytic activity compared with uPA protein expression. Table 1 also reveals that the expression of MMP-1 and MMP-3 mRNA, protein and activities are profoundly and coordiantely inhibited . This effect is consistent with responses to various growth factors and cytokines noted in several cell types that reflect the presence of similar response elements in the promoter regions of the two genes. By contrast, Table 1 indicates that MMP-2 expression by the cultured ESCs is unaffected by progestin treatment. This lack of response reflects the absence of response elements from the MMP-2 promoter, and is consistent with the constitutive expression of MMP-2 in numerous cell types. Moreover, unlike the profound changes seen in PAI-1 expression, that of the MMP inhibitor TIMP-1 is unaffected by the progestin treatment. Note that as was the case with TF expression, Table 1 shows that the expression of all of the progestin-regulated endpoints are blocked by RU 486

In summary, coordinated inhibition of uPA, secondary to PAI-1 regulation, and MMP-1 and MMP-3, independent of TIMP-1 effects, would aid the conversion to the BM type ECM surrounding decidualized ESCs. These changes would stabilize the vasculature, thereby counteracting their tendency to bleed during endovascular trophoblast invasion.

Table 1

Endpoint	P4 effects protein/mRNA	P4 effects activity	RU486 vs. P4
PAI-1	↑↑↑↑	↑↑↑↑	Reversed
uPA	↓	↓↓	Reversed
tPA	↓	↓↓↓↓	Reversed
MMP-1	↓↓↓↓	↓↓↓↓	Reversed
MMP-3	↓↓↓↓	↓↓↓↓	Reversed
MMP-2	0	0	0
TIMP-1	0	N.A.	0

II. Steroid Withdrawal-mediated Menstruation-related Effects in Decidualized Human ESCs

Withdrawal of circulating E2 and P4 elicits menstruation-associated sloughing of the functional layer of the endometium (see Introduction). To determine whether decidualized ESCs are a relevant menstruation model: 1) cultures of ESCs isolated from specimens of cycling endometrium were incubated with E2 + progestin to simulate steroid exposure during the luteal phase; 2) withdrawal was carried out by a switch to either steroid-free control medium, or medium containing the antiprogestins RU 486 or onapristone; 3) parallel cultures were maintained in E2 + progestin.

A. Direct regulation of menstruation-related changes

As expected from the progestin-regulated increase in TF and PAI-1 and inhibited tPA expression in cultured ESCs described above, steroid withdrawal was observed to reverse expression of all of the endpoints. These changes are consistent with a switch from the hemostatic endometrial environment of implantation to the hemorrhagic environment of menstruation. As predicted from their documented antagonism of the progesterone receptor, both RU 486 and onapristone elicited much more potent withdrawal effects than produced by a change to steroid-free control medium.

B. Indirect regulation of menstruation-related changes

Endpoints shown to be inhibited by progestin treatment of cultured ESCs in Table 1, i.e, uPA, MMP-1 and MMP-3, were also observed to be upregulated by the change to steroid-free control medium; greater withdrawal effects were produced by medium containing the antiprogestins RU 486 or onapristone. By contrast, neither MMP-2 nor TIMP-1 expression was affected by steroid withdrawal. The up-regulation of uPA,MMP-1 and MMP-3 is consistent with degradation and destabilization of the ECM surrounding blood vessels. This would increase their fragility and foster bleeding. At the the same time degradation of the ECM throughout the functional layer is expected to promote sloughing.

Interestingly, our in vitro observations were validated by localization of MMP and TIMP mRNA to the stromal and epithelial compartments of specimens of cycling human endometrium by ISH. Thus, Rodgers et al [(1994) J Clin Invest. 94: 946], demonstrated that MMP-3 mRNA was strongly expressed and MMP-1 mRNA was weakly expressed in the stroma of follicular phase endometrium. Both mRNA species were reduced to non detectable levels during the progesterone-dominated luteal phase, then upregulated in correspondence with steroid withdrawal leading to menstruation. By contrast, MMP-2 and TIMP-1 mRNA were maintained at constant levels in the stromal compartment throughout most of the menstrual cycle, with only marginal upregulation evident in the peri-menstrual period.

The diagram in Fig. 1 (at the end of the document) summarizes the key local events regulating endometrial hemostasis and hemorrhage.

III. Regulation of angiogenesis in Human Endometrium
1. The steps of angiogenesis
Proliferation of endometrial glandular and stromal cells during the follicular phase requires re-establishment of a blood supply. Blood vessels lost during menstruation are restored by the process of angiogenesis, which includes: 1) fragmentation of the basement membrane underlying the endothelial cells; 2) endothelial cell migration toward an angiogenic stimulus; 3) endothelial cell proliferation ; 4) laying down of a new basement membrane by newly formed capillaries, 5) tight junction formation between adjacent endothelial cells and creation of a lumen.

2. Potential angiogenic stimuli in human endometrium
Exceedingly low levels of circulating hormones during the peri-menstrual period suggests that non-endocrinolgical mechanisms likely initiate post-menstrual angiogenesis. For example hypoxia has been shown to induce expression of the potent angiogenic stimulus, VEGF, in endometrial glands and stroma. Since the peri-menstrual period is accompanied by acute, local ischemia, this mechanism may be important in the immediate peri-menstrual period. Moreover, the activity of TF-generated thrombin, which is a potent angiogenic agent, is greatly elevated in menstrual endometrium.

Although endothelial cell mitosis has been demonstrated in follicular phase endometrium, the identification of estrogen and/or progesterone receptors by IH staining in the endothelial cells of cycling endometrial sections is equivocal. This suggests that steroid-regulated angiogenesis in human endometrium may be mediated by paracrine factors elaborated by glandular and adjacent stromal cells. To date, the inability to isolate endothelial cells from human endometrium has precluded direct studies of angiogenesis here.

LEGEND TO FIGURE 1

Biochemical mechanisms of menstruation.

Top figure: The concerted actions of estradiol (E2) and progesterone (P) exert several effects on the endometrium that increase hemostasis during the peri-implantational phase (i.e. increasing expression of procoagulant tissue factor (TF) while minimizing fibrinolytic and ECM-degrading protease activity by increasing type-1 plasminogen activator inhibitor (PAI-1) and decreasing urokinase-type and tissue-type PA (uPA and tPA) and matrix metalloproteinase (MMP) expression). Spiral arterial vascular patency and blood flow is maintained by reduced endothelin-1 (ET-1) synthesis and increased ET-1 degradation mediated by enkephalinase (EKase). The resulting endometrial environment is expected to permit endovascular trophoblast invasion in the absence of hemorrhage.

Middle figure: A decline in ovarian steroid levels during the late luteal phase in non-fertile cycles is anticipated to produce increased ECM-degrading protease activity resulting in increased vascular and stromal ECM fragility, greatly reduced hemostatic and enhanced fibrinolytic potential. Progestational withdrawal also enhances ET-1 expression and reduces ET-1 degradation which eventually induces intense spiral artery vasoconstriction with resultant ischemia and free radical formation.

Bottom figure: This process eventually leads to overt hemorrhage secondary to ischemia-induced vascular necrosis with reactive vasodilation and degradation of the perivascular and stromal ECM with sloughing of tissue in the functional layer of the endometrium. The latter is mediated, in part, by increased stromal tPA, uPA and MMP production and by ischemia-induced release of lysosomal proteases.

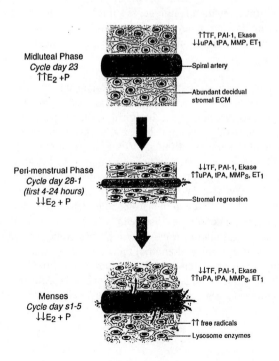

Bibliography

Selected Readings:

Lockwood CJ, Nemerson Y, Guller S, Krikun G, Alvarez M, Hausknecht V, Gurpide E, Schatz F (1993) Progestational regulation of human endometrial stromal cell tissue factor expression during decidualization. J Clin Endocrinol Metab 76:231-236.

Schatz F, Lockwood CJ (1993) Progestin regulation of plasminogen activator inhibitor type I in primary cultures of endometrial stromal and decidual cells. J Clin Endocrinol Metab 77:621-625.

Lockwood CJ, Schatz F (1996) A biological model for the regulation of peri-implantational hemostasis and menstruation. J Soc Gynecol Invest 3:159-165.

LAPAROSCOPIC OVARY DECAPSULATION FOR OVULATION INDUCTION IN WOMEN WITH POLYCYSTIC OVARY SYNDROME RESISTANT TO CLOMIPHENE CITRATE THERAPY

I.V. Surcel, S. Parastie, A. Rosca, D. Muresan, Diana Stefan

1st Dept. Obstet. Gynecol., "Iuliu Hațieganu" University of Medicine and Pharmacy, Cluj-Napoca, Romania

Polycystic ovary syndrome (PCOS) is considered the most common endocrine disturbance in women, and its etiopathology is still subject of debate and hypotheses.

PCOS is characterized by chronic anovulation and hyperandrogenism caused by alterations to the hypothalamo - pituitary - ovary axis, with disturbance of the follicular development and change of the internal hormonal environment of the ovary.

Recent studies bring arguments in favour of the primary affection of the ovary. An abnormal response of the granulosa cells in the polycystic ovaries was evidenced at FSH stimulation (5), as well as of thecal cells at LH stimulation (7), while Rosenfeld *et al.* (1990) suggested an increased activity of Cytochrome P450c-17 alpha, responsible for a great amount of ovarian androgens; Carey *et al.* (1993) evidenced a defect of the gene coding the Cytochrome P450c-17 alpha (3). Hyperandogenism blocks the selection of the dominant follicle and ovulation, and at the hypothalamo-pituitary level it induces an abnormal pattern of gonadotropic hormone secretion, with the increase of LH and decreased of FSH.

Local growth factors - insulin and insulin-like growth factor (ILG-F1) will facilitate the LH action at the level of the theco-stromal structures, which results in hyperthecosis and increased androgen secretion. A vicious circle is thus closed, which starts with the alteration of intraovarian mechanisms regulating follicular development and steroidogenesis and thus explains the lack of response from the ovary to clomiphene stimulation in certain cases of

PCOS (3). In these cases the favourable effect of the partial ovarian resection, devised by Stein and Leventhal back in 1935, is explained by the reduced androgen secretion and the changes of the internal hormonal environment of the ovary with estrogen dominant, which facilitate the selection of a pre-ovulating follicle.

The aim of our study is to assess the efficiency of laparoscopic surgery in the induction of ovulation in patients with PCOS resistant to clomiphene citrate stimulation.

Material and methods

The study included 28 patients, mean age 28.7 years (range 24-38), with primary sterility by anovulation not responding to clomiphene citrate therapy, and who tested positive at progesterone.

The PCOS diagnosis was based on morphological criteria evidenced by ultrasonography such as: enlarged ovaries, hypoechogenic and with cystic structure (follicular cysts <10 mm having the aspect of necklace-like pattern). In 10 of 11 women in which histopathological tests were performed, capsule thickening, follicular cysts and hyperthecosis were evidenced.

Fourteen patients had oligomenorrhea, one was obese and one had hirsutism.

Laparoscopic surgery consisted of the "cold" puncture of the ovaries in 10 patients, electrocautery puncture in 9, and wedge ovary resection in 9.

The follow-up assessed the subsequent menstrual periods, ovulation induction and rate of pregnancies.

Results

Diagnostic laparoscopy evidenced enlarged ovaries, with opaque smooth capsule ("pearly-white") in 20 women. In 8 patients multiple cysts were evidenced, and in 8 it was associated with uterine myoma (3 patients), peritubar adhesions (5 patients), and tubar-distal obstruction (2 patients).

Of the 3 therapeutical procedures performed, the best result was obtained with "cold" puncture (Table 1), which lead to normal periods in all the women with oligomenorrhea, ovulation in 70%, while pregnancy rate was 38% when no other local disturbances were associated.

Surprisingly, the poorest results were obtained in the patients treated by wedge resection.

Table 1: Results

			Pregnancy	
Method of PCOS treatment	Normal periods	Ovulation	PCOS+ (Total)	
"Cold" puncture (43%)	6/6 (100%)	7/10 (20%)	3/10 (30%)	3/7
Electrocautery drill (33%)	5/7 (71%)	6/9 (66%)	3/9 (33%)	2/6
Wedge resection -	-	2/9 (22%)	-	
TOTAL (38%)	13/19 (68%)	15/28 (53%)	6/28 (21%)	5/13

Discussion

Our results, though less good, are comparable with those reported by other authors (Table 2). The explanation is that the main diagnostic criterion was laparoscopic, and the typical aspect of PCOS was found only in 71% of the patients; the histological criterion could only be demonstrated in 34% of the patients. Moreover, the pregnancy rate was also influenced by the associated pelvic pathology in 30% of the cases.

Though the ovulation induction mechanism is not clearly defined, the studies of Sumioki *et al.* (1988) demonstrated a decrease of the LH secretion, of testosterone by 52%, androstendion by 52%, and estrone by 51% following electrocauterization of the ovaries.

Table 2: Comparison between our results and other authors

	Normal periods	Ovulation	Pregnancy
Farhi (1995) Electrocautery (22 patients)	41%	-	-
Armar (1993) Ovarian diathermy (55 patients)	-	86%	66%
Campo (1993) Wedge resection (23 patients)	-	56%	43%
Authors	68%	53%	8%

The better results obtained in our study with "cold" puncture suggest that surgical treatment acts by changing the intraovarian mechanisms regulating folliculogenesis and steroidogenesis, and not by reducing the mass of androgen-producing ovarian tissue.

Laparoscopic surgical treatment, even minimally invasive, entails the risk of adhesions, especially after cautery. However, the advantages are recognized: important minimization of the cost of hormone therapy, repeated ovulation is induced by a single therapeutic procedure, no risk of ovarian hyperstimulation (4,8).

To conclude, we appreciate that laparoscopic surgery is effective as ovulation induction therapy and it represents a therapeutic alternative in women with PCOS resistant to Clomiphene stimulation.

References

1. Armar NA, Lachelin GC. Laparoscopic ovarian diathermy: an effective treatment for anti-estrogen resistant anovulatory infertility in women with the polycystic ovary syndrome. *Br J Obstet Gynecol* 1993; 100: 161-4
2. Campo S Felli *et al.* Endocrine changes and clinical outcome after laparoscopic ovarian resection in women with polycystic ovaries. *Human Reproduction* 1993; 8: 359-63

3. Ciotta L, Carco S, Di Grazia G, Palumbo. La sindrome dell'ovario polichistico: profilo etiopatogenico, problematiche diagnostiche e terapeutiche. *Rivista di Ostetrica e Ginecologia* 1996; 9: 67-76

4. Donesky BW, Adashi EY. Surgically induced ovulation in the polycystic ovary syndrome: wedge resection revisited in the age of laparoscopy. *Fertil Steril* 1995; 63: 439-63

5. Erickson GE, Magoffin DA *et al.* Granulosa cells of polycystic ovaries: are they normal or abnormal? *Human Reproduction* 1992; 7: 293

6. Farhi J, Soule S, Jacobs HS. Effects of laparoscopic ovarian elecrocautery on ovarian response and outcome of treatment with gonadotropins in clomiphene citrate resistant patients with polycystic ovary syndrome. *Fertil Steril* 1995; 64: 930-5

7. Gilling Smith C, Story H, *et al.* Evidence for a primary abnormality of thecal cell steroidogenesis in the polycystic ovary syndrome. *Clin Endocrinol* 1997; 47: 93-9

8. Gjonnaess H. Ovarian electrocautery in the treatment of women with polycystic ovary syndrome (PCOS). Factors affecting the results. *Acta Obstet Gynaecol Scand* 1994; 73: 407-12

9. Rosenfield RL, Barnes RB *et al.* Dysregulation of cytochrome P450c-17 alpha as cause of polycystic ovarian syndrome. *Fertil Steril* 1990; 53: 785-9

10. Sumioki H, Korenaga M *et al.* The effects of laparoscopic multiple puncture resection of ovary on hypothalamo-pituitary axis in polycystic ovary syndrome. *Fertil Steril* 1988; 50: 567-72

ENDOMETRIOSIS AND PELVIC PAIN

M.G. Porpora, M. Natili, S. Colagrande,, J. Piazze and E.V. Cosmi.

2nd Institute of Obstetrics and Gynaecology, "La Sapienza" University of Rome- Italy

INTRODUCTION

Endometriosis is frequently associated with cyclic or acyclic pelvic pain such as dysmenorrhea, chronic pelvic pain and deep dyspareunia. Endometriosis has been found in 38-51% of patients undergoing laparoscopy for chronic pelvic pain (1; 2). Several mechanisms have been proposed to explain the relationship between endometriosis and pain including peritoneal inflammation, release of chemical mediators of pain such as prostaglandins, histamine, interleukin-1 and tumor necrosis factor , infiltration and tissue damage, adhesion and scar formation. Pain symptoms, however, are not consistently present in all women with endometriosis. The relationship between endometriosis and pain is still unclear.

Numerous reports have failed to relate the severity of pelvic pain symptoms to the severity and the type of endometriosis. Different type of endometriosis can be found: peritoneal (typical and atypical implants), ovarian and rectovaginal endometriosis.

Laparoscopic surgeons have suggested that typical and atypical implants can induce different pain symptoms: fresh atypical lesions may cause a functional- type of pain such as dysmenorrhea, whereas old typical pigmented lesions may cause an organic-type of pain such as deep dyspareunia or chronic pain (3).

A positive correlation has been also found between deep endometriosis, particularly of the rectovaginal septum, and severe pain symptoms (2; 4).

The aim of our study was to evaluate if the prevalence and severity of pelvic pain symptoms were related to stage of disease, site, presence typical and/or atypical lesions, adhesions and size of endometriomas.

MATERIALS AND METHODS

From January 1995 to January 1997, 75 patients with suspected endometriosis, 60 patients referred to our centre for pain symptoms and 15 patients without pain but with infertility or clinical and ultrasonographic suspect of ovarian endometriomas, underwent laparoscopy. The age of the patients ranged between 14 to 47 years (mean 29.6 ± 6.06). Preoperatively, the patients completed a questionnaire on the presence, the characteristics and the localization of pain and were requested to grade the severity of the dysmenorrhea, acyclic pelvic pain and deep dyspareunia using a 10-point visual analog scale (VAS), in which 0 indicates the absence of pain and 10 unbearable pain. A score of 1 to 5 was considered mild pain, of 6 to 7 moderate pain, and from 8 to 10 severe pain. At laparoscopy, endometriosis was staged according to the revised American Fertility Society classification (AFSc) (5); the presence and localization of superficial and deep implants, particularly on the uterosacral ligaments, adhesions and size of ovarian endometriomas were recorded.

Data analysis was performed with an unpaired Student's t-test and the rank sum test (Wilcoxon) for the comparison of parametric and nonparametric continuous variables, respectively. For the comparison of more than two numeric variables, an ANOVA test was run, with previous normal distribution testing. The correlation between the presence of typical or atypical implants, stage and the VAS scores were performed with the Spearman's rank correlation test. A p value of <0.05 was considered statistically significant.

RESULTS

According to the VAS, in the 60 patients with pain symptoms, dysmenorrhea was mild in 8 cases (13.3 %), moderate in 35 (58.3%) and severe in 17 (28.3%); acyclic pain was mild in 19 (31.6%), moderate in 25 (41.6) and severe in 16 (26.6%) women. Moderate or severe deep dyspareunia were found in 21 (35 %) and 9 (15%) patients respectively. In the group of patients who did not complain for pain, only 5 women reported a mild dysmenorrhea that rarely required medical treatment. All the patients were distributed according to the revised American Fertility Society classification (AFSc) as follows: eight patients (9.3%) stage I; six patients (8%) stage II; 40 patients (53.3%) stage III; 21 patients (28%) stage IV. Isolated ovarian endometriomas were found in 22 (29.3%) women, ovarian and peritoneal lesions in 45 (60%), peritoneal implants alone in 7 (9.3%), and lesions on the uterosacral ligaments in 35 cases (46.6%). Pelvic adhesions were found in 63 patients: in 39 cases limited to the ovary(ies) and the broad ligament, and 24 also located in the pouch of Douglas. The size of ovarian endometriomas ranged between 1.5 to 11 cm (mean 4.8 ± 2.17 cm). Typical endometrial lesions were observed in 29 patients, atypical implants in 4 patients, and both lesions in 19 women. No endometriosis of the rectovaginal septum was found in this group of patients.

The visual analog score for acyclic pelvic pain and deep dyspareunia significantly correlated with the presence of endometriosis located on the uterosacral ligaments (p<0.002). No correlation was observed between stage of disease, presence and size of ovarian endometriomas, presence of typical and/or atypical peritoneal lesions, presence of adhesions and pain symptom scores.

DISCUSSION AND CONCLUSIONS

The relationship between endometriosis and severity of pain symptoms is still controversial. Vercellini et al. (6) reported that the revised AFS stage per se did not correlate with the frequency and severity of dysmenorrhea and noncyclic pain in 244 patients with pain symptoms. Surprisingly, the severity of deep dyspareunia was inversely correlated with stage of endometriosis. The dysmenorrhea and dyspareunia were less common in patients with endometriosis located only on the ovaries than in patients with lesions at other sites. By contrast, Fedele et al. reported a significant association between ovarian endometriomas and dysmenorrhea and severe pelvic pain (7). Muzii et al. found a significantly correlation between severity of dysmenorrhea, the stage of endometriosis and the presence of ovarian endometriomas (8). In our study, stage of disease did not correlate with the frequency and the severity of any pain symptom, and no correlation was found between the presence and size of ovarian endometriomas and pain symptoms.

The presence of typical or atypical peritoneal endometriosis did not significantly correlate with the severity of pain. Previous reports (9) however showed a significantly correlation between the intensity of dysmenorrhea and the number of endometrial implants in patients with endometriosis.

The uterosacral ligaments are a frequent site for deep infiltrating endometriotic lesions and it has been reported that the depth of penetration correlates with the percentage of patients with pelvic pain. (2; 4; 10) In our study the presence of endometriosis on the uterosacral ligaments was significantly related to the severity of both acyclic pelvic pain and deep dyspareunia.

In conclusion our preliminary data found significant correlation only between pain symptoms and the localization of disease on uterosacral ligaments. However it is possible that laparoscopic evaluation of endometriosis fails to reveal the real extent of the disease. Computer reconstruction of gland histology have enphatized how extensive can be ramifications of what appear to be small lesion at the peritoneal surface (11). Furthermore, patient's assessment of pelvic pain may be influenced by psychological factors (12). Thus, pelvic pain evaluation may be biased by patient's subjectivity. Further studies on a larger number of patients will better clarify the relationship between endometriosis and pain.

REFERENCES

1. Vercellini P, Fedele L, Molteni P et al. Laparoscopy in the diagnosis of gynecological chronic pelvic pain. Int J Gynecol Obstet 1990; 32: 261-5.

2. Konickx P R, Meleuman C, Demeyere S et al. Suggestive evidence that pelvic endometriosis is a progressive disease, whereas deeply infiltrating endometriosis is associated with pelvic pain. Fertil Steril 1991; 55: 759-65.

3. Vercellini P, Bocciolone l, Vendola N et. al. Peritoneal endometriosis. Morphologic appearance in women with chronic pelvic pain. J Reprod Med 1991; 36: 533-6.

4. Cornillie FJ, Oosterlynck D et al. Deeply infiltrating pelvic endometriosis: histology   and clinical significance. Fertil Steril 1990; 53: 978-83.

5. The American Fertility Society. Revised American Fertility Society classification of endometriosis. 1985. Fertil Steril 1985; 43: 351-52.

6. Vercellini P, Trespidi L, De Giorgi O, Cortesi I et al. Endometriosis and pelvic pain: relation to disease stage and localization. Fertil Steril 1996; 65: 299-304.

7. Fedele L, Bianchi S et al. Pain symptoms associated with endometriosis. Obstet Gynecol 1992; 79: 767-9.

8. Muzii L, Marana R, et al. Correlation between endometriosis-associated dysmenorrhea and the presence of typical or atypical lesions. Fertil Steril 1997; 68: 19-22.

9. Perper MM, Nezhat F, Goldstein H et al. Dysmenorrhea is related to the number of implants in endometriosis patients. Fertil Steril 1995; 63: 500-3.

10. Chapron C, Dubuisson JB. Laparoscopoic treatment of deep endometriosis located on the uterosacral ligaments. Hum Reprod 1996; 11:868-73.

11. Donnez J, Nisolle M, Kanakas Roux F. Three dimensional architectures of peritoneal endometriosis. Fertl Steril 1992; 57:980-3.

12. Low W Y, Edelmann R. Psycosocial aspects of endometriosis: a rewiew. J Psycosom Obstet Gynecol 1991; 12; 3-12.

The effect of inhaled nitric oxide on arterial oxygenation is superior after prior alveolar recruitment

D. Gommers, R-J M. Houmes, S.J.C. Verbrugge, and B. Lachmann

Dept. of Anaesthesiology (Room Ee 2393), Erasmus University Rotterdam, P.O. Box 1738, 3000 DR Rotterdam, The Netherlands

In 1987 nitric oxide (NO), an endothelium-derived relaxing factor (EDRF) synthesized from L-arginine by the enzyme NO-synthase, was identified as an important endogenous vasodilator (1). Several years later, Pepke-Zaba and colleagues (2) showed that inhalation of gaseous NO can be used as a selective pulmonary vasodilator without causing systemic vasodilation. By dilating constricted pulmonary vessels selectively in ventilated areas, NO likely diverts pulmonary blood flow from non-ventilated to ventilated lung regions thereby decreasing pulmonary shunt and increasing arterial oxygenation (3). Excess of NO which reaches the bloodstream binds rapidly and avidly to haemoglobin; this eliminates its availability for causing systemic vasodilation (1).

Inhalation of NO, in concentrations ranging from 10 parts per billion (ppb) to 80 parts per million (ppm), has been shown to cause reduction of pulmonary hypertension and to improve pulmonary gas exchange in both neonates with persistent pulmonary hypertension (PPHN) and respiratory distress syndrome (RDS) and in adults with acute respiratory distress syndrome (ARDS) (3-9). The results of these studies showed a great variability in dose-response and an optimal NO concentration could not be demonstrated (3-9). Therefore, the individual dose of NO should be tested and in the light of its potential toxicity, it is suggested that inhaled NO should be administered at the lowest possible concentration (6-8).

Gerlach and colleagues (6) reported that the NO dose-response curves for improving arterial oxygenation and decreasing pulmonary arterial pressure (PAP) are different. In adults with ARDS, there was a continuous, dose-dependent reduction of PAP,

349

whereas the improvement of oxygenation had a maximum at 10 ppm and, at higher doses, drifted back towards the initial blood gas value (6). The authors suggested that at high doses of NO, it also diffuses to badly or non-ventilated lung areas leading to an increase of the ventilation/perfusion mismatch followed by a decrease of arterial oxygenation.

Despite the beneficial effects of inhaled NO on the pulmonary shunt, little attention has been paid to the frequent occurrence of non-responders (10). The exact mechanism of non-response to inhaled NO is not known but it has been suggested that the pathophysiology of the pulmonary hypertension, deterioration of cardiac performance, and severe atelectasis could play a role (10-12). Kinsella and colleagues (10) reported a limited success of NO inhalation on improving blood gases, especially in newborns with reduced lung compliance. They suggested that probably the reduced lung volume will contribute to decreased efficacy of inhaled NO by decreased effective delivery of NO to its site of action in the terminal lung units (10).

This could explain the results of our study in which inhalation of NO was less efficacious to improve arterial oxygenation without prior administration of a low dose of exogenous surfactant (25 mg/kg) in lung-lavaged rabbits (Fig. 1) (13). This was confirmed

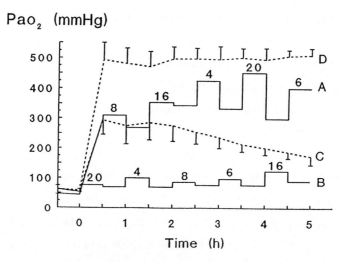

Figure 1 Change in arterial oxygenation (PaO_2) in lung-lavaged rabbits during the 5 h observation period. The solid lines (A, B) are two representative examples of the animals which received NO. A = one animal of the group receiving a low dose of surfactant (25 mg/kg) and inhaling five different NO concentrations (4, 8, 10, 16, 20 ppm). B = one animal of the group which inhaled five different doses of NO directly after the lavage procedure. Between two consecutive inhalations of NO, NO was switched off for 30 min to get a new baseline blood gas value. The broken lines represent the control groups (n=6 per group) which received only exogenous surfactant (C = 25 mg/kg; D = 150 mg/kg).

by the results of Karamanoukian and colleagues (14) who showed that inhalation of 80 ppm of NO for 10 min did not improve oxygenation in congenital diaphragmatic hernia lambs, but when these animals were first treated with exogenous surfactant (50 mg/kg), inhaled NO decreased PAP and improved blood gases. From experimental and clinical observations, it is known that exogenous surfactant therapy leads to recruitment of atelectatic lung regions with improvement of functional residual capacity and arterial oxygenation (15,16). Thus, exogenous surfactant therapy can improve the efficacy of inhaled NO due to alveolar recruitment. Recently, Strüber et al. (17) reported the synergistic effect on lung function of the combination of inhaled NO and exogenous surfactant in an adult patient who developed lung failure postoperatively.

Other strategies designed to recruit atelectatic lungs, such as high-frequency oscillation (HFO) or increased PEEP level, may be as beneficial as surfactant therapy in the delivery of inhaled NO to the target cells. In lung lavaged rabbits, however, no additional effect of inhaled NO was seen on PaO_2 when, instead of exogenous surfactant, PEEP was increased from 6 to 10 cmH_2O to recruit collapsed alveoli (18). In this study, half of the animals developed a pneumothorax during the observation period indicating that the used peak airway pressures were too high. From clinical experience it is known that one of the benefits of surfactant therapy includes lower peak airway pressures with reduced risk of barotrauma (15). Putensen et al. (19) demonstrated, however, that in dogs with oleic acid-induced lung injury, adequate recruitment of the lung by a PEEP of 10 cmH_2O was essential to get an increase in oxygenation after inhaled NO compared with a control group without PEEP. Also in adult patients with ARDS, Puybasset et al. (20) reported that the effect of NO on PaO_2 was potentiated by the application of 10 cmH_2O PEEP, and this only in patients in whom PEEP had induced a significant alveolar recruitment. Thus, it seems realistic to conclude that alveolar recruitment by PEEP can also improve the efficacy of inhaled NO; however, we speculate that in our rabbits (body weight of 3 kg) the used airway pressures were too high, leading to high intra-thoracic pressures, which make dilatation of the pulmonary vasculature impossible due to inhaled NO. This could also be of importance in neonates with RDS and therefore we suggested that alveolar recruitment induced by exogenous surfactant is more beneficial than increased PEEP for improving arterial oxygenation due to inhaled NO because of the use of lower airway pressures (18).

Recruitment of collapsed alveoli can further be achieved by instillation of perfluorocarbons (PFC) (21-24). In lung lavaged rabbits, we have shown that intratracheal administration of PFC combined with conventional mechanical gas ventilation (this technique is called partial liquid ventilation) resulted in dose-dependent improvement of arterial oxygenation, which is confirmed by recent pilot studies in patients (21,22,25). The dose-dependent improvement in oxygenation results from filling of the collapsed atelectatic alveoli in the dependent part of the lung by the non-compressible PFC, preventing the alveoli from end-expiratory collapse which one could call 'fluid-PEEP' (21). We could demonstrate that the combination of PFC and inhaled NO has a cumulative effect on improving gas exchange in lung-lavaged pigs (26). In this study, all animals received four incremental doses of 5 mL of PFC per kg body weight and between each dose 4 different doses of NO (10, 20, 30, and 40 ppm) were inhaled (Fig. 2) (27). Inhaled NO had no effect on improving arterial oxygenation in two animals in which the first low dose of PFC had no effect on arterial oxygenation. But when arterial oxygenation increased after the second dose of PFC, inhaled NO resulted in a further improvement of arterial oxygenation.

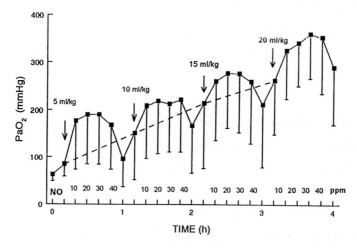

Figure 2 Change in arterial oxygenation (PaO_2) after four incremental doses of 5 mL/kg perfluorocarbons (PFC) in lung lavaged pigs. Between each dose of PFC, 4 different doses of NO (10, 20, 30, and 40 ppm) were inhaled each time for 10 min. NO was switched off for 10 min each time before the next dose of PFC was installed. The dotted line represents the change of arterial oxygenation in relation to four incremental doses of PFC. Data are presented as mean±SD.

The successful combination of PFC and inhaled NO was confirmed by Wilcox et al. (28). In congenital diaphragmatic hernia lambs, arterial oxygenation increased from 110±22 torr to 185±46 torr after inhalation of 80 ppm NO for 10 min and decreased when NO was switched off (28).

In both experimental studies, we have shown that after a low dose of PFC or exogenous surfactant, PaO_2 can be further increased by inhalation of NO (18,27). Similar improvement of gas exchange can also be achieved by increasing the amount of PFC or exogenous surfactant (16,22). This means that it may be possible to save PFC or exogenous surfactant by a combination therapy with NO inhalation.

REFERENCES

1. Palmer RMJ, Ferrige AG, Moncada S. Nitric oxide release accounts for the biological activity of endothelium-derived relaxing factor. Nature 1987; 327: 524-6
2. Pepke-Zaba J, Higenbottam T, Dihn-Xuan AT, Stone D, Wallwork J. Inhaled nitric oxide as a cause of selective pulmonary vasodilation in pulmonary hypertension. Lancet 1991; 338: 1173-4
3. Kinsella JP, Neish SR, Shaffer E, Abman SH. Low-dose inhalational nitric oxide in persistent pulmonary hypertension of the newborn. Lancet 1992; 340:819-20
4   Roberts JD, Polaner DM, Lang P, Zapol WM. Inhaled nitric oxide in persistent pulmonary hypertension of the newborn. Lancet 1992; 340: 818-9
5. Rossaint R, Falke KJ, López F, Slama K, Pison U, Zapol WM. Inhaled nitric oxide for the adult respiratory distress syndrome. N Engl J Med 1993; 328: 399-405
6. Gerlach H, Rossaint R, Pappert D, Falke KJ. Time-course and dose-response of nitric oxide inhalation for systemic oxygenation and pulmonary hypertension in patients with adult respiratory distress syndrome. Eur J Clin Invest 1993; 23:499-502
7. Bigatello LM, Hurford WE, Kacmarek RM, Roberts JD, Zapol WM. Prolonged inhalation of low concentrations of nitric oxide in patients with severe adult respiratory distress syndrome. Anesthesiology 1994; 80: 761-70
8. Puybasset L, Rouby JJ, Mourgeon E, Stewart TE, Cluzel P, Arthaud M, Poète P, Bodin L, Korinek AM, Viars P. Inhaled nitric oxide in acute respiratory failure: dose-response curves. Intensive Care Med 1994; 20: 319-27
9. Finer NN, Etches PC, Kamstra B, Tierney AJ, Peliowski A, Ryan A. Inhaled nitric oxide in infants referred for extracorporeal membrane oxygenation: dose response. J Pediatr 1994; 124: 302-8
10. Kinsella JP, Abman SH. Efficacy of inhalational nitric oxide therapy in the clinical management of persistent pulmonary hypertension of the newborn. Chest 1994; 105: 92S-4S
11. Peacock A. Vasodilators in pulmonary hypertension. Thorax 1993; 48: 1196-9
12. Abman SH. Inhaled nitric oxide therapy in neonatal and pediatric cardiorespiratory disease In: Tibboel D, van der Voort E (eds) Update in intensive care and emergency medicine vol. 25; Intensive care in childhood. Springer-Verlag, Berlin Heidelberg New York, 1996; 322-36
13. Gommers D, Houmes R-JM, Olsson SG, So KL, Lachmann B. Exogenous surfactant and nitric oxide have a synergetic effect in improving respiratory failure. Am J Respir Crit Care Med 1994; 149(Part 2): A568
14. Karamanoukian HL, Glick PL, Wilcox DT, Rossman JE, Holm BA, Morin FC. Pathophysiology of congenital diaphragmatic hernia VIII: inhaled nitric oxide requires exogenous surfactant therapy in the lamb model of congenital diaphragmatic hernia. J Pediatr Surg 1995; 30: 1-4
15. Gommers D, Lachmann B. Surfactant therapy: does it have a role in adults? Clin Intensive Care 1993; 4: 284-95
16. Gommers D, Vilstrup C, Bos JAH, Larsson A, Werner O, Hannappel E, Lachmann B. Exogenous surfactant therapy increases static lung compliance, and cannot be assessed by measurements of dynamic compliance alone. Crit Care Med 1993; 21: 567-74
17. Strüber M, Brandt M, Cremer J, Harringer W, Hirt SW, Haverich A. Therapy for lung failure using nitric oxide inhalation and surfactant replacement. Ann Thorac Surg 1996; 61: 1543-5

18. Gommers D, Hartog A, van 't Veen A, Lachmann B. Improved oxygenation by nitric oxide is enhanced by prior lung aeration with surfactant, rather than positive end-expiratory pressure, in lung lavaged rabbits. Crit Care Med 1997; 25: 1868-73
19. Putensen C, Räsänen J, López FA, Downs JB. Continuous positive airway pressure modulates effect of inhaled nitric oxide on the ventilation-perfusion distributions in canine lung injury. Chest 1994; 106: 1563-9
20. Puybasset L, Rouby J-J, Mourgeon E, Cluzel P, Souhil Z, Law-Koune J-D, Stewart T, Devilliers C, Lu Q, Roche S, Kalfon P, Vicaut E, Viars P. Factors influencing cardiopulmonary effects of inhaled nitric oxide in acute respiratory failure. Am J Respir Crit Care Med 1995; 152: 318-8
21. Verbrugge S, Gommers D, Lachmann B. Liquid ventilation as an alternative ventilatory support. Current Opinion Anaesthesiology 1995; 8: 551-6
22. Tütüncü AS, Faithfull NS, Lachmann B. Intratracheal perfluorocarbon administration combined with artificial ventilation in experimental respiratory distress syndrome: dose-dependent improvement of gas exchange. Crit Care Med 1993; 21: 962-9
23. Tütüncü AS, Faithfull NS, Lachmann B. Comparison of ventilatory support with intratracheal perfluorocarbon administration and conventional mechanical ventilation in animals with respiratory failure. Am Rev Respir Dis 1993; 148: 785-92
24. Tütüncü AS, Akpir K, Mulder P, Erdmann W, Lachmann B. Intratracheal perfluorocarbon administration as an aid in the ventilatory management of respiratory distress syndrome. Anesthesiology 1993; 79: 1083-93
25. Hirschl RB, Pranikoff T, Gauger P, Schreiner RJ, Dechert R, Barlett RH.1995 Liquid ventilation in adults, children, and full-term neonates. Lancet 1995; 346: 1201-2
26. Houmes R-JM, Verbrugge S, Lachmann B. Effects of nitric oxide administration on gas exchange and hemodynamics during perflubron partial liquid ventilation during induced respiratory insufficiency. Am J Resp Crit Care Med 1995; 151(Part 2): A446
27. Houmes RJM, Hartog A, Verbrugge SJC, Böhm S, Lachmann B. Combining partial liquid ventilation with nitric oxide to improve gas exchange in acute lung injury. Intensive Care Med 1996; 23: 163-9
28. Wilcox DT, Glick PL, Karamanoukian HL, Leach C, Morin FC, Fuhrman BP. Perfluorocarbon-associated gas exchange improves pulmonary mechanics, oxygenation, ventilation, and allows nitric oxide delivery in the hypoplastic lung congenital diaphragmatic hernia lamb model. Crit Care Med 1995; 23: 1858-63

Author index